EMERGENCY AND INTENSIVE CARE MEDICINE

ABDOMINAL INJURIES

RISK FACTORS, MANAGEMENT AND PROGNOSIS

EMERGENCY AND INTENSIVE CARE MEDICINE

Additional books in this series can be found on Nova's website under the Series tab.

Additional e-books in this series can be found on Nova's website under the e-book tab.

EMERGENCY AND INTENSIVE CARE MEDICINE

ABDOMINAL INJURIES

RISK FACTORS, MANAGEMENT AND PROGNOSIS

CHAD L. BARRETT
EDITOR

NOVA BIOMEDICAL
New York

Library of Congress Cataloging-in-Publication Data

ISBN: 978-1-63482-590-0
Library of Congress Control Number: 2015936698

Published by Nova Science Publishers, Inc. † New York

Contents

Preface

Severe trauma represents one of the biggest issues threatening modern healthcare systems across the globe. Traumatic injury is the leading cause of lost life years worldwide, responsible for an excess of 5 million deaths every year.

The role of laparoscopy in trauma has not paralleled its popularity in other areas of general surgery for several reasons including the emergent nature of many of the operations, the lack of expertise and comfort level of some surgeons and the fear of missed injuries. In this book, the possible indications and pitfalls of integrating minimally invasive surgical techniques into the management of abdominal injuries are examined. Furthermore, post-traumatic haemorrhage is likely to represent the principle cause of preventable deaths amongst patients sustaining major traumatic injuries. Management of these patients and techniques (both old and emerging) are discussed, which may be able to more accurately identify early coagulopathy and enable goal-directed, targeted therapy.

The third chapter of the book describes currently accepted classifications of pelvic trauma to examine the link between mechanism of injury and factors predictive of mortality. Recent advances made in services, protocols, imaging, instrumentation and management of pelvic trauma are examined, specifically looked at to determine whether any of it has served to improve the historically poor prognosis. Lastly, pancreatic injury in childhood is rare, constituting 0.3% to 0.7% of all trauma admissions at large pediatric trauma centers. Nonetheless, they do occur. The authors explore pancreatic duct ruptures in children, the subsequent diagnosis and treatment options, which usually require surgery or other interventional therapy and carry a significant risk of morbidity.

Chapter 1 – Minimally invasive surgery has progressed quickly since its inception and integration into the practice of general surgery, and there is an emerging body of data describing the management of some abdominal injuries using laparoscopic techniques. However, the use of laparoscopy for trauma remains controversial. There are limitations to the use of laparoscopy in the treatment of abdominal injuries; however, appropriately selected patients can be treated using some laparoscopic techniques. Using diagnostic laparoscopy and minimally invasive surgical techniques can help identify hollow viscous injuries that can be difficult to diagnose clinically and with imaging. Using this modality can mitigate the morbidity of nontherapeutic laparotomy in the evaluation of the abdominal wall and viscera in certain patients. Laparoscopic techniques can be therapeutic as well as diagnostic. Following detection, injuries of the abdominal wall, diaphragm, stomach, and bowel can often be repaired without the morbidity of a laparotomy. Laparoscopic techniques have also been used with success in the diagnosis and treatment of diaphragm injuries. Despite its narrow scope, there is a developing role for laparoscopy in the management of various abdominal injuries. In this chapter, the authors discuss the experience, possible indications, and pitfalls of integrating minimally invasive surgical techniques into the management of abdominal injuries.

Chapter 2 – Severe trauma represents one of the biggest issues threatening modern healthcare systems across the globe. Traumatic injury is the leading cause of lost life years worldwide, responsible for in excess of 5 million deaths every year. Not only does this represent an already huge burden on healthcare delivery systems, current health projections predict that this number will increase to over 8 million by the year 2020. Amongst patients sustaining significant traumatic injury, the biggest causes of mortality are traumatic brain injury and major, uncontrolled post-traumatic haemorrhage, which is responsible for approximately 30-40% of cases of trauma related mortality and accounting for up to 50% of deaths in the initial 24 hour period. Post-traumatic haemorrhage is likely to represent the principle cause of preventable deaths amongst patients sustaining major traumatic injuries.

Key stages in the management of these patients involves rapidly identifying sources of bleeding and the instigation of measures to reduce blood loss, with the overall aim of re-establishing tissue perfusion and stabilisation of haemodynamic status. A relatively recent, but now well-recognised phenomenon related to post-traumatic haemorrhage is that of trauma-related, or trauma-induced coagulopathy (TIC). This describes an impairment of clotting both in the early and ongoing stages following injury, with a multifactorial underlying pathophysiology. The importance of TIC lays in the fact that despite between 25-35% bleeding trauma patients presenting with a degree of coagulopathy on admission, awareness of the phenomenon and pathophysiology is low. More importantly, the presence of TIC is associated with increased transfusion requirements (and the corresponding risk), greater risk of organ injury, septic complications and longer stays both in critical care and overall hospital stay. It is independently associated with both the need for massive transfusion and increased mortality, with mortality in some studies reported as up to 50%.

One of the fundamental stages in the management of traumatic haemorrhage is in the early recognition and identification of coagulopathy. Management is largely based around the transfusion of blood products and specific clotting components, which has traditionally been guided both by clinical judgement and standard laboratory tests (prothrombin time [PT], international normalised ratio [INR], activated partial thromboplastin time [APTT], platelet counts and fibrinogen levels). However, conventional laboratory tests are inadequate for the rapid identification of trauma-induced coagulopathy since they only reflect the initial phase of coagulation (less than 4% of total thrombin production), and give no information regarding the clot stability or any hyperfibrinolysis occurring, which has been recognised as an important factor in TIC. Furthermore, average turnaround times of these tests range from approximately 30-60 minutes, which is simply not fast enough to adequately guide management of the ever changing trauma patient.

A renewed interest in measures of the viscoelastic properties of blood as a point of care test using techniques such as thromboelastography (TEG) or rotational thromboelastometry (ROTEM) has opened up an interesting avenue in the investigation and management of trauma patients, enabling more rapid identification of clotting derangements as well as near real time measures of factors predictive of mortality and transfusion requirements. Dogma regarding management of these patients is constantly being rewritten and redressed and there is still little consensus on the optimum transfusion protocols in these patients. With ongoing research, it is hoped that these techniques may be able to more accurately identify early coagulopathy and enable goal-directed, targeted therapy to these patients to not only improve patient survival and reduce risk of harm, but also increase efficiency of utilisation of these valuable and limited resources.

Chapter 3 – The pelvic cavity, surrounded by the pelvic bones, protects and transmits the vessels and organs of digestion, excretion, reproduction and ambulation. The pelvis contains the inferior aspect of the retroperitoneal and intraperitoneal spaces; disruption of the pelvis may therefore result in not only the loss of structural stability but may jeopardise structures contained within its volume.

Breaking the pelvic ring, with its associated vascular bed, may result in catastrophic haemorrhage and remote organ sequelae, such as brain damage, and is the cause of early death. Late death is usually associated with overwhelming sepsis and multi-organ failure.

Despite the advent of specialised Major Trauma Centers, together with adoption of standardised resuscitation protocols developed to ensure the appropriate and timely use of pelvic stabilisation, interventional radiology and damage control surgery, we are yet to witness the anticipated leap in improving mortality associated with pelvic trauma. Major pelvic trauma was associated with a 10% risk of mortality in the 1980s, yet in spite of the advances in technology and service provision, recent studies show this still to be the case. Indeed, a recent consecutive series performed by O'Sulivan et al. of 174 patients reveals it stands closer to 20%.

Survival following pelvic trauma is still fraught with increased morbidity. Henderson et al. suggest that 80% of survivors who sustained unstable pelvic injuries report some degree of disability, compared with only 13% of those who sustained stable pelvic disruption. Common complaints include: ongoing pain, neurological injuries, sphincter disturbance, impaired gait, sexual dysfunction and vascular injuries, all of which have a profound impact on activities of daily living.

Pelvic fractures encompass a broad spectrum of injuries, from low-energy osteoporotic fractures to high-energy disruptions of the pelvic ring. The prompt and accurate appreciation of a patient's injury pattern and its severity is crucial to the planning of early and effective management.

This chapter will describe currently accepted classifications of pelvic trauma and examine the link between mechanism of injury and factors predictive of mortality. The authors will discuss the relevance of trauma scoring systems being used to identify patients at high risk and the impact this has on management.

Ultimately, pelvic anatomy remains constant; saving life and preventing deformity following trauma to this region still poses a real challenge to the modern day trauma team. This chapter will explore recent advances made in services, protocols, imaging, instrumentation and management of pelvic trauma and examine whether any of it has served to improve the historically poor prognosis.

Chapter 4 – Pancreatic duct ruptures in children are predominantly caused by bicycle handlebar injuries. Acute onset of abdominal symptoms and subsequent pancreatic pseudocyst formation occur within hours or days after the injury. Pancreatic duct ruptures are diagnosed by contrast-enhanced computer tomography (CT), magnetic resonance pancreaticography (MRP), or endoscopic retrograde pancreaticography (ERP). Pancreatic duct ruptures usually require surgery or other interventional therapy and carry a significant risk of morbidity. ERP-guided stent placement of the proximal pancreatic duct, with or without stenting of the rupture site, has been reported recently.

Case Report: Two boys, aged 6 and 6.5 years, sustained pancreatic duct ruptures in handlebar injuries when riding their bicycles. In both cases, free abdominal fluid was noted using ultrasonographic imaging, and levels of serum amylase on admission were 251 U/L and 398 U/L (normal range: <100 U/L), respectively. Octreotide (2 x 0.025 mg/day) was administered intravenously starting on day 1 and day 7, respectively. Both pancreatic duct ruptures (American Association for the Surgery of Trauma [AAST] grade 3) were confirmed with abdominal contrast-enhanced CT scans on the day of admission and 8 days after the injury. Both children underwent ERP-guided stent placement (5.0 French, 8.0 and 7.0 cm in length, respectively) of the major pancreatic duct. In both boys, oral nutrition was started 1 day after the endoscopic intervention and was well tolerated thereafter. The two boys returned home 2 days and 7 days after the intervention. In both patients, peripancreatic fluid accumulation resolved after 2 days and 4 weeks, respectively. Stents were removed by endoscopy after 4 and 9 weeks. Follow-up for 87 and 82 months was uneventful.

Conclusion: ERP-guided stent placement represents a safe and efficient treatment option for pancreatic duct injuries AAST grade 3 in children and may replace more complex surgical treatment in selected cases. Further studies are required to confirm the authors' findings.

In: Abdominal Injuries
Editor: Chad L. Barrett

ISBN: 978-1-63482-590-0

Chapter 1

The Use of Laparoscopy in Abdominal Trauma

Elizabeth Acquista, MD, Julian Maendel, MD and William W. Hope, MD*

Department of Surgery
New Hanover Regional Medical Center
Wilmington, North Carolina, NC, US

Abstract

Minimally invasive surgery has progressed quickly since its inception and integration into the practice of general surgery, and there is an emerging body of data describing the management of some abdominal injuries using laparoscopic techniques. However, the use of laparoscopy for trauma remains controversial. There are limitations to the use of laparoscopy in the treatment of abdominal injuries; however, appropriately selected patients can be treated using some laparoscopic techniques. Using diagnostic laparoscopy and minimally invasive surgical techniques can help identify hollow viscous injuries that can be difficult to diagnose clinically and with imaging. Using this modality can mitigate the morbidity of nontherapeutic laparotomy in the evaluation of

* Corresponding Author: Department of Surgery, New Hanover Regional Medical Center, 2131 South 17th Street, PO Box 9025, Wilmington, NC 28401, Email: William.Hope@seahec.net

the abdominal wall and viscera in certain patients. Laparoscopic techniques can be therapeutic as well as diagnostic. Following detection, injuries of the abdominal wall, diaphragm, stomach, and bowel can often be repaired without the morbidity of a laparotomy. Laparoscopic techniques have also been used with success in the diagnosis and treatment of diaphragm injuries. Despite its narrow scope, there is a developing role for laparoscopy in the management of various abdominal injuries. In this chapter, we discuss the experience, possible indications, and pitfalls of integrating minimally invasive surgical techniques into the management of abdominal injuries.

Keywords: laparoscopy, trauma, abdominal, injuries, diagnostic

Introduction

Since the introduction and widespread adoption of laparoscopic cholecystectomy, minimally invasive surgical techniques have been adopted in many aspects of general surgery and have become the standard for many surgical procedures. The role of laparoscopy in trauma has not paralleled its popularity in other areas of general surgery for several reasons including the emergent nature of many of the operations, the lack of expertise and comfort level of some surgeons, the added time for equipment set-up, the difficulty assessing the retroperitoneum, and the fear of missed injuries [1]. With improvements in laparoscopic training, techniques, and technology, there has been some increased enthusiasm for the role of laparoscopy in trauma, and its use has increased for both the diagnosing and treatment of trauma patients.

History of Laparoscopic Surgery in Trauma

Prompt and accurate diagnosis of abdominal injuries is essential to achieve good outcomes in trauma patients. Several modalities exist to assist the surgeon in identifying traumatic injuries to the abdomen. These range from noninvasive methods such as physical examination, hemodynamic monitoring, and imaging studies to more invasive methods such as paracentesis, diagnostic peritoneal lavage, diagnostic laparoscopy, and ultimately exploratory laparotomy [1]. The initial role of laparoscopy in trauma involved evaluating for peritoneal penetration in hemodynamically stable patients [2, 3]. With increased knowledge and training, indications broadened, and laparoscopy is now used as a diagnostic as well as a therapeutic tool in blunt and penetrating trauma. Ivatury et al. were among the first to define the role of laparoscopy in trauma. This prospective study reported that laparoscopy was accurate for the detection of hemoperitoneum, solid organ injuries, diaphragmatic lacerations, and retroperitoneal hematomas [4]. The authors however reported laparoscopy had a low sensitivity for gastrointestinal injuries and concluded that the major role of laparoscopy in patients with penetrating abdominal trauma was in the avoidance of unnecessary laparotomies and in evaluation of the diaphragm [4]. Although there has been ongoing concern regarding the rate of missed bowel injuries with the use of laparoscopy, Kawahara et al. reported that, using a standard laparoscopic examination, the rate of missed small bowel injury can be minimized in patients with penetrating trauma [5]. In this chapter, we review the evolution of the use of laparoscopy in evaluation and treatment of abdominal trauma.

Patient Selection

The minimally invasive approach to abdominal injuries should be reserved for potential diagnostic and therapeutic interventions in hemodynamically stable patients. Of course, Advanced Trauma Life Support (ATLS) protocols developed by the American College of Surgeons Committee on Trauma should guide the initial care of the injured patient. The majority of cases in which laparoscopy can be useful are low energy penetrating injuries, such as abdominal or thoraco-abdominal stab wounds. Occasionally, minimally invasive techniques can be used in the management of blunt trauma patients, and, less frequently, patients with abdominal gunshot wounds can be selectively managed with laparoscopy.

Laparoscopy As a Diagnostic Tool

Exploratory Laparoscopy / Diagnostic Laparoscopy

Patients with either blunt or penetrating abdominal trauma, who are determined to be hemodynamically stable and at risk for injury to the abdominal wall, diaphragm or intra-abdominal viscera can be candidates for diagnostic laparoscopy. Minimally invasive surgical techniques allow for thorough inspection of the anterior abdominal wall for identification of violated peritoneum. Depending on the trajectory of the missile or blade, both abdominal and thoraco-abdominal entrance wounds can relate to diaphragm injuries. The left diaphragm rather than the right diaphragm is more easily inspected for injury and potentially more easily repaired. However, there are reports of minimally invasive repair of the right diaphragm using thoracoscopy as well as laparoscopy. We recommend the use of a 10-mm, 30-degree scope to assess the anterior abdominal wall with the addition of two working ports to assist with manipulating the colon and viscera to obtain an unobstructed view. The bladder can be inspected for intraperitoneal injury. Additionally, the patient can be positioned in reverse Trendelenburg and tilted to inspect the diaphragms thoroughly. When a previously undiagnosed diaphragm injury is identified, a tube thoracostomy must be placed and careful attention paid to maintaining moderate to low pressure insufflation of the peritoneal cavity.

Injuries to the abdominal viscera can also be diagnosed during diagnostic laparoscopy. If there are entrance and exit wounds, one can take advantage of the trajectory to thoroughly explore that region. However, a systematic approach to exploring the entirety of the peritoneal cavity is recommended [6-8]. It is important to remember that bullets can take an unusual course due to ricochet phenomena, and injuries to the hollow abdominal viscera can be elusive. The presence or absence of hemoperitoneum, ascites, bile, or succus entericus should be noted. The liver, gallbladder, and spleen should be inspected for lacerations, contusions, or missile injuries. The anterior wall of the stomach, pylorus, and small bowel from the ligament of Treitz to the terminal ilium should be inspected carefully. The stomach can be insufflated with air via a nasogastric tube to assist in identifying very small injuries that are not immediately obvious. The ascending, transverse, and descending colon as well as the rectum should be inspected carefully for lacerations or perforations.

Laparoscopy has been found to be a useful tool in the kit of the contemporary surgeon. Diagnostic laparoscopy is safe, efficient, and low risk. It is particularly valuable in the management of hemodynamically stable patients with penetrating abdominal injuries [2].

Morbidity of Laparotomy

When deciding to operate on an injured patient, the morbidity of exploring the abdomen and finding no injury is weighed against the risk of not exploring and missing an injury.

Routine abdominal exploration in the care of an injured patient has been abandoned due to the high rate of nontherapeutic laparotomy. In recent surgical history, there are well studied series of the morbidity of negative laparotomy in trauma patients. This recent history is woven across the past few decades as diagnostic peritoneal lavage, computed tomography scanning, and focused abdominal ultrasound have been incorporated into the care of injured patient. This evolution in the evaluation of the injured brought the nontherapeutic laparotomy rate from as high as 40% to 7-10% [9]. The decline in routine laparotomy has been accompanied by a decrease in the perioperative complications associated with it, such as pneumonia, deep venous thrombosis (DVT), and gastrointestinal (GI) bleeds [9-12]. This time span has also brought changes in recommendations for DVT prophylaxis and GI prophylaxis.

Additionally, there is a notable but unsurprising increase in the length of hospital stay for patients who are recovering from a nontherapeutic trauma laparotomy compared with patients with similar injury patterns who have not been explored [11].

Thus, as the nontherapeutic laparotomy rate decreases, complications and length of hospitalization also decrease.

In 1995 Ross and colleagues [10] evaluated 476 trauma laparotomies and found that 50 of these interventions, 10% of the total laparotomies, were negative laparotomies. Further, they found that the morbidity of nontherapeutic laparotomy in blunt trauma was higher than the morbidity of negative laparotomy in penetrating trauma patients, and the most frequent indication for exploration leading to a nontherapeutic laparotomy was stab injuries.

Of the 50 patients with negative laparotomies, the morbidity was often minor (e.g., wound infection or atelectasis). One in 50 patients developed a small bowel obstruction, and other major complications included ARDS, pneumonia, sepsis, and venous thromboembolism. However, it is unclear if these major complications were more related to the severity of injury or to the nature of polytrauma than to the procedure itself. The morbidity attributed to laparotomy alone in patients without injuries outside of the abdomen is significantly lower than the morbidity of laparotomy in patients with other injuries.

It is critically important that patients are evaluated for their injuries and that the concern for a nontherapeutic laparotomy does not dominate the decision to operate.

A delay in care is a greater risk for a patient than a potentially nontherapeutic intervention. With the addition of minimally invasive techniques to the repertoire of the surgeon, the nontherapeutic laparotomy rate is likely to decline further.

Laparoscopy As a Therapeutic Tool

Injuries of the Abdominal Wall

Laparoscopy is well-suited for intracorporeal assessment of the abdominal wall, particularly for detection of peritoneal violation in the setting of hemodynamically stable penetrating trauma. When there is a question of peritoneal violation, imaging is often unhelpful, and local wound exploration can be inconclusive, particularly when dealing with a tangential wound tract and/or a thick abdominal wall. In this case, laparoscopy provides a definitive answer, as it is relatively easy to insert a laparoscope and, in absence of dense adhesions, gain a clear view of the peritoneum (Figure 1.). After peritoneal violation has been excluded, no further exploration is necessary, saving the patient a nontherapeutic laparotomy [13, 14].

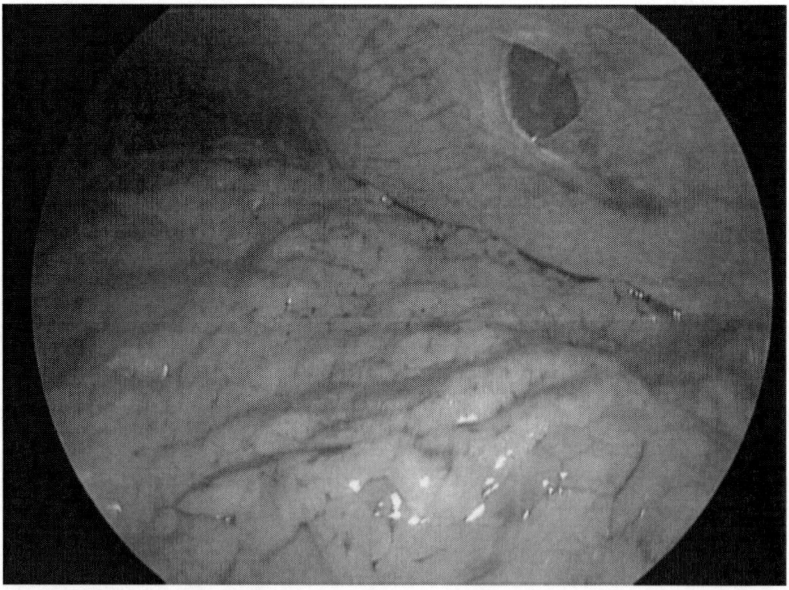

Figure 1. Laparoscopic view of abdominal wall showing peritoneal violation from a stab wound.

Less well defined is the therapeutic role of laparoscopy in abdominal wall trauma. Small peritoneal or facial rents can be repaired primarily either by intracorporeal suturing or use of a suture-passer, and abdominal wall bleeding can be controlled similarly. However, larger abdominal wall defects are probably best repaired via laparotomy, which allows a more thorough inspection of the viscera as well as more secure facial closure.

Injuries of the Diaphragm

Diaphragmatic injuries present a particular diagnostic and therapeutic challenge, because they are difficult to diagnose using conventional imaging and their repair involves equal consideration of both abdominal and thoracic sequelae. Diagnostic laparoscopy is most directly indicated in cases of blunt or penetrating trauma in patients who are hemodynamically stable and have a suspected diaphragmatic injury in the absence of other obvious intraabdominal injury [15]. In this scenario, laparoscopy allows careful visualization of the diaphragm, anterior abdominal wall, and visceral organs and identification or exclusion of associated injuries, while potentially avoiding the complications and increased length of stay associated with nontherapeutic laparotomy [11]. Use of a 30- or 40-degree angle 10-mm scope facilitates exploration. In the event that diaphragmatic injuries are identified, particular attention must be given to maintaining low to moderate inflation pressures to minimize the possibility of inducing a tension pneumothorax.

Diaphragmatic injuries most amenable to the laparoscopic approach include smaller, anteriorly and centrally located defects that are not anterior to or in direct communication with the esophageal hiatus [16]. Particular attention must be paid to the degree of tension needed to achieve adequate approximation, as undue tension compromises the integrity of the repair. In this case consideration must be made for open repair, possibly using mesh. Most authors advocate the use of simple interrupted, figure-of-eight, or mattress sutures using 0 or 1 nonabsorbable braided suture (Figures 2 and 3). Laparoscopic staples have been described as an alternative; however, concerns remain regarding the long term integrity of such repairs.

Traditional teaching has stipulated that chronic diaphragmatic injuries be repaired via the transthoracic approach due to interval development of dense pleural adhesions. More recently, however, studies have found that the transabdominal approach to these chronic defects is equally effective and indeed may have a role for laparoscopy as well [17].

Injuries of the Viscera

As general surgeons develop and maintain advanced laparoscopic skills, the management of identified injuries has not been limited to the abdominal wall, anterior gastrotomies, and diaphragm injuries [8]. Case reports and series to date include descriptions of successful management of injuries to the liver and gallbladder, spleen, stomach, small bowel, colon, and bladder [7, 8, 18-20] (Figures 4 and 5).

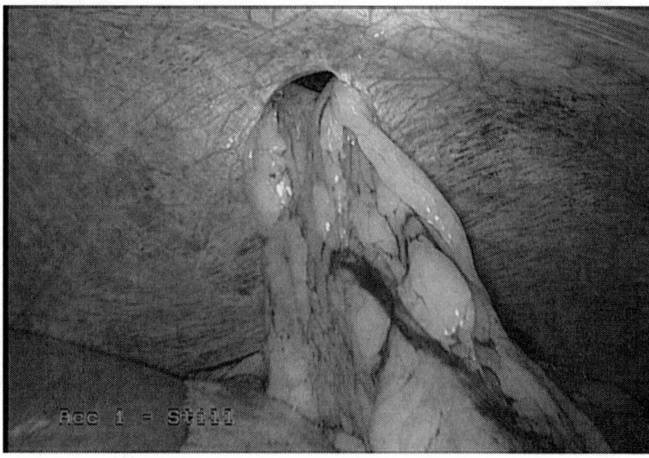

Figure 2. Laparoscopic view of anterior left diaphragm injury with omentum in the chest.

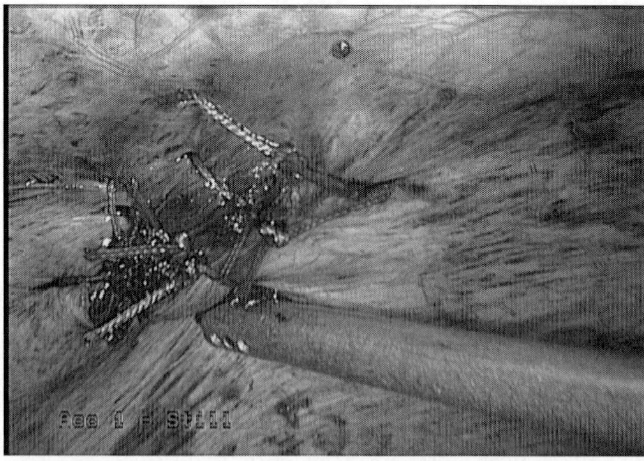

Figure 3. Laparoscopic reduction of omentum and repair of diaphragm injury using intracorporeal suturing.

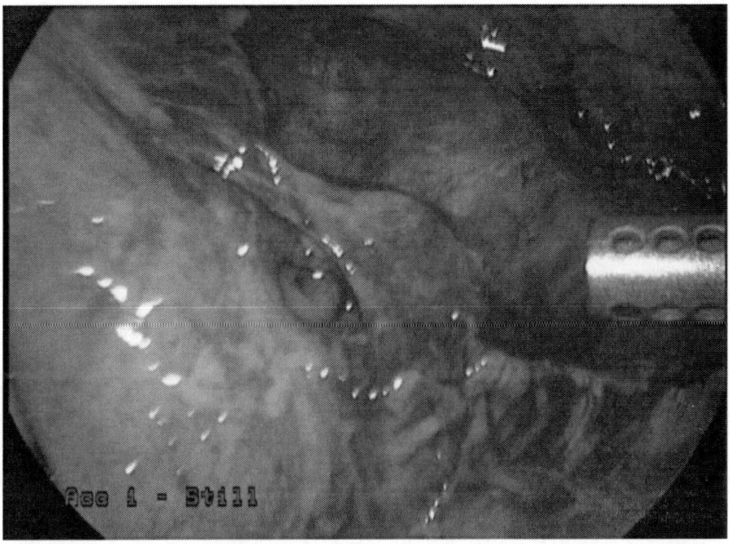

Figure 4. Diagnostic laparoscopy showing colon injury from penetrating trauma.

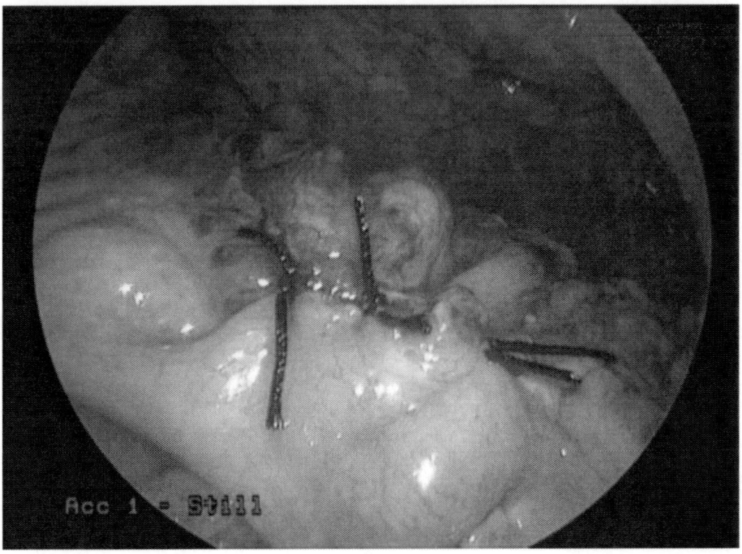

Figure 5. Laparosocpic suture repair of isolated colonic injury from penetrating trauma using intracorporeal suturing.

These cases and series emphasize the skillset and comfort level of the surgeon. Bowel resection and intracorporeal suturing techniques are advanced skills that are being maintained as acute care and trauma surgeons have tended to maintain concurrent elective surgery practices (Figures 6-9). In addition, in smaller hospitals, trauma call rosters are often comprised of capable surgeons with special interests in minimally invasive surgery.

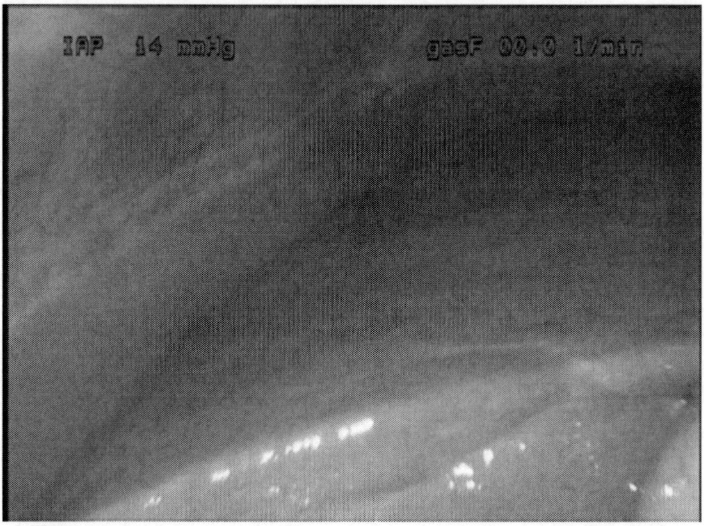

Figure 6. Diagnostic laparoscopy showing succus around the liver from small bowel injury from blunt trauma.

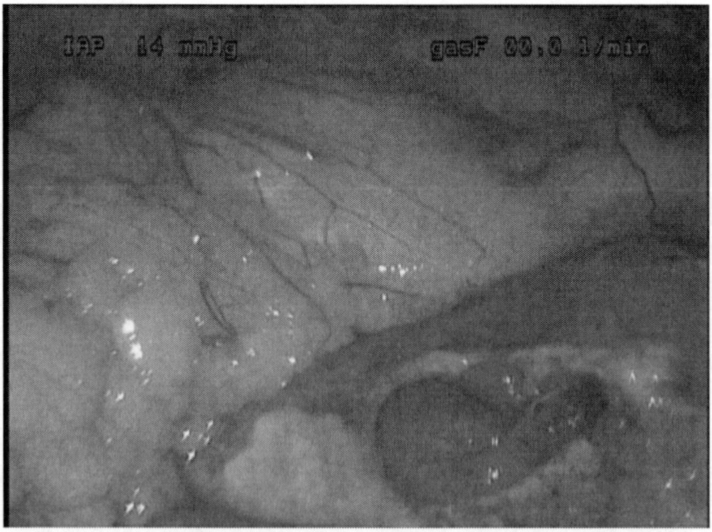

Figure 7. Diagnostic laparocopy showing isolated small bowel injury from blunt trauma.

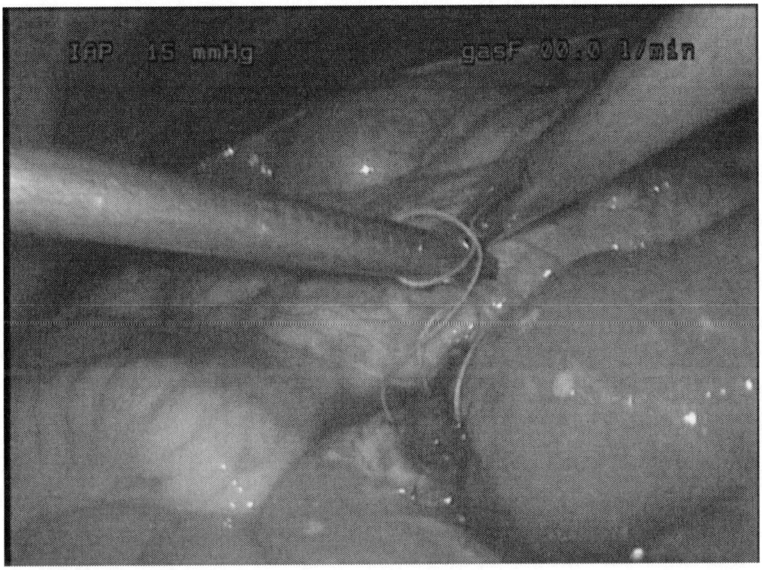

Figure 8. Laparoscopic repair of isolated small bowel injury from blunt trauma with intracorporeal suturing.

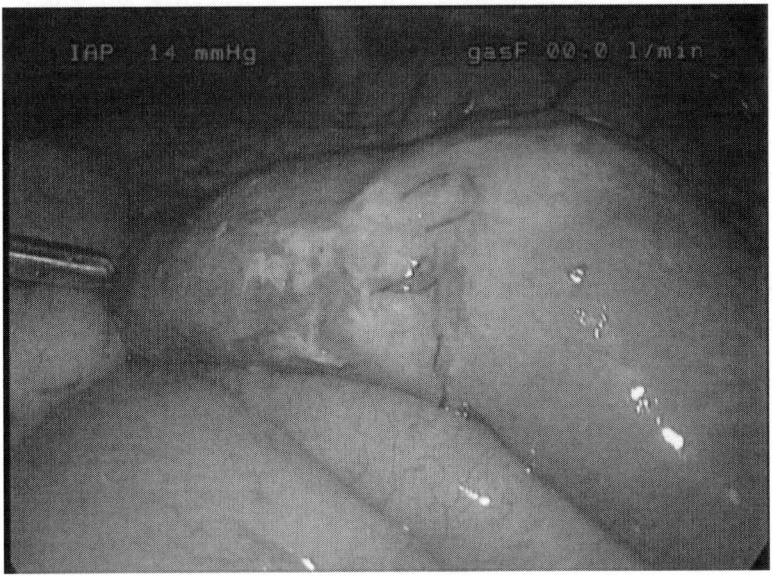

Figure 9. Laparoscopic 2 layer repair of small bowel injury.

Obstacles and Limitations

The obstacles and limitations of laparoscopic evaluation of the patient with an injured abdomen are twofold. There are intrinsic risks of laparoscopy alone under any circumstance as well as specific complication risks associated with laparoscopy and traumatic injuries. Particular concerns include the risk for the development of pneumothorax or tension pneumothorax and the risk of transient elevations in intracranial pressure (ICP) due to elevated intra-abdominal pressure during insufflation [21-24]. Previous concerns regarding cost have largely been debunked after demonstrating that diagnostic laparoscopy can be cost effective [25].

Insufflation during laparoscopy to pressures of 15 mm Hg and above can lead to tension pneumothorax and obstructive shock culminating in cardiac arrest. In polytrauma patients, caution must be used in the approach to abdominal injuries in patients with head injuries. Traumatic brain injury can be complicated by transient elevations of ICP due to elevated intra-abdominal pressure during insufflation [23]. Additionally, bowel injuries continue to be elusive and difficult to diagnose. Finally, in any definitive repair that is undertaken irrespective of approach, there is a certain propensity to fail. However, reports of injuries to the viscera managed by intracorporeal techniques have had very good success with few reports of morbidity [8, 18, 19].

While minimally invasive surgery is very safe, there are series of injuries associated with trocar placement including injuries to the bowel and vasculature. Perioperative and delayed complications include wound infection and hernia. The development of tension pneumothorax due to abdominal insufflation has also been described in both animal models and in case reports and reviews [21, 24]. In particular, in the management of patients with thoracoabdominal trauma or those noted to have a traumatic diaphragm injury, care must be taken to prevent the pressure of abdominal insufflation from overcoming the central venous pressure or the relatively flexible right atrial wall. A tube thoracostomy should be placed in these cases as soon as possible to prevent tension phenomena. Signs that there is a tension pneumothorax can include abdominal ballooning of the hemidiaphragm, increased heart rate and airway pressure, elevated exhaled carbon dioxide, decreased tidal volume, and hypoxia. Thus, close communication should be maintained with anesthesia colleagues. Abdominal insufflation also causes elevation in ICP. This has been noted in case series and animal models. Thus, management of intra-abdominal injury in patients with associated head injury is relatively contraindicated, depending on the severity of the head injury [23]. Additionally, laparoscopic management of any identified injuries has the potential to fail, such as in anastomotic breakdown after repair or a leaking repair of a bladder injury. And worse, there may be a false sense of security after exploratory laparoscopy; a bowel injury is easily missed.

Conclusion

Laparoscopy in the care of the injured patient is still a somewhat controversial intervention, although minimally invasive surgery has, indeed, made great strides since its inception and integration into the practice of general surgery. While there are limitations to the use of laparoscopy in the diagnosis and treatment of abdominal injuries, it can be advantageous to manage a carefully selected group of patients this way. Minimally invasive surgical techniques can be therapeutic as well as diagnostic, and once identified, injuries are frequently repaired without the added morbidity of a laparotomy. The morbidity of nontherapeutic laparotomy can also be circumvented in cases when no injuries are identified. In hemodynamically stable patients at risk for peritoneal injury, a surgeon with sound judgment can potentially diagnose and manage injuries taking advantage of minimally invasive techniques, or decide that the best course is to proceed with laparotomy. Information will continue to emerge as this skill is incorporated into clinical care under the guidance of skilled general surgeons.

References

[1] Rozycki GS, Root HD. The diagnosis of intraabdominal visceral injury. *J. Trauma.* May;68(5):1019-23. Epub 2010/05/11.

[2] Fabian TC, Croce MA, Stewart RM, Pritchard FE, Minard G, Kudsk KA. A prospective analysis of diagnostic laparoscopy in trauma. *Ann. Surg.* 1993 May;217(5):557-64; discussion 64-5. Epub 1993/05/01.

[3] Smith RS. Cavitary endoscopy in trauma: 2001. *Scand J. Surg.* 2002;91(1):67-71. Epub 2002/06/22.

[4] Ivatury RR, Simon RJ, Stahl WM. A critical evaluation of laparoscopy in penetrating abdominal trauma. *J. Trauma.* 1993 Jun;34(6):822-7; discussion 7-8. Epub 1993/06/01.

[5] Kawahara NT, Alster C, Fujimura I, Poggetti RS, Birolini D. Standard examination system for laparoscopy in penetrating abdominal trauma. *J. Trauma.* 2009 Sep;67(3):589-95. Epub 2009/09/11.

[6] Chelly MR, Major K, Spivak J, Hui T, Hiatt JR, Margulies DR. The value of laparoscopy in management of abdominal trauma. *Am. Surg.* 2003 Nov;69(11):957-60. Epub 2003/11/25.

[7] Barzana DC, Kotwall CA, Clancy TV, Hope WW. Use of laparoscopy in trauma at a level II trauma center. *JSLS.* 2011 Apr-Jun;15(2):179-81. Epub 2011/09/10.

[8] Zantut LF, Ivatury RR, Smith RS, Kawahara NT, Porter JM, Fry WR, et al. Diagnostic and therapeutic laparoscopy for penetrating abdominal trauma: a multicenter experience. *J. Trauma.* 1997 May;42(5):825-9; discussion 9-31. Epub 1997/05/01.

[9] Weigelt JA, Kingman RG. Complications of negative laparotomy for trauma. *Am. J. Surg.* 1988 Dec;156(6):544-7. Epub 1988/12/01.

[10] Ross SE, Dragon GM, O'Malley KF, Rehm CG. Morbidity of negative coeliotomy in trauma. *Injury.* 1995 Jul;26(6):393-4. Epub 1995/07/01.

[11] Renz BM, Feliciano DV. The length of hospital stay after an unnecessary laparotomy for trauma: a prospective study. *J. Trauma.* 1996 Feb;40(2):187-90. Epub 1996/02/01.

[12] Schnuriger B, Lam L, Inaba K, Kobayashi L, Barbarino R, Demetriades D. Negative laparotomy in trauma: are we getting better? *Am. Surg.* 2012 Nov;78(11):1219-23. Epub 2012/10/24.

[13] Uranues S, Popa DE, Diaconescu B, Schrittwieser R. Laparoscopy in Penetrating Abdominal Trauma. *World J. Surg.* 2014 Dec 2. Epub 2014/12/03.

[14] O'Malley E, Boyle E, O'Callaghan A, Coffey JC, Walsh SR. Role of laparoscopy in penetrating abdominal trauma: a systematic review. *World J. Surg.* 2013 Jan;37(1):113-22. Epub 2012/10/12.

[15] Matthews BD, Bui H, Harold KL, Kercher KW, Adrales G, Park A, et al. Laparoscopic repair of traumatic diaphragmatic injuries. *Surg Endosc.* 2003 Feb;17(2):254-8. Epub 2002/10/26.

[16] Crandall M, Popowich D, Shapiro M, West M. Posttraumatic hernias: historical overview and review of the literature. *Am. Surg.* 2007 Sep;73(9):845-50. Epub 2007/10/18.

[17] Murray JA, Weng J, Velmahos GC, Demetriades D. Abdominal approach to chronic diaphragmatic hernias: is it safe? *Am. Surg.* 2004 Oct;70(10):897-900. Epub 2004/11/09.

[18] Hope WW, Christmas AB, Jacobs DG, Sing RF. Definitive laparoscopic repair of penetrating injuries to the colon and small intestine: a case report. *J. Trauma*. 2009 Mar;66(3):931-2. Epub 2009/03/12.
[19] Woo K, Margulies DR, Gaon MD, Cunneen SA. Intracorporeal laparoscopic management of mesenteric avulsion in a blunt trauma patient. *J. Trauma*. 2009 Oct;67(4):E104-7. Epub 2008/09/26.
[20] Wright JL, Porter JR. Laparoscopy and the management of blunt bladder trauma. *J. Trauma*. 2007 Nov;63(5):1165-6. Epub 2007/05/22.
[21] Machairiotis N, Kougioumtzi I, Dryllis G, Katsikogiannis N, Katsikogianni F, Courcoutsakis N, et al. Laparoscopy induced pneumothorax. *Journal of thoracic disease*. 2014 Oct;6(Suppl 4):S404-6. Epub 2014/10/23.
[22] Guth AA, Pachter HL. Laparoscopy for penetrating thoracoabdominal trauma: pitfalls and promises. *JSLS*. 1998 Apr-Jun;2(2):123-7. Epub 1999/01/07.
[23] Kamine TH, Papavassiliou E, Schneider BE. Effect of abdominal insufflation for laparoscopy on intracranial pressure. *JAMA surgery*. 2014 Apr;149(4):380-2. Epub 2014/02/14.
[24] Wiedeman JE, Knolmayer TJ, Bowyer MW. Is tension pneumothorax a threat in trauma laparoscopy? *J. Trauma*. 1998 Oct;45(4):677-83. Epub 1998/10/23.
[25] Marks JM, Youngelman DF, Berk T. Cost analysis of diagnostic laparoscopy vs laparotomy in the evaluation of penetrating abdominal trauma. *Surg. Endosc*. 1997 Mar;11(3):272-6. Epub 1997/03/01.

In: Abdominal Injuries
Editor: Chad L. Barrett

ISBN: 978-1-63482-590-0

Chapter 2

Coagulopathy in Major Trauma

S. Fleming[1,•], R. Bird[1], V. Perkins[1] and B. Patel[1,*]

[1]The Royal London Hospital and Barts Cancer Institute,
Queen Mary University, Old Anatomy Building,
Charterhouse Square, London, UK

Abstract

Severe trauma represents one of the biggest issues threatening modern healthcare systems across the globe. Traumatic injury is the leading cause of lost life years worldwide, responsible for in excess of 5 million deaths every year. Not only does this represent an already huge burden on healthcare delivery systems, current health projections predict that this number will increase to over 8 million by the year 2020. Amongst patients sustaining significant traumatic injury, the biggest causes of mortality are traumatic brain injury and major, uncontrolled post-traumatic haemorrhage, which is responsible for approximately 30-40% of cases of trauma related mortality and accounting for up to 50% of deaths in the initial 24 hour period. Post-traumatic haemorrhage is likely to represent the principle cause of preventable deaths amongst patients sustaining major traumatic injuries.

Key stages in the management of these patients involves rapidly identifying sources of bleeding and the instigation of measures to reduce

• E-mail: simonsfleming@doctors.org.uk.

* Tel: +44 (0)20 7882 2081, Fax: +44 (0) 207 882 3888, E-mail: b.patel@qmul.ac.uk. www.bci.qmul.ac.uk.

blood loss, with the overall aim of re-establishing tissue perfusion and stabilisation of haemodynamic status. A relatively recent, but now well-recognised phenomenon related to post-traumatic haemorrhage is that of trauma-related, or trauma-induced coagulopathy (TIC). This describes an impairment of clotting both in the early and ongoing stages following injury, with a multifactorial underlying pathophysiology. The importance of TIC lays in the fact that despite between 25-35% bleeding trauma patients presenting with a degree of coagulopathy on admission, awareness of the phenomenon and pathophysiology is low. More importantly, the presence of TIC is associated with increased transfusion requirements (and the corresponding risk), greater risk of organ injury, septic complications and longer stays both in critical care and overall hospital stay. It is independently associated with both the need for massive transfusion and increased mortality, with mortality in some studies reported as up to 50%.

One of the fundamental stages in the management of traumatic haemorrhage is in the early recognition and identification of coagulopathy. Management is largely based around the transfusion of blood products and specific clotting components, which has traditionally been guided both by clinical judgement and standard laboratory tests (prothrombin time [PT], international normalised ratio [INR], activated partial thromboplastin time [APTT], platelet counts and fibrinogen levels). However, conventional laboratory tests are inadequate for the rapid identification of trauma-induced coagulopathy since they only reflect the initial phase of coagulation (less than 4% of total thrombin production), and give no information regarding the clot stability or any hyperfibrinolysis occurring, which has been recognised as an important factor in TIC. Furthermore, average turnaround times of these tests range from approximately 30-60 minutes, which is simply not fast enough to adequately guide management of the ever changing trauma patient.

A renewed interest in measures of the viscoelastic properties of blood as a point of care test using techniques such as thromboelastography (TEG) or rotational thromboelastometry (ROTEM) has opened up an interesting avenue in the investigation and management of trauma patients, enabling more rapid identification of clotting derangements as well as near real time measures of factors predictive of mortality and transfusion requirements. Dogma regarding management of these patients is constantly being rewritten and redressed and there is still little consensus on the optimum transfusion protocols in these patients. With ongoing research, it is hoped that these techniques may be able to more accurately identify early coagulopathy and enable goal-directed, targeted therapy to these patients to not only improve patient survival and reduce risk of harm, but also increase efficiency of utilisation of these valuable and limited resources.

1. Introduction – The Problem of Coagulopathy in Trauma

Severe trauma represents one of the biggest issues threatening modern healthcare systems across the globe. Traumatic injury, being the leading cause of death in under-40s, is the leading cause of lost life years worldwide and is responsible for in excess of 5 million deaths every year. Not only does this represent an already huge burden on healthcare delivery systems, current health projections predict that this number will increase to over 8 million by the year 2020 [1, 2]. Whilst difficult to quantify exactly the financial cost of this to worldwide healthcare providers, it is estimated that in the NHS alone, trauma expenditure is in the region of £0.3-0.4 billion [3]. Amongst patients sustaining significant traumatic injury, the biggest causes of mortality are traumatic brain injury and major, uncontrolled post-traumatic haemorrhage, which is responsible for approximately 30-40% of cases of trauma related mortality and accounting for up to 50% of deaths in the initial 24 hour period [4]. Post-traumatic haemorrhage is likely to represent the principle cause of preventable deaths amongst patients sustaining major traumatic injuries.

Key stages in the management of these patients involves rapidly identifying sources of bleeding and the instigation of measures to reduce blood loss, with the overall aim of re-establishing tissue perfusion and stabilisation of haemodynamic status. In addition to the surgical bleeding caused directly by traumatic injuries, both blunt and penetrating, a relatively recent, but increasingly more well recognised contributing phenomenon is that of trauma related coagulopathy. This is a multifactorial pathological process that occurs early in the post-injury period culminating in derangement of the coagulation cascade and potentiation, and potentially increased severity of ongoing haemorrhage [5].

It is estimated that between 25-35% of trauma patients on admission to hospital present with coagulopathy, with the risk higher as the injury severity score increases. Furthermore, coagulopathy in trauma is associated with an increased number of transfusions (along with its own potential complications and which independently is a risk factor for coagulopathy) and increased likelihood of need for massive transfusion (defined variably including replacement of entire circulating volume or transfusion of $\geq$10 units packed red cells within 24 hours, or in the more acute setting, transfusion of $\geq$5 units within 4 hours) [6], greater risk of organ injury and septic complications, and longer stays in critical care facilities, as well as having a mortality rate of up to

50% and an increased risk of developing a late, secondary hypercoagulable state, with risk of thromboses [7-10]. Those patients presenting with bleeding in addition to what is known as the 'lethal triad' of acidosis, hypothermia and coagulopathy will have a mortality rate approaching 90% [11].

Increasing awareness and recognition of traumatic coagulopathy has revolutionised the management of trauma patients over the last 10 years, shifting the resuscitation paradigm from restoration of the circulating volume with aggressive crystalloid infusion and packed red cell transfusion, alongside attempts at primary definitive surgical intervention, to a 'damage-control resuscitation' approach. This includes practices such as permissive hypotension, identification of coagulopathy and haemostatic resuscitation measures to correct it, as well as lifesaving, damage limitation surgical intervention where necessary, delaying definitive procedures until the patient is more stable [12, 13].

Unfortunately, whilst our understanding of pathophysiological mechanisms that accompany trauma have undoubtedly increased and our management strategies have evolved to adapt to this increased knowledge, awareness of the phenomenon of traumatic coagulopathy, whilst on the up, is still comparatively low amongst clinicians, or that it is often seen as an inevitable consequence of other resuscitative procedures, that can be managed as a secondary consideration. Early recognition and diagnosis of traumatic coagulopathy remains low. In terms of the management of active bleeding and our 'lethal triad' of coagulopathy, hypothermia and acidosis, management of coagulopathy features minimally in comparison to the other aspects of resuscitation in current guidelines and protocols, such as those delivered by ATLS, and in any case focus mainly on the later stages of management, which may have detrimental effects on the outcomes of these patients. In order to remedy this, in 2013, a multidisciplinary, pan-European task force pioneered a campaign known as 'STOP the Bleeding Campaign' which aims to increase awareness of the problem of coagulopathy and develop guidelines on its management. The acronym represents Search for patients at risk of developing coagulopathy, Treat any identified bleeding and coagulopathy as soon as they develop, Observe for response and Prevent secondary bleeding and coagulopathy [14].

After highlighting the magnitude of the problem of trauma associated coagulopathy, it is these vital steps, in addition to the pathophysiology underlying this phenomenon that we hope to cover in the following chapter.

2. The Pathophysiology of Trauma Related Coagulopathy

Whilst our understanding of trauma associated coagulation has rapidly expanded over the last decade, it is only relatively recently that much of our comprehension of the pathophysiological mechanisms underlying it has been elucidated. Major haemorrhage is, after severe traumatic brain injury, the biggest cause of death following traumatic injury, and much of this bleeding is attributable to coagulopathy as opposed to, or in conjunction with surgical bleeding. It is therefore obvious that if we are to save lives we need to develop better ways of treating traumatic coagulopathy. This challenge can only be faced by developing and nurturing our understanding of the mechanisms underpinning traumatic coagulopathy.

The traditional concept of traumatic coagulopathy was largely attributed to acidosis and hypothermia (two key components of our lethal triad) as well as the phenomenon of dilution, not only of the haematocrit secondary to rapid infusion of large volumes of crystalloid solution (then a key part of the ATLS guidelines), but also of components of the coagulation cascade, after transfusion with packed red cells, lacking in clotting factors and fibrinogen. Indeed, it is for these reasons that traumatic coagulopathy was often seen to be a largely iatrogenic event and perhaps understandably so. After all, these patients sustain significant injuries and may well be taken to theatre, both leading to exposure which may precipitate the development of hypothermia as well as being infused and transfused with fluids deplete in coagulation factors, often in large volumes and without prior warming. This coupled with the fact that these patients are by default already sick and likely to be acidotic (due to lactate production and potentially exacerbated by the hyperchloraemic acidosis that may occur after infusion with large volumes of 0.9% saline) leads to a potentially very dangerous situation, where the chances of developing a life threatening coagulopathy in the most seriously injured patients can be up to 98% [11, 15-17].

However, whilst there may certainly be a degree of iatrogenic contribution to the problem of coagulopathy for the above reasons, recent studies and advancement in our understanding of the mechanisms underlying traumatic coagulopathy show that this does not explain the full story. As already alluded to, around a quarter of major trauma patients already have a degree of coagulopathy upon presentation, when many of the potentially exacerbating iatrogenic factors have yet to occur and this is associated with a four-fold increase in mortality, compared to patients with similar injuries but no coagulopathy [18, 19]. In one of these key studies by Brohi *et al.* it was demonstrated that the presence of coagulopathy was correlated with the injury severity score, regardless of the age and mechanism. The overall mortality rate was 19.5%, but mortality in the group of coagulopathic patients was 46% compared with 10.9% in the non-coagulopathic cohort. Moreover, this increase in mortality was statistically independent from the injury severity score, so the presence of coagulopathy and increase in mortality cannot simply be attributed to these patients just being the most severely injured [7].

Several studies have confirmed the presence of this acute traumatic coagulopathy that are not attributable to iatrogenic mechanisms but more likely to be due to endogenous processes related directly and indirectly to the injury and can develop in the absence of hypothermia or haemodilution. These endogenous processes lead to the rapid development of clinically significant coagulopathy, which is often termed acute traumatic coagulopathy (ATC) and can be thought of as the endogenous precursor to trauma related coagulopathy as a whole, which is exacerbated by iatrogenic and other factors. This early coagulopathy is demonstrated in a study by Floccard *et al.* who showed that of 45 patients who had blood samples taken at the injury scene, 56% were coagulopathic after only 25 minutes [7, 18, 20, 21]. The main theories to explain the pathophysiology underlying trauma related coagulopathy are as follows:

2.1. Hypoperfusion

Shock and hypoperfusion appear along with tissue trauma to be some of the most significant factors in the initiation of traumatic coagulopathy. Shock is a well-known independent risk factor for predicting adverse outcomes amongst trauma patients [22, 23] and multiple studies have demonstrated a correlation between the degree of hypoperfusion and the level of coagulopathy on arrival at hospital as measured by standard laboratory tests such as prothrombin time (PT), international normalised ratio (INR) and activated partial thromboplastin time (APTT) [24, 25].

Studies by Brohi, Frith and Cohen *et al.* demonstrated the overriding importance of hypoperfusion in the initiation of ATC by showing that in their study of patients who had suffered traumatic brain injury (TBI), nobody without evidence of hypoperfusion (i.e., those who had a normal base deficit) had deranged coagulation tests, based on the PT/APTT, regardless of the severity of their initial injury according to the injury severity score. However, prolongation of the PT/APTT i.e., the degree of coagulopathy, was significantly correlated with the extent of hypoperfusion evidenced by increasing base deficit, with only 2% of patients who had a base deficit under 6mEq/L demonstrating coagulopathy, compared with 20% of those with a base deficit greater than 6mEq/L. In these patients, the injury severity score was also predictive of the severity of the coagulopathy. The importance of hypoperfusion in addition to trauma in the pathogenesis of ATC had also been confirmed in animal studies [5, 25, 26]. These changes all occurred in the absence of any fluid administration and fibrinogen and platelets levels were all within normal range. Coagulopathy is rarely present even in severely injured patients in the absence of shock and so clearly shock is key factor in the development of traumatic coagulopathy.

2.2. Trauma, Inflammation and Hyperfibrinolysis

The exact mechanisms underlying the significance of hypoperfusion on the development of coagulopathy are not entirely clear and are likely to be multifactorial. The resulting acidaemia is almost certainly a contributing factor, but other mechanisms related to endothelial disruption and the subsequent inflammatory response is also likely to account for this phenomenon. Tissue damage is an inherent component of trauma but varies hugely with the mechanism of injury and the severity of the trauma. For example, high velocity, blunt force trauma to the chest or abdomen can cause significant internal injury load and widespread tissue disruption, as do explosion related injuries or gunshot injuries, whilst perhaps as potentially lethal penetrative injuries such as knife wounds cause relatively localised trauma only.

However, they may all still result in trauma related coagulopathy, although as we have already established, the higher the injury severity score, the more likely coagulopathy is to be present.

The mechanisms responsible for the initiation of coagulopathic processes in response to tissue trauma are still not fully understood, though it increases all the time. Tissue trauma and damaged endothelium results in the exposure of tissue factor to the bloods components including platelets and von Willebrand factor, leading to formation of the platelet plug and initiation of aspects of the coagulation cascade. The tissue factor complexes with activated factor VII, and this complex in turn generates a small amount of thrombin.

This initiates a chain reaction in which platelet activation and thrombin generation is amplified and propagated by various interactions between platelets, clotting factors and other components. Thrombin is responsible for the conversion of fibrinogen to fibrin, which forms a mesh-like structure that is rendered stable and insoluble by factor XIIIa (figure 1) [27, 28].

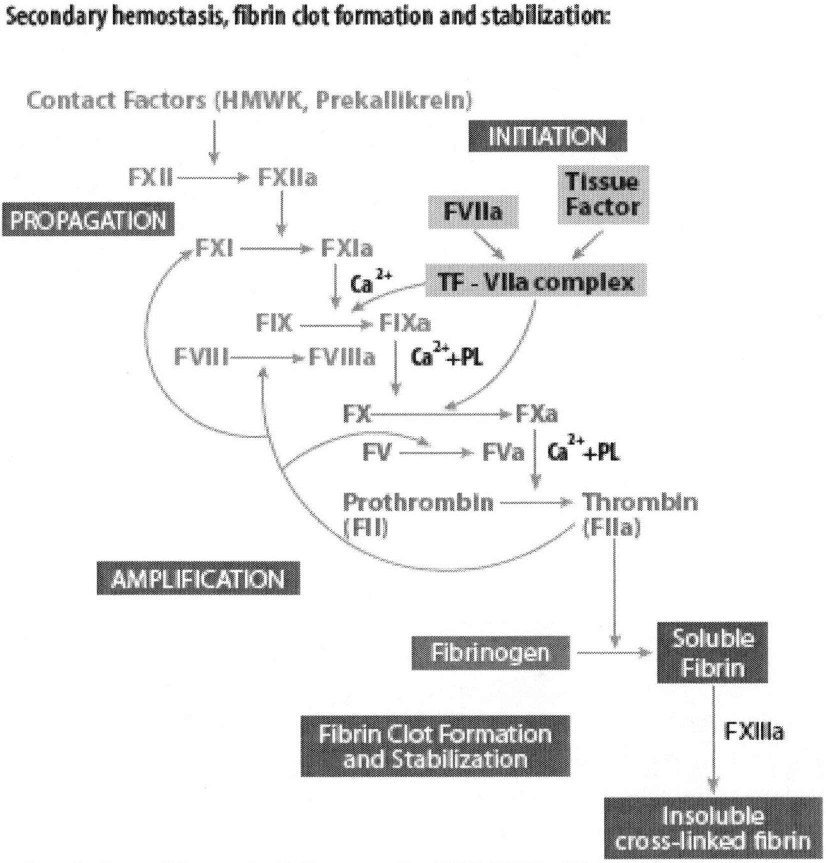

Reproduced from Lin and Selby et al. ORBCON. Bloody Easy, Coagulation Simplified. 2013. [27].

Figure 1. The traditional view of the coagulation cascade, with its intrinsic component driven by substrates already present within blood and the extrinsic pathway, dependent on endothelial damage and tissue trauma for its activation, all culminating in the common pathway which results in the formation of fibrin due to conversion of fibrinogen by thrombin and its subsequent crosslinking by factor XIII to produce a stable clot (PL – phospholipid, HMWK – high molecular weight kininogen).

In order to prevent a never ending propagation of coagulation and extension of clot beyond the area of injury to areas of healthy, non-damaged tissues and vessels, it is necessary that there exists an inherent system to counteract the ongoing activation and generation of thrombin and fibrin. This is known as the fibrinolytic system and occurs after tissue injury due to the release of tissue type plasminogen activator (tPA), which, as the name suggests, activates plasminogen to active plasmin. Plasmin then works to break down the fibrin mesh formed by the coagulation cascade and also activates various matrix metalloproteinases (MMPs) which breakdown the extracellular matrix of the clot. This results in the generation of so called fibrin degradation products, such as D-dimer. Many complex systems beyond the scope of this work exist in order to regulate the balance between clot formation and breakdown, so that and appropriate response to tissue injury occurs [29].

In major trauma, there is a propensity towards hyperfibrinolysis i.e., anticoagulation via the dampening of clot formation and promotion of the breakdown of already formed clot, which may contribute to trauma related coagulopathy. This is evidenced in various studies by the presence of elevated D-dimer levels compared to those which might be expected [26, 30, 31]. In one prospective study, Raza *et al.* showed that levels of plasmin antiplasmin (PAP) complex, a sensitive marker of fibrinolytic activity, demonstrated the presence of at least moderate fibrinolysis in over 60% of 303 patients presenting to a single major trauma centre from 2007 to 2009 [32]. Moreover, the presence of fulminant hyperfibrinolysis is correlated with a massive increase in mortality: in a study by Tauber *et al*, it was shown that mortality in patients with fulminant hyperfibrinolysis was 87.5%, compared with a mortality of 11.1% in those trauma patients with low grade fibrinolysis [33].

The pathophysiology of hyperfibrinolysis in trauma is likely to be multifactorial. It is thought that both direct and indirect tissue trauma in combination with systemic hypoperfusion and shock are the main drivers behind hyperfibrinolysis. tPA is released from damaged tissues directly as a result of injury and ischaemia, with greater amounts released as the severity of the injury increases. Hypoperfusion in trauma has been shown to lead to a reduction in the levels of plasmin activator inhibitor 1 (PAI-1), a substance which inhibits tPA. tPA levels in these patients can be twice as high as those in trauma patients with a comparable injury severity score without any evidence of shock, thus worsening the degree of fibrinolysis. It has also been postulated that hypoperfusion during trauma leads to the upregulation of thrombomodulin production by endothelial cells, which binds with thrombin and results in the upregulation of the activation of protein C, a compound that then in turn promotes an anticoagulant pathway by preventing the cleavage of factor V to factor Va, subsequently promoting an anticoagulant pathway. Activated protein C is also known to consume and further decrease levels of PAI-1 (exacerbating the direct effect of hypoperfusion of PAI-1 levels and further potentiating lack of tPA inhibition). However, it is unclear that increased activation of protein C contributes significantly to the hyperfibrinolysis seen in trauma patients, especially in the presence of normal platelets counts, which has been shown to attenuate the anticoagulant effect of even large increases in activated protein C. Furthermore, levels of circulating PAI-1 massively outweigh those of activated protein C and so it is unlikely that PAI-1 levels would be significantly repressed by this mechanism [26, 34-37]. Another theory on the reduced levels of fibrinogen present in traumatic injury and the hyperfibrinolysis it that it represents part of a spectrum of disseminated intravascular coagulation (DIC) where widespread activation of the clotting system leads to depletion of clotting factors and ultimately coagulopathy and in some ways there are a lot of similarities [38, 39]. However, histological evidence does not support the presence of microvascular thromboses that are characteristic of DIC in relation to trauma. Furthermore, there is little in the way of supporting evidence for the consumption of clotting factors in the same way that occurs as part of DIC. Acute traumatic coagulopathy is therefore thought to represent a separate entity to DIC, with its own pathogenesis [19, 40]. What is clear though, is that hyperfibrinolysis is clearly implicated in the mechanism of coagulopathy of trauma, with strong evidence of hyperfibrinolysis and critical depletion of fibrinogen which occurs rapidly after the onset of major trauma [41, 42]. This has, with great clinical importance, been further underlined by the results of the large, multi-centre CRASH-2 trial, which demonstrated significantly improved survival in trauma patients suffering major haemorrhage when treated with tranexamic acid, an antifibrinolytic agent that inhibits activation of plasminogen to plasmin and thus the breakdown of fibrin clots, without significant associated risks [43]. So revolutionary was this study that it is now gold-standard clinical practice to administer tranexamic acid in such settings [44].

2.3. Hypothermia

Hypothermia commonly occurs in trauma patients and as already mentioned, increases mortality in this group [45]. This may be due to environmental exposure, heat loss through open wounds, traumatic brain injury and subsequent lack of temperature autoregulation, haemorrhage, hypoperfusion of muscles or infusion with room temperature fluids and blood products in an attempt at resuscitation. Indeed, the infusion of 2L of room temperature crystalloid solution will require more energy to warm the patient than can be delivered by conventional means (hot air blankets, airway warming etc.) in 1 hour [46]. Moderate hypothermia (core body temperature 28-32°C) due to exposure alone is associated with a mortality rate of around 21%, as demonstrated in one multicentre study of over 400 patients [47]. However, Jurkovich *et al.* showed that hypothermia of <32°C in severely traumatically injured patients when compared with patients with exposure related hypothermia, is approaching 100%, independent of the degree of hypoperfusion or the severity of the initial injury, or indeed how much fluid the patients had received [48]. However, this does not necessarily imply that the hypothermia is independently associated with such a high mortality, for how do we know that this degree of hypothermia is not simply a marker of severity of hypoperfusion and shock in these patients, factors which we have already established are independently associated with mortality in trauma [49]. Despite this, the importance prognostically of hypothermia in trauma patients has resulted in adjusted parameters for classifying the degree of hypothermia in this group to acknowledge the fact that mortality is indeed higher in these groups, regardless of whether this is independent of other mechanisms (table 1):

Table 1. The difference in classification between the non-injured and traumatically injured hypothermic patients

Degree of hypothermia	Traditional classification (°C)	Trauma classification (°C)
Mild	32-35	34-36
Moderate	28-32	32-34
Severe	<28	<32

In relation to the coagulopathy of trauma, hypothermia is associated in a linear fashion with a reduction of tissue factor-factor VIIa complex which is responsible for primary thrombin production and initiation of fibrin clot formation. It is also decreases the activation and plugging of platelets, by decreasing the ability of vWF to bind with platelet surface complexes. Additionally, hypothermia shifts the oxygen disassociation curve to make oxygen less readily available, which potentiates acidosis, another component of our lethal triad [50-52].

Clinically significant effects of hypothermia can be seen in temperatures below 34°C on coagulation, bleeding and platelet function, however, hypothermia is a weak independent predictor of mortality and moderate and mild hypothermia (the majority of trauma patients) it is unlikely that hypothermia contributes in a clinically significant manner to the coagulopathy that is seen in these patients, but rather it is mainly attributable to other mechanisms, such as shock and endothelial activation [18, 49].

2.4. Acidaemia

Acidaemia in trauma is mainly as a result of shock and hypoperfusion, leading to a shift towards anaerobic metabolism in insufficiently perfused tissues and the accumulation of lactic acid. Furthermore, resuscitation with 0.9% (or "normal") saline leads to an increased chloride load and can precipitate a hyperchloraemic acidosis, which has the additional effect of potentiating any existing lactic acidosis [53]. Acidaemia has a detrimental effect on the function of various proteases involved in the coagulation pathways: animal and human *in vivo* studies have demonstrated that when lowering pH from normal levels to around 7.1 and 6.8 respectively, coagulation is impaired by depletion of clotting factors, thrombin generation inhibition and reduction of clot stability, as well as degradation of fibrinogen. In the human study, clot formation time was increased by 168% at a pH of 6.8 compared to that at a pH of 7.4 [54, 55].

In vitro studies suggest that clinically relevant inhibition of proteases involved in the coagulation cascade only occurs below a pH of around 7.2 [56]. However, despite the impairment of coagulation as a result of administration of acidic solutions and the generation of acidaemia, treatment of acidaemia by the administration of buffer solutions does not seem to reverse the associated coagulopathy, implying that it is not as simple as the inhibition of coagulation proteases that is responsible for coagulopathy in a state of acidaemia. Whilst the effect of acidosis on coagulation cannot be denied, it is difficult to separate out the independent effects of pH from the more global issue of hypoperfusion, which exacerbates acidaemia, and endothelial damage, triggered by the mechanisms discussed above and indeed contributed to by systemic acidosis.

2.5. Haemodilution

In the initial management of patients who have sustained major trauma, fluid resuscitation is often one of the earliest therapies to be initiated, usually with crystalloid solutions but occasionally with colloids and of course packed red cells. Intuitively, you would presume by adding a solution devoid of any coagulation components (including clotting factors, platelets and fibrinogen) to the patients circulating volume, you will cause a direct dilutional effect of these constituents, thus precipitating coagulopathy. In addition to the dilutional effects of fluid administration as an iatrogenic cause of haemodilution in trauma, endogenous physiological mechanisms also contribute. Reduced hydrostatic pressure in the intravascular space results (by virtue of Starling forces) in the shift of fluid from the intracellular and interstitial spaces into the intravascular compartment; of course, these fluids are also devoid of any procoagulant components.

In vitro studies do indeed seem to support a directly proportionate dilutional effect related to the volume of fluid that has been infused, although with mild-moderate haemodilution, this effect does not seem to be as significant [57-59]. However, it is more difficult to translate these findings into *in vivo* settings, as a result of the complexity of interactions that also modify the coagulation response. As already covered, the degree of tissue trauma, inflammation and hypoperfusion can affect the endothelial release of clotting components, as can the neuroendocrine response to traumatic injury, such as release of adrenaline and anti-diuretic hormone (vasopressin). Secondly, platelets sequestered in the body in secondary stores may be mobilised in response to traumatic injury and this can confound the levels that are seen and make it difficult to quantify the haemodilutional effect and subsequent deleterious result on coagulation [60].

As alluded to earlier, in the seminal paper by Brohi *et al.* looking at the incidence of and mortality in acute traumatic coagulopathy on a group of 1,088 trauma patients who presented to one major trauma unit in London, they found that whilst a quarter of patients were coagulopathic on arrival, this bore no relation to the amount of fluid administered prior to their arrival [7]. However, another study conducted in Germany in which average fluid administration prior to arrival was much higher, identified a statistically significant dilutional effect, showing that of people who had received >3L prior to arrival, the presence of coagulopathy was around 50% [10]. Interestingly, the primary difference between these studies was that the choice of IV fluid used for resuscitation in the German studied included a much greater proportion of colloid, which may suggest that colloids are more inclined to precipitate a coagulopathic effect, whether by haemodilution (which may be more pronounced in the use of colloids, given that their very purpose is to pull in and retain more fluid in the intravascular compartment) or another mechanism, such as interference with clot formation and/or stabilisation of the fibrin plug. This theory tends to be supported by studies which show very little to no effect of crystalloid infusion of coagulopathy in healthy volunteers and indeed, even in *in vitro* studies, the use of colloids seems to have far greater coagulopathic effects than crystalloid solutions [61, 62].

2.6. Consumption and Depletion of Clotting Factors

In a similar vein of thinking as the effect of dilution on potential coagulopathy, it is easy to envisage that a loss of clotting factors occurs, either as a direct result of haemorrhage and subsequent loss of clotting factors onto the floor(!) or because of consumption of these factors during widespread coagulation and clot formation, both within vessels and extravascular clotting. *In vitro* studies have shown an inverse correlation between haematocrit and bleeding time, once the haematocrit falls below about 30% [63]. It was previously widely believed that consumption of clotting factors was a major contributing factor to trauma related coagulopathy in a similar picture to DIC, seen, for example, in sepsis. However, studies in elective surgical settings involving the pre-administration of additional clotting factors, platelets and fibrinogen appear not to support a significant role for consumption/depletion of clotting factors or platelets as a significant mechanism in the development of trauma related coagulopathy. Furthermore, as already stated, there is no significant evidence in post-mortem studies of trauma patients of widespread thrombus formation as would be seen in a consumptive coagulopathy/DIC-type picture [40, 64].

2.7. Immune Activation

Multiple, complicated immune mechanisms may contribute to trauma related coagulopathy, but in the scope of this chapter, they represent a relatively small component of the wider aetiology underlying the pathology. Tissue damage and hypoperfusion results in widespread release of various cytokines and immune activators, such as tumour necrosis factor, interleukin-1 and CD-40 ligand, all of which can further activate endothelial cells and potentiate the release of tPA, which results in increased fibrinolysis. Immune stimulation also leads to release of a variety of damage-associated molecular patterns (DAMPs) which further exacerbate tissue damage via the activation of various proteases and oxidative stress [21, 65].

3. Identification and Prediction of Traumatic Coagulopathy

Transfusion of blood products is currently guided by clinical judgment and standard laboratory tests, these are usually activated partial thromboplastin time (aPTT), prothrombin time (PT), international normalized ratio (INR), platelet count, and plasma fibrinogen. However, routine coagulation tests only reflect the initiation phase of haemostasis at the point of testing and consequently are unsuitable, inaccurate monitors for coagulopathy in the ever-changing trauma patient.

None of these tests were developed to predict bleeding or to guide coagulation management in the surgical or trauma setting, the major limitations being lack of real-time monitoring, with reported median turnaround time for testing of 78-88 minutes making results quickly historical. They have an inability to identify or differentiate between singular or multiple coagulation factor deficiencies; and provide no rapid assessment of fibrinolysis, platelet dysfunction, or haemostatic response to injury. In trauma, timely availability of blood and component therapy is vital but we should still aim for patient tailored haemostatic resuscitation to avoid exposure to risk.

ROTEM is a point of care (POC) testing device measuring the viscoelastic properties on multiple aspects of blood coagulation using a sample of citrated whole blood. Measurements are made on the interactions of coagulation factors, inhibitors and cellular components during the phases of clotting in whole blood. It can therefore identify coagulopathies secondary to dilution, consumption, deficiencies and hyper-fibrinolysis. Thus it becomes possible to make a timely distinction between surgical bleeding and bleeding caused by coagulopathy. The equipment is easy to use by adequately trained non-laboratory personnel as a POC test in both the perioperative and emergency setting. The device is a mobile unit that can be easily transported to the operating theatre for regular reassessment of clotting during massive transfusion. It provides fast information on the cause of bleeding, and thus allows guided coagulation management and optimum blood product usage. This has the positive effect of reducing transfusion-related risks and provides improved patient health outcomes, which in turn has the potential to reduce transfusion requirements, re-exploration rates, health resources consumption and healthcare costs. By using ROTEM, haemostatic therapy can be individualized according to the patient's actual needs, potentially reducing the risks of both under-transfusion (increased risk of bleeding) and over-transfusion (increased risk of ARDS, acute lung injury, sepsis and multi-organ failure).

Testing Procedure

The system has four independent measurement channels, which enable the simultaneous independent tests and with an integrated computer producing automatic analysis. The two tests are normally performed together for each patient:-

EXTEM: coagulation is activated by a small amount of tissue factor to monitor the coagulation process via the extrinsic pathway.

FIBTEM: coagulation is activated, as in *EXTEM*, to monitor the clot firmness after blocking the platelet contribution.

Together, these allow differentiation between low fibrinogen and low platelet functionality as a cause of reduced clot strength.

FIBTEM is always used in conjunction with *EXTEM*. Therefore, the resulting clot is only dependent on the fibrin formation and fibrin polymerisation.

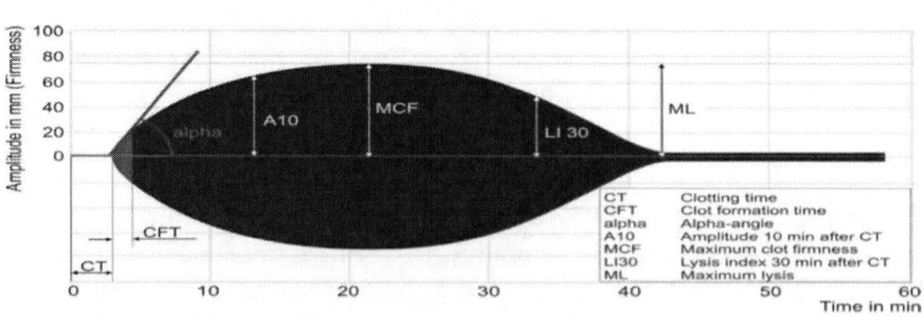

Figure taken from TEM training material.

Figure 2. Illustration of a TEMogram showing clot initiation (clotting time), clot dynamics (a angle, clot formation time) and clot firmness (max clot firmness).

Normal Values for different Assays

ROTEM TEST	CT (s)	CFT (s)	MCF (mm)	ML (% MCF)
Extem	40-80	34-160	50-72	<15
Fibtem	-	-	9-25	-

CT=clotting time
CFT=clot formation time
MCF=maximum clot firmness
ML=maximum lysis
In FIBTEM analysis, MCF<9mm: reduced fibrinogen level or impaired polymerisation, a
MCF>25mm, indicates increased fibrinogen level.

Analysis and Use of the Tests

The time taken for testing using ROTEM is typically between 10 and 20 minutes and the analyses can be repeated 10 minutes after administration of coagulation factors or blood products to guide further management.

ROTEM produces rapid, easily interpretable graphical and numerical results which represent the three different phases of cell-based haemostasis which result in clot formation. Analysis of the structural changes in the clot have shown that the reaction time (CT) corresponds to the initiation phase, the clot formation time (CFT) reflects the amplification phase. It has been demonstrated that the 'thrombin burst' is reflected by the α-angle, which determines the clot strength and stability of the clot. The ability of the graph to reflect thrombin generation has profound clinical utility, because secondary coagulation factor deficiencies, for example massive bleeding, dilution, consumption and thrombocytopenia result in impaired thrombin generation and impaired clot strength and maximum clot firmness (MCF). The whole blood-based trace, therefore, reveals the contribution of all circulating plasma and cellular components to clot formation. Enhanced fibrinolysis contributes significantly to bleeding in trauma patients, and this condition is readily identified by clot lysis. The results from this system therefore allows clinicians to determine the precise cause of bleeding and improves the diagnosis and subsequent management of patients who experience unexplained blood loss resulting from surgery or trauma.

Since the validity and efficacy of the test relies heavily on the interpretation of the results by involved health professionals, the tests should be performed by trained staff, who are able to analyse and interpret the results accurately to ensure the consistency of application.

In order to standardise the interpretation, an algorithmic approach is often used to guide clinicians in their interpretation and management of appropriate blood product usage when running ROTEM tests.

4. Management Strategies for Trauma Related Coagulopathy: Haemostatic Resuscitation Methods

The ideal resuscitation strategy in major trauma patients has been debated for decades and much has changed over the years to reflect our increasing understanding of mechanisms of and physiological responses to trauma. Even with our improved knowledge, as we have discussed, trauma is still the leading cause of death worldwide in what should be a healthy, productive demographic, and massive haemorrhage is probably within this group the leading cause of potentially preventable mortality.

Paradoxically, much of our progressive understanding in the field of trauma management and the preservation of life comes from the field of combat. This is largely to do with the sheer numbers of patients seen in these settings, who rather than being distributed amongst many trauma centres separated both geographically and administratively, tend to be channelled to a limited number of centres, thereby making standardisation and data collection simpler.

Trauma in a civilian setting, however, represents a fortunately smaller proportion of patients admitted overall. Despite recent advances in our understanding of coagulopathy in trauma, and the evolution of resuscitation strategies, without the widespread usage of point of care testing such as those discussed above, much of the current management relies on empirical transfusion protocols of various blood components and gestalt impressions of the treating medical staff [66].

4.1. General Resuscitative Principles

In terms of the immediate management of the trauma patient, the most pressing measure is to avoid at all costs (or reverse where already developed) the "lethal triad" of acidosis, hypothermia and coagulopathy. Since haemorrhage is the leading cause of potentially reversible death, it stands to reason that an immediate aim of trauma resuscitation should be directed at control of obvious sources of bleeding. This approach can be applied both in the pre-hospital and emergency department settings with the use of splinting, tourniquets and wound packing or surgical and endovascular approaches to arresting of bleeding. Over the past 15 years or so (though the concept has been described prior to this) management of these patients has shifted from early attempts at definitive surgical management to a "damage control surgery" strategy, which traditionally was focussed on the arrest of major haemorrhage and control of bleeding points. With the resuscitative focus on avoiding or reversing the lethal triad and stabilising the patient's physiological parameters, these two elements have recently been reconciled to form a more holistic "damage control resuscitation" approach. This has been defined by Hodgetts *et al.* as "*a systematic approach to major trauma, combining the [(catastrophic haemorrhage) Airway, Breathing, Circulation] paradigm with a series of clinical techniques from point of wounding to definitive treatment, in order to minimise blood loss, maximise tissue oxygenation and optimise outcome*", a strategy which incorporates all of the above physiological and surgical aims to optimise the care of the injured patient [67-69].

Current aims of this strategy include avoidance of hypothermia by warming of fluids and blood components prior to administration, minimising exposure of the patient, rapid control of obvious haemorrhage, covering the patient with air warmed blankets and increasing the room temperature of environments where trauma victims are cared for e.g., resuscitation rooms and trauma theatres (these should be uncomfortably warm for the staff!). Continuous arterio-venous rewarming has also been shown to reduce mortality in severely injured trauma patients. This involves creating a circuit whereby blood is removed via the femoral artery and passed through a warming circuit before being reinfused via the femoral vein [70, 71]. Acidosis should also be avoided by the judicious use of buffer solutions, such as bicarbonate, although tri-hydroxymethylaminomethane (THAM) may be used preferentially (especially by the US military) as it appears to have less effect on oxygen dissociation than bicarbonate and rapidly lowers PaCO2 to restore the acid-base balance [12, 72].

It terms of volume resuscitation in trauma, it has long been recognised that after major haemorrhage it is preferential to restore volume with blood components as opposed to crystalloid or colloid, to maximise the oxygenation carrying capacity and prevent tissue hypoxia. This also avoids the issues identified above of haemodilution potentially contributing to the aetiology of trauma related coagulopathy. Traditionally, an aggressive volume resuscitation strategy was employed, aimed at restoring intravascular volumes to those prior to injury. However, this has the unwanted potential of elevating hydrostatic pressures to such levels that may disrupt clots formed in bleeding vessels, thus potentiating ongoing haemorrhage. In the 1990s, Bickell *et al.* described an innovative approach to delayed resuscitation, bringing about the concept of "permissive hypotension", that is, volume resuscitation to maintain a systolic blood pressure of around 80-90mmHg, enough, in theory, to maintain cerebral and vital organ perfusion without increasing the risk of rebleeding, a concept also described in animal models [73, 74].

This hypotensive strategy has been employed by both civilian and military bodies but it has the obvious downside of prolonging potential tissue hypoperfusion and acidosis as well as being one of the driving factors in trauma related coagulopathy, so clearly a balance must be struck. In one meta-analysis of resuscitation strategies in animal models, there was shown to be a universal increase in survival in animals resuscitated with a hypotensive approach, however, some argue that the study designs, including the injury mechanisms, are biased to favour this approach, and that different injury mechanism may warrant different resuscitation strategies [75, 76]. There are some studies which have shown there to be no difference in survival between hypotensive and normotensive approaches to resuscitation or even that hypotensive resuscitation results in an adverse effect on mortality [77, 78]. Rapid control of haemorrhage and a fast, reliable method of assessment of the patient's physiology are therefore required to optimise the outcome in major trauma.

4.2. Current Limitations and Controversies around the Treatment of Trauma Related Coagulopathy

Whilst our evolution of our understanding of trauma related coagulopathy has increased exponentially over the past decade, treatment is still largely based around empirical regimes, and guided by standard laboratory tests which are woefully inadequate in terms of their ability to accurately guide in a timely manner the ongoing management of the rapidly changing severely injured major trauma patient. There is also ongoing international debate surrounding the optimum treatment strategy for these patients and there is often little or no consensus even between trauma centres of the same country as to how to manage trauma related coagulopathy. Part of the problem lies in the fact that we still lack a complete definition as to what exactly constitutes both acute traumatic coagulopathy and the broader concept of trauma related coagulopathy as a whole. Again, this is largely due to our incomplete understanding of the underlying mechanisms. Initiatives such as "Advanced Bleeding Care in Trauma", a multidisciplinary, international task force which aims to rationalise the current evidence and make recommendations on best practise have gone some way to addressing these issues [79].

Most of our current definitions of traumatic coagulopathy are based around conventional standard laboratory tests, which as we have already addressed, are inadequate when it comes to the diagnosis and management of traumatic coagulopathy. Arbitrary figures have been used across international literature to "define" trauma related coagulopathy, such as prothrombin time (PT) more than 18 seconds [7], international normalised ratio (INR) >1.5 [80] or INR >1.2 [81]. These tests fail to accurately reflect and respond to the underlying pathophysiological changes happening during trauma related coagulopathy, which is one of the other limitations to its management. Not only is it time consuming to diagnose via these methods in the first place (as well as potentially inaccurate) but there are also further issues surrounding monitoring the response to treatment strategies. This is partly why there has been such resurgence in the interest in viscoelastic haemostatic assays in trauma, such as ROTEM and TEG, as they give information regarding actual clot formation and strength, as well as fibrinolysis, as opposed to traditional tests which only give limited information about the initiation of coagulation, without reflecting the whole process [82].

Further controversies exist still with regards to the exact thresholds in trauma patients that should trigger the administration of various blood components. The trend towards earlier transfusion with red cells has largely been adopted in preference to crystalloid/colloid infusions which may potentiate coagulopathy and have no oxygen carrying capacity (thereby also contributing to acidosis and ongoing coagulopathy), however, in terms of ongoing transfusion requirements, it was shown that in trauma patient enlisted in the Transfusion Requirements in Critical Care (TRICC) trial (where patients with a low haemoglobin were randomised to either a restrictive or liberal transfusion group), it appears safe to opt for a more restrictive transfusion approach, that is, transfusing to maintain a haemoglobin of between 7-10g/dL. This approach does not seem to have any detrimental effects on mortality, but did show some evidence to support a reduced pro-inflammatory profile that has been associated with red blood cell transfusions in trauma patients, though further high powered studies are needed to confirm these findings [83]. Controversy also exists in the ideal administration of other blood products, including when to administer them and in what ratios should they be given, as we shall cover in more detail shortly.

4.3. Transfusion and the Treatment of Trauma Related Coagulopathy

4.3.1. Transfusion Components

Differing transfusion strategies utilise blood components in different ways and many hospitals have developed protocols to guide the delivery, including massive haemorrhage/transfusion protocols, massive haemorrhage/transfusion being inconsistently defined in various different ways; a replacement of total circulating volume over 24 hours, transfusion of ≥10 units of packed red cells, blood loss of more than 150ml/min, transfusion of more than 4 units in one hour or replacement of 50% of the circulating volume in 3 hours [76]. There is currently no universal or even nationwide consensus on the optimum combinations and ratios of these components, however, it is increasingly recognised that all components have to be utilised in a haemostatic approach to resuscitation, that is, with the aim of restoring circulating volume and arresting coagulopathy and ongoing haemorrhage.

- *Packed red cells* (PRCs) – The erythrocyte component of whole blood, washed of plasma to reduce the presence of plasma proteins. Erythrocytes as the oxygen carrying component of blood help to reduce coagulopathy following trauma by increasing the oxygen delivery to tissues, resulting in a decrease in anaerobic respiration and lactic acid generation, and an overall attenuation of hypoxia induced acidaemia. They also contribute to the coagulation mechanism by the marginalisation of platelets (in basic terms, the flow of erythrocytes pushes the platelets to the edges of the vessels, in closer contact with the endothelium, which if then breached will result in platelet plugging), promotion of thrombin generation and the activation of platelets [84, 85].
- *Platelets* – Integral to the initiation of the clotting cascade, they form the initial platelet plug at the site of endothelial injury and then activate subsequent clotting cascades, ultimately resulting in fibrin deposition and organisation into the stable mesh. Much of the support for transfusion thresholds for platelets is based on general clinical

consensus rather than hard clinical evidence. In the context of coagulopathy in trauma, much less research has been performed on investigating the optimum transfusion triggers and requirements for platelets. A generally held level of 50 x 10^9/l is often used as a cut off for platelet transfusion, although higher levels, 100 x 10^9/l have been advocated in major brain injury or in significant haemorrhage [79, 86].

- *Fresh frozen plasma* (FFP) – Each unit contains around 200-250mls of plasma and is a source of coagulation factors (with the exception of factor VIII as this rapidly breaks down). There is wealth of evidence to suggest that larger volumes of FFP should be administered in major trauma than were used in traditional approaches, and that this should be given empirically, without waiting for the results of standard laboratory tests of coagulation, to avoid and treat trauma related coagulopathy. However, as with much of the literature, there is no consensus on exactly how much should be given and how early this should be [87, 88].
- *Other components – Fibrinogen concentrates* may be given where conventional treatment with FFP has been insufficient to increase levels of fibrinogen in order to attenuate coagulopathic bleeding. In areas where prepared fibrinogen concentrates are not readily available, *cryoprecipitate* can be utilised instead. In the context of coagulopathy (in in-vitro and clinical studies) administration of fibrinogen concentrate can increase the total fibrinogen levels and improve clot firmness [89, 90]. There has also been considerable interest in the use of *recombinant factor VIIa*, which is used to potentiate thrombin generation and subsequent clot formation. It is licensed for use in major bleeding associated with congenital deficiency of factor VII and in some cases of haemophilia, however, studies investigating its potential therapeutic use in coagulopathy of trauma have shown inconclusive results, with some authors purporting to show a reduction in the need for red cell transfusion when using rFVIIa, whilst others have observed no change in the overall mortality. Additionally, it seems as though the risk of thromboembolic events is significantly elevated in patients receiving rFVIIa [91-93]. *Prothrombin complex concentrate (PCC)* contains factors II, VII, IX and X (as well as proteins C & S) and had been widely used in the management of congenital disorders of coagulation as well as for the rapid reversal of anti-coagulant agents. Its use in traumatic

coagulopathy has been postulated, however, meaningful data is lacking and currently it is not part of the recommended practice for the management of trauma related coagulopathy, according to the latest European guidelines. However, some animal studies have shown a potential reversal of coagulopathy with the use of PCC and significantly improved haemostasis, so this may well be an avenue that is investigated by further trials in the near future [79, 94]. *Factor XIII* has been demonstrated to be a significant contributor to the development of clot firmness and even relatively minor deficiencies in FXIII have been associated with increased bleeding tendencies in surgical patients [95, 96]. However, robust research into this avenue of therapy is also currently lacking, though one recent *in vitro* study has shown some benefit of administration of FXIII in coagulopathy associated with significant dilution [97]. More work is clearly needed though before this translates into any clinical practice.

4.3.2. Complications of Transfusions

The complications of transfusions are numerous and well recognised, and so it is important that patients are not transfused indiscriminately. The most widely occurring complication associated with transfusion is that of compatibility mismatching, which is almost always related to human error. Whilst rigorous protocols are in place for the checking and rechecking of blood products, errors do happen, and the results can be fatal. Mistransfusion rates are thought to be somewhere in the region of 1 in 18,000 units of packed red cells, in the United Kingdom, although more recent data is lacking. Fatality due to error in ABO matching occurs in the transfusion of around 1 in 800,000 units [98, 99]. Transmission of infective diseases, incorporating viral, bacterial, protozoan and prion diseases is another area of great concern in transfusion practice. In the developed world, donor screening both via questionnaires and screening of blood has resulted in a drastic reduction in the transmission of blood borne infections such as hepatitis and HIV. In patients who are immunocompromised, blood products specifically tested as negative for specific viruses such as cytomegalovirus (CMV) may be required to prevent infection in these susceptible individuals. This adds a further layer of complexity to the transfusion protocol in these cases. The risk of bacterial contamination and subsequent infection is much higher in the case of platelets, as these are stored at a temperature of 20-24°C, an ideal temperature for the proliferation of bacteria. Even across the relatively short storage lifespan of platelets (5 days), this is more than enough time for a very limited bacterial count to multiply to very high levels. It is estimated that platelet transfusion related sepsis may be responsible for up to 1000 cases of severe or fatal sepsis in the United States [100]. In some centres, culturing of platelets is performed prior to transfusion in an attempt to ameliorate this risk.

Transfusion of red blood cells in the trauma setting has been independently associated with post-injury multi-organ failure (MOF) as has the age of the red blood cells, with those older than 14 days carrying a substantially increased risk, as well as the occurrence of post-injury infection. The exact mechanisms behind this are unclear, but it is thought to originate from complex immunomodulatory mechanisms, as well as contributed to by the presence of white blood cells. Studies comparing the rates of infection between transfusion with leucocyte depleted packed red cells and non-leucocyte depleted packed red cells are, however, inconclusive. Since 1999, all allogenic blood components in the UK are leucocyte deplete, regardless [101-103].

Transfusion related acute lung injury (TRALI) is another widely known, but thankfully uncommon (although likely underdiagnosed) complication related to transfusion. It occurs within 4 hours post-transfusion and results in a non-cardiogenic pulmonary oedema casing dyspnoea and hypoxia and, though the exact mechanism behind it is unclear, it is thought to have a multifactorial aetiology with immune-mediated alteration of the permeability of pulmonary capillaries [100, 104]. Despite the obvious clinical advantages associated with transfusion and its overall clinical importance, the risks cannot be ignored and so it is imperative that this resource is utilised in a carefully controlled manner, to aid haemostatic control resuscitation whilst minimising the subsequent risk of transfusion related complications to the patient.

4.3.3. Current Transfusion Strategies and Massive Transfusion Protocols

Historically, large volume blood loss was treated with the aim of normalising circulating volume and this was initially achieved via the infusion of large volumes of crystalloid/colloid solutions. As concerns regarding dilution, tissue perfusion and oxygenation mounted, the trend moved towards early transfusion with packed red cells, but now, with our ever increasing awareness of trauma related coagulopathy, practice has further evolved to incorporate a haemostatic resuscitative approach in massively injured patients.

Previously, transfusion of red blood cells occurred early during resuscitation, and the administration of other components such as FFP and platelets would be delayed until any coagulopathy was confirmed by conventional laboratory tests (PT, INR, APTT etc.) or one blood volume had been lost. However, as we have already established, as many as 25% of patients already have significant coagulopathy on arrival at the hospital and conventional laboratory tests are poor indicators and prognosticators of trauma associated coagulopathy so this approach leads to significant delays in correcting a person's coagulopathic status. This realisation that acute traumatic coagulopathy often complicates issues in major trauma has led to many trauma centres developing massive transfusion protocols (MTPs) in an attempt to not only restore sufficient circulating volume and achieve adequate perfusion of tissues, but to additionally correct any coagulopathy, all as part of damage control/haemostatic control resuscitation. In both military and civilian studies, the use of a pre-defined, set protocol for guiding administration of blood products has been shown to be associated with an overall decrease in the amount of blood products transfused and a reduction in overall mortality [105, 106].

With the general acceptance of the need for MTPs, the next issue has been in identifying the ideal component ratios for transfusion. The paradigm of massive transfusion has gradually shifted over the years towards a strategy of early administration of plasma in order to address the early coagulopathy that has been shown to occur in trauma and indeed, may already be present on arrival [107].

The debate surrounding timing and dosing of plasma, however, is still hotly contested. The vast majority of emerging research, including early mathematical models of major haemorrhage and the increasing body of both military and civilian studies, supports earlier administration of higher ratios of FFP to PRCs, i.e., ≥1:2 [108-114]. Of these, Borgman *et al.* were perhaps the first to show a direct relationship between mortality and FFP administration, demonstrating a mortality of 65% in casualties who received FFP:PRCs in rations of <1:4 compared to a mortality of 19% in those receiving a ratio of 1:1 [113].

In a retrospective analysis of prospective data gathered by the German Society of Trauma Surgery, Maegele *et al.* showed that higher FFP:PRC ratios were associated with decreased mortality, with mortality rates in the 'low' (FFP:PRC <0.9), 'medium' (0.9–1.1), and 'high' (>1.1) ratio groups of 25, 10, and 3.5%, respectively [114].

One of the major drawback of the studies supporting high ratios FFP:PRCs is that they are all retrospective in nature, and data is lacking from any large scale, prospective randomised controlled trials (RCTs). One small prospective study looking at optimal ratios failed to show an improved outcome in patients transfused with a 1:1 ratio [115]. It has been speculated that the main confounding factor in studies suggesting high ratios of FFP improves mortality is that of "survival bias", meaning that the patients who were more likely to survive to begin with were the ones who survived long enough to receive FFP transfusion, thereby making it seem as though it was the administration of FFP that improved survival rates, when in reality, those patients would have survived regardless. However, many people feel that this is unlikely to account for the improved results seen with high ratios of FFP, since the injury severity is similar between groups receiving different ratios of FFP:PRC in these studies and furthermore, it cannot explain the increased survival in studies where FFP was immediately available (i.e., pre-thawed FFP was available) [116].

Less extensive research has been done into the ideal transfusion of platelets in trauma related coagulopathy, however, their role and importance in the coagulation pathway means that they cannot be ignored. Whilst their role in thrombin generation is felt to be one of the most important factors in the formation of the stable clot, it is not yet fully appreciated what their other roles may be in the context of trauma related coagulopathy. Some advocate early administration of platelets in addition to FFP in a 1:1:1 ratio [109] though this strategy has not been universally accepted and in the face of current scientific evidence may be unjustified until more research is done on the matter [82].

Whilst it is not clear yet what the precise optimum ratio of FFP:PRC:platelets should be, it is generally accepted that earlier and higher ratios of FFP should be given empirically in the context of coagulopathy in trauma, in contrast to the "old way" of waiting for the results of standard laboratory measures of coagulopathy that do not reflect the true *in vivo* status of coagulation in the trauma patient. Current European guidelines recommend early administration of FFP in a ratio of at least 1:2 with administration of platelets guided by laboratory values, aiming to maintain platelet counts of greater than 50 x 10^9/l or >100 x 10^9/l if there is ongoing major bleeding. The antifibrinolytic, tranexamic acid should also be administered as early as possible and calcium gluconate should also be administered to maintain plasma calcium concentrations within the normal range (since administration of citrated blood products chelates the plasma calcium. Hypocalcaemia in major trauma has also been independently associated with increased mortality) [79, 117].

Clearly more work needs to be done to accurately define optimum ratios of blood products in trauma, and the Pragmatic, Randomized Optimal Plasma and Platelet Ratio (PROPPR) Study in North America, a large, multi-centre

RCT with the aim of comparing outcomes in different ratio groups of severely bleeding major trauma patients aims to do just that. Data analysis is currently underway and the results once available should hopefully address these issues [118].

4.3.4. The Next Step: Point of Care Testing and Goal Directed Management

Whilst the above work has been instrumental in guiding transfusion strategies in trauma patients, and the use of MTPs clearly has conveyed significant benefit on mortality, clearly a "one size fits all" policy cannot address the subtleties and differences in presentation between individual patients. There are a multitude of variables affecting the degree of coagulopathy in trauma, many of which we do not fully understand: age of the patient, underlying pre-existing health conditions, mechanism of injury, severity of injury, individual genetic factors underlying propensity towards coagulopathy, physiological reserves of the patient etc. Coagulopathy in trauma is a dynamic condition and it is not always easy to appreciate this. Surely an ideal approach would be one in which we could individually monitor coagulopathy in these patients and then tailor their management specifically towards their particular clinical condition at any one point in time? This would not only ensure that the patients were transfused according to their requirements, but it would ameliorate over-transfusion and its associated risks.

The use of thromoboelastometry such as TEG or ROTEM provides us with a dynamic, real time measure of whole blood clotting and can be used to rapidly identify coagulopathy in the trauma patient, as we have already discussed.

Prompt haemostatic resuscitative measure can then be undertaken to correct disturbances of coagulation as they occur, with administration of FFP, platelets, fibrinogen concentrates, recombinant FVIIa or other coagulation factors, or it can even be used to predict an individual's need for massive transfusion and guide preventative transfusion strategies.

In some European centres, the use of ROTEM to monitor and guide management of trauma related coagulopathy has not only been associated with a reduction in mortality, but also an overall reduction in blood product usage – meaning a lower potential for transfusion associated adverse effects conservation of what is a valuable and limited resource [119, 120]. Its use in trauma as standard protocol is yet to be fully validated, but this is likely to represent the most promising method we have in the diagnosis and management of trauma related coagulopathy, and would eliminate the debate surrounding optimum transfusion triggers and ratios, allowing goal directed and management optimally and individually tailored to each patient.

References

[1] Murray C. J., Lopez A. D. Alternative projections of mortality and disability by cause 1990-2020: Global Burden of Disease Study. *Lancet,* 1997; 349(9064):1498-504.

[2] NCEPOD. Trauma: Who Cares? 2007.

[3] National Audit Office. Major Trauma Care in England. The Stationery Office; 2010.

[4] Johansson P. I. Coagulation monitoring of the bleeding traumatized patient. *Curr. Opin. Anaesthesiol.*, 2012; 25(2):235-41.

[5] Frith D., Goslings J. C., Gaarder C., Maegele M., Cohen M. J., Allard S., et al. Definition and drivers of acute traumatic coagulopathy: clinical and experimental investigations. *J. Thromb Haemost.,* 2010; 8(9):1919-25.

[6] Mitra B., Cameron P. A., Gruen R. L., Mori A., Fitzgerald M., Street A. The definition of massive transfusion in trauma: a critical variable in examining evidence for resuscitation. *Eur. J. Emerg. Med.,* 2011; 18(3): 137-42.

[7] Brohi K., Singh J., Heron M., Coats T. Acute traumatic coagulopathy. *J. Trauma,* 2003; 54(6):1127-30.

[8] MacLeod J. B., Lynn M., McKenney M. G., Cohn S. M., Murtha M. Early coagulopathy predicts mortality in trauma. *J. Trauma,* 2003; 55(1): 39-44.

[9] Holcomb J. B., Wade C. E., Brasel K. J., Vercruysse G., MacLeod J., Dutton R. P., et al. Defining present blood component transfusion practices in trauma patients: papers from the Trauma Outcomes Group. *J. Trauma,* 2011; 71(2 Suppl. 3):S315-7.

[10] Maegele M., Lefering R., Yucel N., Tjardes T., Rixen D., Paffrath T., et al. Early coagulopathy in multiple injury: an analysis from the German Trauma Registry on 8724 patients. *Injury,* 2007; 38(3):298-304.

[11] Ferrara A., MacArthur J. D., Wright H. K., Modlin I. M., McMillen M. A. Hypothermia and acidosis worsen coagulopathy in the patient requiring massive transfusion. *Am. J. Surg.*, 1990; 160(5):515-8.

[12] Byers R. An upshot of war - damage control resuscitation. *Int. Emerg. Nurs.*, 2010; 18(4):221-5.

[13] Holcomb J. B., Jenkins D., Rhee P., Johannigman J., Mahoney P., Mehta S., et al. Damage control resuscitation: directly addressing the early coagulopathy of trauma. *J. Trauma,* 2007; 62(2):307-10.
[14] Rossaint R., Bouillon B., Cerny V., Coats T. J., Duranteau J., Fernández-Mondéjar E., et al. The STOP the Bleeding Campaign. *Crit. Care,* 2013; 17(2):136.
[15] Cosgriff N., Moore E. E., Sauaia A., Kenny-Moynihan M., Burch J. M., Galloway B. Predicting life-threatening coagulopathy in the massively transfused trauma patient: hypothermia and acidoses revisited. *J. Trauma,* 1997; 42(5):857-61; discussion 61-2.
[16] Schreiber M. A. Coagulopathy in the trauma patient. *Curr. Opin. Crit. Care,* 2005; 11(6):590-7.
[17] Thomas D., Wee M., Clyburn P., Walker I., Brohi K., Collins P., et al. Blood transfusion and the anaesthetist: management of massive haemorrhage. *Anaesthesia,* 2010; 65(11):1153-61.
[18] Brohi K., Cohen M. J., Davenport R. A. Acute coagulopathy of trauma: mechanism, identification and effect. *Curr. Opin. Crit. Care,* 2007; 13(6):680-5.
[19] Hess J. R., Brohi K., Dutton R. P., Hauser C. J., Holcomb J. B., Kluger Y., et al. The coagulopathy of trauma: a review of mechanisms. *J. Trauma,* 2008; 65(4):748-54.
[20] Floccard B., Rugeri L., Faure A., Saint Denis M., Boyle E. M., Peguet O., et al. Early coagulopathy in trauma patients: an on-scene and hospital admission study. *Injury*, 2012;43(1):26-32.
[21] Cap A., Hunt B. J. The pathogenesis of traumatic coagulopathy. *Anaesthesia,* 2015; 70 Suppl. 1:96-e34.
[22] Siegel J. H., Rivkind A. I., Dalal S., Goodarzi S. Early physiologic predictors of injury severity and death in blunt multiple trauma. *Arch. Surg.*, 1990; 125(4):498-508.
[23] Davis J. W., Parks S. N., Kaups K. L., Gladen H. E., O'Donnell-Nicol S. Admission base deficit predicts transfusion requirements and risk of complications. *J. Trauma,* 1996; 41(5):769-74.
[24] Niles S. E., McLaughlin D. F., Perkins J. G., Wade C. E., Li Y., Spinella P. C., et al. Increased mortality associated with the early coagulopathy of trauma in combat casualties. *J. Trauma*, 2008;64(6):1459-63; discussion 63-5.

[25] Cohen M. J., Brohi K., Ganter M. T., Manley G. T., Mackersie R. C., Pittet J. F. Early coagulopathy after traumatic brain injury: the role of hypoperfusion and the protein C pathway. *J. Trauma,* 2007; 63(6):1254-61; discussion 61-2.

[26] Brohi K., Cohen M. J., Ganter M. T., Matthay M. A., Mackersie R. C., Pittet J. F. Acute traumatic coagulopathy: initiated by hypoperfusion: modulated through the protein C pathway? *Ann. Surg.,* 2007; 245(5): 812-8.

[27] Network ORBC. Bloody Easy. Coagulation Simplified. 2013. Available from: http://thrombosiscanada.ca/wp-content/uploads/2013/08/Bloody_Easy_Coag_2013.pdf.

[28] Adams R. L., Bird R. J. Review article: Coagulation cascade and therapeutics update: relevance to nephrology. Part 1: Overview of coagulation, thrombophilias and history of anticoagulants. *Nephrology,* (Carlton). 2009; 14(5):462-70.

[29] Collen D. The plasminogen (fibrinolytic) system. *Thromb Haemost.,* 1999; 82(2):259-70.

[30] Innes D., Sevitt S. COAGULATION AND FIBRINOLYSIS IN INJURED PATIENTS. *J. Clin. Pathol., 1*964; 17:1-13.

[31] Gando S., Tedo I., Kubota M. Posttrauma coagulation and fibrinolysis. *Crit. Care Med.*, 1992; 20(5):594-600.

[32] Raza I., Davenport R., Rourke C., Platton S., Manson J., Spoors C., et al. The incidence and magnitude of fibrinolytic activation in trauma patients. *J. Thromb Haemost.*, 2013; 11(2):307-14.

[33] Tauber H., Innerhofer P., Breitkopf R., Westermann I., Beer R., El Attal R., et al. Prevalence and impact of abnormal ROTEM(R) assays in severe blunt trauma: results of the 'Diagnosis and Treatment of Trauma-Induced Coagulopathy (DIA-TRE-TIC) study'. *Br. J. Anaesth.,* 2011; 107(3):378-87.

[34] Schneiderman J., Adar R., Savion N. Changes in plasmatic tissue-type plasminogen activator and plasminogen activator inhibitor activity during acute arterial occlusion associated with severe ischemia. *Thromb Res.*, 1991; 62(5):401-8.

[35] Brohi K., Cohen M. J., Ganter M. T., Schultz M. J., Levi M., Mackersie R. C., et al. Acute coagulopathy of trauma: hypoperfusion induces systemic anticoagulation and hyperfibrinolysis. *J. Trauma,* 2008; 64(5):1211-7; discussion 7.

[36] Campbell J. E., Meledeo M. A., Cap A. P. Comparative response of platelet fV and plasma fV to activated protein C and relevance to a model of acute traumatic coagulopathy. *PLoS One,* 2014;9(6):e99181.

[37] Lijnen H. R. Pleiotropic functions of plasminogen activator inhibitor-1. *J. Thromb Haemost.*, 2005; 3(1):35-45.

[38] Sawamura A., Hayakawa M., Gando S., Kubota N., Sugano M., Wada T., et al. Disseminated intravascular coagulation with a fibrinolytic phenotype at an early phase of trauma predicts mortality. *Thromb Res.,* 2009; 124(5):608-13.

[39] Gando S., Sawamura A., Hayakawa M. Trauma, shock, and disseminated intravascular coagulation: lessons from the classical literature. *Ann. Surg.*, 2011; 254(1):10-9.

[40] Rizoli S., Nascimento B., Key N., Tien H. C., Muraca S., Pinto R., et al. Disseminated intravascular coagulopathy in the first 24 hours after trauma: the association between ISTH score and anatomopathologic evidence. *J. Trauma,* 2011; 71(5 Suppl. 1):S441-7.

[41] Rourke C., Curry N., Khan S., Taylor R., Raza I., Davenport R., et al. Fibrinogen levels during trauma hemorrhage, response to replacement therapy, and association with patient outcomes. *J. Thromb Haemost.,* 2012; 10(7):1342-51.

[42] Kashuk J. L., Moore E. E., Sawyer M., Wohlauer M., Pezold M., Barnett C., et al. Primary fibrinolysis is integral in the pathogenesis of the acute coagulopathy of trauma. *Ann. Surg.,* 2010; 252(3):434-42; discussion 43-4.

[43] Shakur H., Roberts I., Bautista R., Caballero J., Coats T., Dewan Y., et al. Effects of tranexamic acid on death, vascular occlusive events, and blood transfusion in trauma patients with significant haemorrhage (CRASH-2): a randomised, placebo-controlled trial. *Lancet,* 2010; 376 (9734):23-32.

[44] Roberts I., Shakur H., Afolabi A., Brohi K., Coats T., Dewan Y., et al. The importance of early treatment with tranexamic acid in bleeding trauma patients: an exploratory analysis of the CRASH-2 randomised controlled trial. *Lancet,* 2011; 377(9771):1096-101, 101.e1-2.

[45] Tsuei B. J., Kearney P. A. Hypothermia in the trauma patient. *Injury,* 2004; 35(1):7-15.

[46] Gentilello L. M. Advances in the management of hypothermia. *Surg. Clin. North Am.,* 1995; 75(2):243-56.

[47] Danzl D. F., Pozos R. S., Auerbach P. S., Glazer S., Goetz W., Johnson E., et al. Multicenter hypothermia survey. *Ann. Emerg. Med.,* 1987; 16(9):1042-55.

[48] Jurkovich G. J., Greiser W. B., Luterman A., Curreri P. W. Hypothermia in trauma victims: an ominous predictor of survival. *J. Trauma,* 1987; 27 (9):1019-24.

[49] Shafi S., Elliott A. C., Gentilello L. Is hypothermia simply a marker of shock and injury severity or an independent risk factor for mortality in trauma patients? Analysis of a large national trauma registry. *J. Trauma,* 2005; 59(5):1081-5.

[50] Wolberg A. S., Meng Z. H., Monroe D. M., Hoffman M. A systematic evaluation of the effect of temperature on coagulation enzyme activity and platelet function. *J. Trauma,* 2004; 56(6):1221-8.

[51] Kermode J. C., Zheng Q., Milner E. P. Marked temperature dependence of the platelet calcium signal induced by human von Willebrand factor. *Blood,* 1999; 94(1):199-207.

[52] Davis P. R., Byers M. Accidental hypothermia. *J. R. Army Med. Corps.,* 2005; 151(4):223-33.

[53] Brill S. A., Stewart T. R., Brundage S. I., Schreiber M. A. Base deficit does not predict mortality when secondary to hyperchloremic acidosis. *Shock,* 2002; 17(6):459-62.

[54] Martini W. Z., Dubick M. A., Wade C. E., Holcomb J. B. Evaluation of tris-hydroxymethylaminomethane on reversing coagulation abnormalities caused by acidosis in pigs. *Crit. Care Med.,* 2007; 35(6): 1568-74.

[55] Engström M., Schött U., Romner B., Reinstrup P. Acidosis impairs the coagulation: A thromboelastographic study. *J. Trauma,* 2006; 61(3):624-8.

[56] Meng Z. H., Wolberg A. S., Monroe D. M., Hoffman M. The effect of temperature and pH on the activity of factor VIIa: implications for the efficacy of high-dose factor VIIa in hypothermic and acidotic patients. *J. Trauma,* 2003; 55(5):886-91.

[57] Bolliger D., Szlam F., Molinaro R. J., Rahe-Meyer N., Levy J. H., Tanaka K. A. Finding the optimal concentration range for fibrinogen replacement after severe haemodilution: an in vitro model. *Br. J. Anaesth.,* 2009; 102(6):793-9.

[58] Bolliger D., Szlam F., Levy J. H., Molinaro R. J., Tanaka K. A. Haemodilution-induced profibrinolytic state is mitigated by fresh-frozen plasma: implications for early haemostatic intervention in massive haemorrhage. *Br. J. Anaesth.*, 2010; 104(3):318-25.

[59] Brazil E. V., Coats T. J. Sonoclot coagulation analysis of in-vitro haemodilution with resuscitation solutions. *J. R. Soc. Med.,* 2000; 93 (10): 507-10.

[60] Bolliger D., Gorlinger K., Tanaka K. A. Pathophysiology and treatment of coagulopathy in massive hemorrhage and hemodilution. *Anesthesiology*, 2010; 113(5):1205-19.

[61] Brummel-Ziedins K., Whelihan M. F., Ziedins E. G., Mann K. G. The resuscitative fluid you choose may potentiate bleeding. *J. Trauma,* 2006; 61(6):1350-8.

[62] Coats T. J., Brazil E., Heron M., MacCallum P. K. Impairment of coagulation by commonly used resuscitation fluids in human volunteers. *Emerg. Med. J.,* 232006. p. 846-9.

[63] Eugster M., Reinhart W. H. The influence of the haematocrit on primary haemostasis in vitro. *Thromb Haemost.,* 2005; 94(6):1213-8.

[64] Martin D. J., Lucas C. E., Ledgerwood A. M., Hoschner J., McGonigal M. D., Grabow D. Fresh frozen plasma supplement to massive red blood cell transfusion. *Ann. Surg.*, 1985; 202(4):505-11.

[65] Hunt B. J., Jurd K. M. Endothelial cell activation. A central pathophysiological process. *BMJ*, 1998; 316(7141):1328-9.

[66] Davenport R., Manson J., De'Ath H., Platton S., Coates A., Allard S., et al. Functional definition and characterization of acute traumatic coagulopathy. *Crit. Care Med.*, 2011; 39(12):2652-8.

[67] Holcomb J. B., Helling T. S., Hirshberg A. Military, civilian, and rural application of the damage control philosophy. *Mil. Med.,* 2001; 166(6): 490-3.

[68] Schwab C. W. Introduction: damage control at the start of 21st century. *Injury,* 35. England 2004. p. 639-41.

[69] Hodgetts T. J., Mahoney P. F., Kirkman E. Damage control resuscitation. *J. R. Army Med. Corps.*, 2007; 153(4):299-300.

[70] Tieu B. H., Holcomb J. B., Schreiber M. A. Coagulopathy: its pathophysiology and treatment in the injured patient. *World J. Surg.*, 2007; 31(5):1055-64.

[71] Gentilello L. M., Jurkovich G. J., Stark M. S., Hassantash S. A., O'Keefe G. E. Is hypothermia in the victim of major trauma protective or harmful? A randomized, prospective study. *Ann. Surg.,* 1997; 226(4):439-47; discussion 47-9.
[72] Revell M., Porter K., Greaves I. Fluid resuscitation in prehospital trauma care: a consensus view. *Emerg. Med. J.,* 2002; 19(6):494-8.
[73] Bickell W. H., Wall M. J., Jr., Pepe P. E., Martin R. R., Ginger V. F., Allen M. K., et al. Immediate versus delayed fluid resuscitation for hypotensive patients with penetrating torso injuries. *N. Engl. J. Med.,* 1994; 331(17):1105-9.
[74] Stern S. A., Dronen S. C., Birrer P., Wang X. Effect of blood pressure on hemorrhage volume and survival in a near-fatal hemorrhage model incorporating a vascular injury. *Ann. Emerg. Med.,* 1993; 22(2):155-63.
[75] Mapstone J., Roberts I., Evans P. Fluid resuscitation strategies: a systematic review of animal trials. *J. Trauma*, 2003; 55(3):571-89.
[76] Midwinter M. J., Woolley T. Resuscitation and coagulation in the severely injured trauma patient. *Philos. Trans. R. Soc. Lond. B. Biol. Sci.,* 2011; 366(1562):192-203.
[77] Dutton R. P., Mackenzie C. F., Scalea T. M. Hypotensive resuscitation during active hemorrhage: impact on in-hospital mortality. *J. Trauma,* 2002; 52(6):1141-6.
[78] Garner J., Watts S., Parry C., Bird J., Cooper G., Kirkman E. Prolonged permissive hypotensive resuscitation is associated with poor outcome in primary blast injury with controlled hemorrhage. *Ann. Surg.,* 2010; 251 (6):1131-9.
[79] Spahn D. R., Cerny V., Coats T. J., Duranteau J., Fernandez-Mondejar E., Gordini G., et al. Management of bleeding following major trauma: a European guideline. *Crit. Care*, 2007; 11(1):R17.
[80] Rugeri L., Levrat A., David J. S., Delecroix E., Floccard B., Gros A., et al. Diagnosis of early coagulation abnormalities in trauma patients by rotation thrombelastography. *J. Thromb Haemost.,* 2007; 5(2):289-95.
[81] Davenport R. Pathogenesis of acute traumatic coagulopathy. *Transfusion,* 2013; 53 Suppl. 1:23S-7S.
[82] Stahel P. F., Moore E. E., Schreier S. L., Flierl M. A., Kashuk J. L. Transfusion strategies in postinjury coagulopathy. *Curr. Opin. Anaesthesiol.,* 2009; 22(2):289-98.

[83] McIntyre L., Hebert P. C., Wells G., Fergusson D., Marshall J., Yetisir E., et al. Is a restrictive transfusion strategy safe for resuscitated and critically ill trauma patients? *J. Trauma,* 2004; 57(3):563-8; discussion 8.

[84] Joist J. H., Bauman J. E., Sutera S. P. Platelet adhesion and aggregation in pulsatile shear flow: effects of red blood cells. *Thromb Res.,* 1998; 92(6 Suppl. 2):S47-52.

[85] Peyrou V., Lormeau J. C., Herault J. P., Gaich C., Pfliegger A. M., Herbert J. M. Contribution of erythrocytes to thrombin generation in whole blood. *Thromb Haemost.,* 1999; 81(3):400-6.

[86] Guidelines for the use of platelet transfusions. *Br. J. Haematol.,* 2003; 122(1):10-23.

[87] O'Shaughnessy D. F., Atterbury C., Bolton Maggs P., Murphy M., Thomas D., Yates S., et al. Guidelines for the use of fresh-frozen plasma, cryoprecipitate and cryosupernatant. *Br. J. Haematol.,* 2004; 126(1):11-28.

[88] Rossaint R., Cerny V., Coats T. J., Duranteau J., Fernandez-Mondejar E., Gordini G., et al. Key issues in advanced bleeding care in trauma. *Shock*, 2006; 26(4):322-31.

[89] Fries D., Innerhofer P., Reif C., Streif W., Klingler A., Schobersberger W., et al. The effect of fibrinogen substitution on reversal of dilutional coagulopathy: an in vitro model. *Anesth. Analg.*, 2006; 102(2):347-51.

[90] Fenger-Eriksen C., Anker-Møller E., Heslop J., Ingerslev J., Sørensen B. Thrombelastographic whole blood clot formation after ex vivo addition of plasma substitutes: improvements of the induced coagulopathy with fibrinogen concentrate. *Br. J. Anaesth.,* 2005; 94(3):324-9.

[91] Johansson P. I., Ostrowski S. R. Evidence supporting the use of recombinant activated factor VII in congenital bleeding disorders. *Drug Des. Devel. Ther.,* 2010; 4:107-16.

[92] Boffard K. D., Riou B., Warren B., Choong P. I., Rizoli S., Rossaint R., et al. Recombinant factor VIIa as adjunctive therapy for bleeding control in severely injured trauma patients: two parallel randomized, placebo-controlled, double-blind clinical trials. *J. Trauma,* 2005; 59(1):8-15; discussion -8.

[93] Hauser C. J., Boffard K., Dutton R., Bernard G. R., Croce M. A., Holcomb J. B., et al. Results of the CONTROL trial: efficacy and safety of recombinant activated Factor VII in the management of refractory traumatic hemorrhage. *J. Trauma,* 2010; 69(3):489-500.

[94] Dickneite G., Doerr B., Kaspereit F. Characterization of the coagulation deficit in porcine dilutional coagulopathy and substitution with a prothrombin complex concentrate. *Anesth. Analg.*, 2008; 106(4):1070-7, table of contents.

[95] Lorand L. Factor XIII: structure, activation, and interactions with fibrinogen and fibrin. *Ann. N Y Acad. Sci.*, 2001; 936:291-311.

[96] Chandler W. L., Patel M. A., Gravelle L., Soltow L. O., Lewis K., Bishop P. D., et al. Factor XIIIA and clot strength after cardiopulmonary bypass. *Blood Coagul. Fibrinolysis*, 2001; 12(2):101-8.

[97] Winstedt D., Thomas O. D., Nilsson F., Olanders K., Schött U. Correction of hypothermic and dilutional coagulopathy with concentrates of fibrinogen and factor XIII: an in vitro study with ROTEM. *Scand. J. Trauma Resusc. Emerg. Med.*, 2014; 22(1):73.

[98] Williamson L. M., Lowe S., Love E. M., Cohen H., Soldan K., McClelland D. B., et al. Serious hazards of transfusion (SHOT) initiative: analysis of the first two annual reports. *BMJ*, 1999; 319 (7201):16-9.

[99] Sazama K. Reports of 355 transfusion-associated deaths: 1976 through 1985. *Transfusion*, 1990; 30(7):583-90.

[100] Goodnough L. T. Risks of blood transfusion. *Crit. Care Med.*, 2003; 31(12 Suppl.):S678-86.

[101] Moore F. A., Moore E. E., Sauaia A. Blood transfusion. An independent risk factor for postinjury multiple organ failure. *Arch. Surg.*, 1997; 132(6):620-4; discussion 4-5.

[102] Claridge J. A., Sawyer R. G., Schulman A. M., McLemore E. C., Young J. S. Blood transfusions correlate with infections in trauma patients in a dose-dependent manner. *Am. Surg.*, 2002; 68(7):566-72.

[103] Joint United Kingdom (UK) Blood Transfusion and Tissue Transplantation Services Professional Advisory Committee. Guidelines for the Blood Transfusion Services in the UK. 8th Edition. Publisher: The Stationery Office. 2013.

[104] Toy P., Lowell C. TRALI--definition, mechanisms, incidence and clinical relevance. *Best Pract. Res. Clin. Anaesthesiol.*, 2007; 21(2):183-93.

[105] Cotton B. A., Au B. K., Nunez T. C., Gunter O. L., Robertson A. M., Young P. P. Predefined massive transfusion protocols are associated with a reduction in organ failure and postinjury complications. *J. Trauma*, 2009; 66(1):41-8; discussion 8-9.

[106] Cotton B. A., Gunter O. L., Isbell J., Au B. K., Robertson A. M., Morris J. A., Jr., et al. Damage control hematology: the impact of a trauma exsanguination protocol on survival and blood product utilization. *J. Trauma,* 2008; 64(5):1177-82; discussion 82-3.

[107] Stansbury L. G., Dutton R. P., Stein D. M., Bochicchio G. V., Scalea T. M., Hess J. R. Controversy in trauma resuscitation: do ratios of plasma to red blood cells matter? *Transfus. Med. Rev.*, 2009; 23(4):255-65.

[108] Holcomb J. B., Zarzabal L. A., Michalek J. E., Kozar R. A., Spinella P. C., Perkins J. G., et al. Increased platelet:RBC ratios are associated with improved survival after massive transfusion. *J. Trauma*, 2011; 71(2 Suppl. 3):S318-28.

[109] Holcomb J. B., Wade C. E., Michalek J. E., Chisholm G. B., Zarzabal L. A., Schreiber M. A., et al. Increased plasma and platelet to red blood cell ratios improves outcome in 466 massively transfused civilian trauma patients. *Ann. Surg.,* 2008; 248(3):447-58.

[110] Ho A. M., Dion P. W., Cheng C. A., Karmakar M. K., Cheng G., Peng Z., et al. A mathematical model for fresh frozen plasma transfusion strategies during major trauma resuscitation with ongoing hemorrhage. *Can. J. Surg.,* 2005; 48(6):470-8.

[111] Sperry J. L., Ochoa J. B., Gunn S. R., Alarcon L. H., Minei J. P., Cuschieri J., et al. An FFP:PRBC transfusion ratio >/=1:1.5 is associated with a lower risk of mortality after massive transfusion. *J. Trauma,* 2008; 65(5):986-93.

[112] Spinella P. C., Perkins J. G., Grathwohl K. W., Beekley A. C., Niles S. E., McLaughlin D. F., et al. Effect of plasma and red blood cell transfusions on survival in patients with combat related traumatic injuries. *J. Trauma,* 2008; 64(2 Suppl.):S69-77; discussion S-8.

[113] Borgman M. A., Spinella P. C., Perkins J. G., Grathwohl K. W., Repine T., Beekley A. C., et al. The ratio of blood products transfused affects mortality in patients receiving massive transfusions at a combat support hospital. *J. Trauma,* 2007; 63(4):805-13.

[114] Maegele M., Lefering R., Paffrath T., Tjardes T., Simanski C., Bouillon B., et al. Red-blood-cell to plasma ratios transfused during massive transfusion are associated with mortality in severe multiple injury: a retrospective analysis from the Trauma Registry of the Deutsche Gesellschaft für Unfallchirurgie. *Vox Sang,* 2008; 95(2):112-9.

[115] Scalea T. M., Bochicchio K. M., Lumpkins K., Hess J. R., Dutton R., Pyle A., et al. Early aggressive use of fresh frozen plasma does not improve outcome in critically injured trauma patients. *Ann. Surg.,* 2008; 248(4):578-84.

[116] Johansson P. I., Stensballe J., Ostrowski S. R. Current management of massive hemorrhage in trauma. *Scand. J. Trauma Resusc. Emerg. Med.,* 2012; 20:47.

[117] Gaunt C., Woolley T. Management of haemorrhage in major trauma. Continuing Education in Anaesthesia, Critical Care and Pain. 2014.

[118] Baraniuk S., Tilley B. C., del Junco D. J., Fox E. E., van Belle G., Wade C. E., et al. Pragmatic Randomized Optimal Platelet and Plasma Ratios (PROPPR) Trial: Design, rationale and implementation. *Injury,* 2014; 45 (9):1287-95.

[119] Johansson P. I., Stensballe J. Effect of Haemostatic Control Resuscitation on mortality in massively bleeding patients: a before and after study. *Vox Sang.,* 2009; 96(2):111-8.

[120] Schöchl H., Nienaber U., Hofer G., Voelckel W., Jambor C., Scharbert G., et al. Goal-directed coagulation management of major trauma patients using thromboelastometry (ROTEM)-guided administration of fibrinogen concentrate and prothrombin complex concentrate. *Crit. Care,* 2010; 14(2):R55.

In: Abdominal Injuries
Editor: Chad L. Barrett

ISBN: 978-1-63482-590-0

Chapter 3

Pelvic Trauma

S. Fleming*[*]*, J. Berwin and B. Patel
The Royal London Hospital and Barts Cancer Institute,
Queen Mary University London, London, UK

Abstract

The pelvic cavity, surrounded by the pelvic bones, protects and transmits the vessels and organs of digestion, excretion, reproduction and ambulation. The pelvis contains the inferior aspect of the retroperitoneal and intraperitoneal spaces; disruption of the pelvis may therefore result in not only the loss of structural stability but may jeopardise structures contained within its volume [1, 2].

Breaking the pelvic ring, with its associated vascular bed, may result in catastrophic haemorrhage and remote organ sequelae, such as brain damage, and is the cause of early death. Late death is usually associated with overwhelming sepsis and multi-organ failure [3].

Despite the advent of specialised Major Trauma Centers, together with adoption of standardised resuscitation protocols developed to ensure the appropriate and timely use of pelvic stabilisation, interventional radiology and damage control surgery, we are yet to witness the anticipated leap in improving mortality associated with pelvic trauma [4].

[*] Corresponding author: Simon Fleming. The Royal London Hospital and Barts Cancer Institute. Queen Mary University London, Old Anatomy Building, Charterhouse Square, London EC1M 6BQ. Tel: +44 (0)20 7882 2081, fax: +44 (0) 207 882 3888, E-mail: simonsfleming@doctors.org.uk.

Major pelvic trauma was associated with a 10% risk of mortality in the 1980s [1], yet in spite of the advances in technology and service provision, recent studies show this still to be the case. Indeed, a recent consecutive series performed by O'Sulivan et al. of 174 patients reveals it stands closer to 20% [2].

Survival following pelvic trauma is still fraught with increased morbidity. Henderson et al. suggest that 80% of survivors who sustained unstable pelvic injuries report some degree of disability, compared with only 13% of those who sustained stable pelvic disruption [1]. Common complaints include: ongoing pain, neurological injuries, sphincter disturbance, impaired gait, sexual dysfunction and vascular injuries, all of which have a profound impact on activities of daily living [1, 3].

Pelvic fractures encompass a broad spectrum of injuries, from low-energy osteoporotic fractures to high-energy disruptions of the pelvic ring. The prompt and accurate appreciation of a patient's injury pattern and its severity is crucial to the planning of early and effective management [3].

This chapter will describe currently accepted classifications of pelvic trauma and examine the link between mechanism of injury and factors predictive of mortality. We will discuss the relevance of trauma scoring systems being used to identify patients at high risk and the impact this has on management.

Ultimately, pelvic anatomy remains constant; saving life and preventing deformity following trauma to this region still poses a real challenge to the modern day trauma team. This chapter will explore recent advances made in services, protocols, imaging, instrumentation and management of pelvic trauma and examine whether any of it has served to improve the historically poor prognosis.

Injuries of the Pelvis

To manage patients with pelvic injury, one must consider bony and soft tissue damage as both may occur concurrently. Indeed the more serious complications associated with pelvic fractures occur following damage to the pelvic contents, particularly following major haemorrhage from large vessels or injuries of the lower urinary tract.

Pelvic Fractures

Biomechanics

The adult innominate bone is formed following fusion of the ilium, ischium and pubis. Ossification of these bones occurs between the seventh and eighth year of life. Together with the sacrum, sacroiliac joints, the pubic symphysis and surrounding ligamentous attachments, a ring is formed enabling the pelvis to perform its main function of load transfer from the spine to the lower extremities. In biomechanical terms, the pelvis can be divided into anterior and posterior segments of the ring [5] (*The pelvic girdle book).*

Due to a 55-60° inclination of the pelvis in the horizontal plane and the sinusoidal shape of the erect spine in the lateral plan, the bodies point of balance when standing lies in front of the spine meaning it is easily affected by rotational forces. The center of rotation of the pelvis is located just posterior to the centers of the femoral heads. Rotational forces are balanced by an intact pubic symphysis and posterior ligamentous structures. When walking, forces are therefore constantly interchanging between compression and traction [6].

Destabilisation of the pelvis results from fractures of the posterior pelvic ring but not of the anterior pelvic ring. The reason for this is the dramatic alteration to the tension of the ring, which significantly changes the spatial arrangement of the pelvis. Fractures of the posterior pelvic ring are therefore more disruptive to the mechanical distribution of forces within the pelvis as well as its kinematics [6].

Epidemiology

Despite considerable variation in the reported incidence of pelvic fractures, a review of current literature suggests that pelvic fractures remain relatively uncommon injuries. Balogh et al. report figures as low as 23 per 100,000 [7], which seems to support recent texts quoting a range of 20-37 per 100,000 [6]. Others, such as a series reported by Demetriades et al. of 14,568 patients admitted over an 8-year period to a level 1 Los Angeles trauma center, have demonstrated that the incidence of pelvic fractures in adults is 10.0%, but that for paediatric patients (less than 16 years old) the incidence was 4.6% [8]. The explanation for lower incidences of paediatric pelvic injuries is that the pelvic ring is more elastic and therefore has higher restoring forces [9].

Current literature also struggles to discern whether the mortality associated with pelvic ring fractures is caused solely by the fracture or, whether in the context of polytrauma, mortality ultimately occurs following life threatening vascular, cardiothoracic or neurological injuries.

A 12 month prospective study by Balogh et al. looking at the outcomes of all patients with pelvic trauma treated at their level 1 trauma center report an overall mortality of 23% but go on to say that 60% of those patients died in the pre-hospital setting and that the pelvic ring fracture related mortality was only 7% [7]. Another study by Demetriades et al. of 16,630 trauma registry patients with blunt trauma reports an overall mortality of 13.5% but attribute only 0.8% of deaths as a direct result of pelvic fracture [8].

In a later article published by Demetriades et al., they attribute a 2.9% incidence of mortality from exsanguination related to pelvic fracture. Interestingly, there were no reported deaths in the paediatric group [9].

In a 12-month population-based study of the epidemiology of pelvic ring fractures treated in a level 1 trauma center found that high-energy pelvic ring fractures were more likely to occur in males, young people, patients with a higher Injury Severity Score (ISS), as well as those with a lower blood pressure. See table 1.

In this same study by Balogh et al., the mechanism of injury for low-energy pelvic ring fractures was exclusively a fall from height less than 1metre. The mechanism for the high-energy pelvic ring fracture and pre-hospital death groups were predominantly related to road traffic collisions, with 31% of injuries attributed to motorbike crashes, 27% in car crashes, 22% were pedestrians hit by a car. Injuries sustained following agricultural, bicycle, and horse accidents as well as falls from a height greater than 10ft were each responsible for pelvic ring fractures in 5% or less of cases [7].

Patients who suffer high-energy pelvic ring fractures are less likely to sustain this injury isolation. Balogh et al. found that only 12% of this cohort had an isolated injury, and that patients with pelvic ring fractures that died in the pre-hospital setting sustained facial injuries in 61% of cases, chest injuries in 89% of cases and intraperitoneal organ injuries in 39% of cases.

Table 1. Data from the epidemiological study by Balough et al. They treated 138 patients with a pelvic ring fracture in 12 months [7]

Patient Group	Number of patients	Male (%)	Age (yr)	ISS	SBP (mmHg)	Tile A/B/C (%)
All	138	43	59 +/- 2	20 +/- 2	N/A	61/26/13
High-energy	59	64	41 +/- 3	23 +/- 3	111 +/- 1	41/41/18
Low-energy	61	20	83 +/- 1	6 +/- 1	153 +/- 1	98/2/0
Pre-hospital death	18	50	41 +/- 6	61 +/- 4	N/A	0/53/47

For patients with high-energy pelvic ring fractures who survived the pre-hospital setting, 5% sustained facial injuries, 44% sustained chest injuries and 15% sustained intraperitoneal organ injuries [7].

Indeed, due to the high energy required to cause Type C fractures, there is a higher incidence of concomitant injury as well as a higher rate of mortality. Arnold et al. suggest that 50-70% of patients with type C fractures were polytraumatised and that they have a fourfold higher associated mortality compared to those suffering an isolated pelvic fracture [6].

High-energy injuries are more likely to yield a more unstable fracture pattern requiring operative reduction and stabilisation.

Table 2 shows that Type C Pelvic fractures are associated with a greater necessity for operative fixation, but that evidence of radiological healing as well as reported clinical outcomes following surgery are lower in this group compared to Type B fractures.

Pelvic Injuries

Injury to the pelvis is often divided into pelvic ring injuries and acetabular fractures. The former can then be classified as isolated osseous or ligamentous injuries, with or without associated pelvic instability or as complex pelvic trauma with concomitant soft tissue injuries.

Pelvic Ring Injuries

Pelvic ring injury usually result from high-energy trauma impacting either directly or, indirectly via energy transferred from the femur.

Table 2. Data from two different studies of objective and subjective clinical outcomes following operative fixation for pelvic fracture

Author	No. Patients	Fracture Type (%)			Operative Fixation (%)			Reported Pain Free after Fixation (%)			Radiological Healing (%)			Clinical Result Reported as "good/ excellent" (%)		
		A	B	C	A	B	C	A	B	C	A	B	C	A	B	C
Pohlemann, T., et al. [10]	1722	63.6	21.0	15.5	3.99	37.3	54.3	55	41	27	-	90.8	74.6	-	74	54
Siegmeth, A., et al. [11]	126	-	41	59	-	50	56	-	-	-	-	80	23	-	53.4	15.5

As the pelvic ring is primarily formed by the sacrum and two innominate bones, disruption of the ring will only result from fractures or dislocations occurring at two points approximately opposite from each other [6].

Classifying Pelvic Ring Injuries

To accurately classify pelvic ring fractures, adequate plain films using anteroposterior, inlet, and outlet views as well as thin-cut (3mm) CT scans are required. Currently, the three main classification systems used are all adapted from the work of Pennal and Tile and are designed to help with developing a management strategy as well as predicting associated injuries and prognosis [12].

Tile

The pelvis is divided into anterior and posterior arches relative to the acetabulum. The fracture pattern is dictated by the stability of the posterior arch, which contains the sacroiliac complex.

Injuries are on a stability scale, from stable (Type A fractures) to unstable (Type C fractures). As table 3 describes, these fractures are further subdivided to describe the plane and extent of instability.

Table 3. Describes the Tile Classification for pelvic fractures [6, 12]

Type	Description	
Type A	Stable	
A1	Avulsion injuries, not involving the pelvic ring	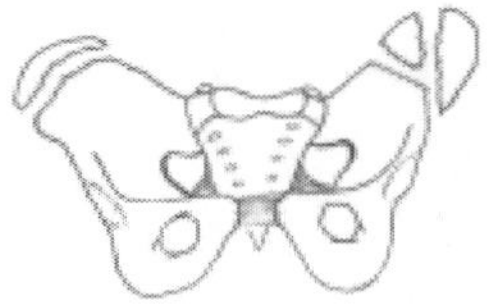
A2	Minimal displacement of the ring but stable. e.g., iliac wing or stable, minimally displaced anterior arch fractures	
A3	Stable, transverse fractures of the sacrum or coccyx.	
Type B	Partially stable (Rotationally unstable; vertically stable)	

Type	Description	
B1	Open book injury, external rotation instability	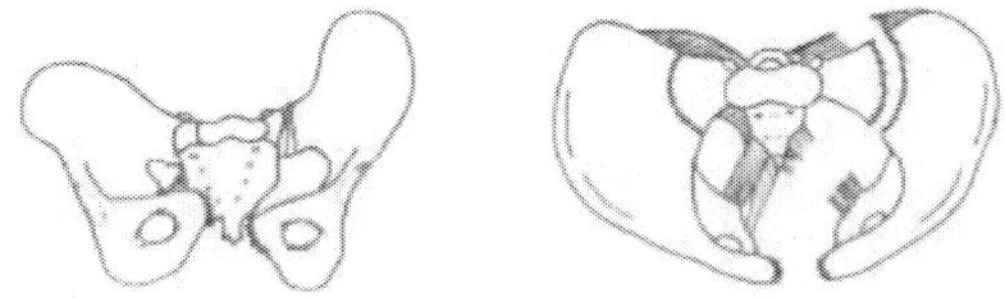
B2	Lateral Compression injury; ipsilateral internal rotational instability B2-1: Anterior arch is disruption is ipsilateral to the compression fracture posteriorly B2-2: Anterior arch disruption is contralateral to the compression fracture. Gives rise to 'Bucket Handle' injury	
B3	Lateral Compression injury; bilateral rotational instability B3-1: Bilateral open-book injuires B3-2: Bilateral lateral-compression injuries B3-3: Combination of the above	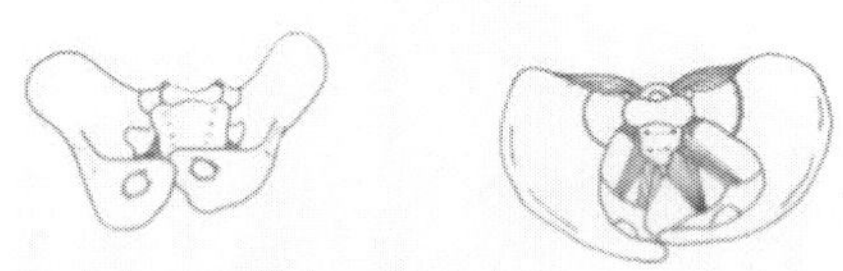
Type C	Rotationally and vertically unstable	
C1	Unilateral injury; unilateral instability	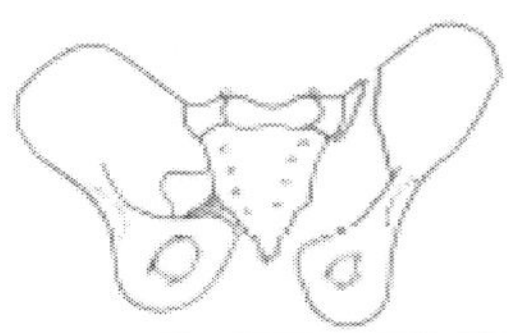
C2	Bilateral injury; unilateral instability (type C) with contralateral partial stability (type B)	
C3	Bilateral injury; bilateral rotational and vertical instability, with associated acetabular fracture	

Young-Burgess

This system was derived from retrospective analysis of clinical and radiographic appearances of pelvic fractures. It describes three vectors of energy transfer to the pelvic girdle that give rise to fracture.

Table 4. Describes the Young-Burgess Classification for pelvic fractures [6, 12]

Category	Description	
Anteroposterior Compression	Open book injury, external rotation of the hemipelvis. Damages anterior structures e.g., symphyseal diastasis or vertically oriented rami fractures and causes varying degrees of injury severity posteriorly	
I	<2.5cm widening of symphyseal or anterior SI joint; stretched but intact SI, sacrotuberous and sacrospinous ligaments; intact posterior SI ligaments	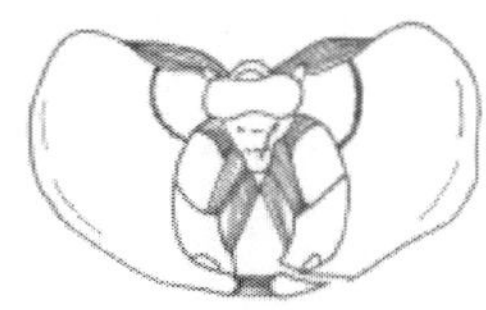
II	>2.5cm symphyseal diastasis; widened anterior SI joint; disrupted anterior SI, sacrotuberous, and sacrospinous ligaments; intact posterior SI ligaments	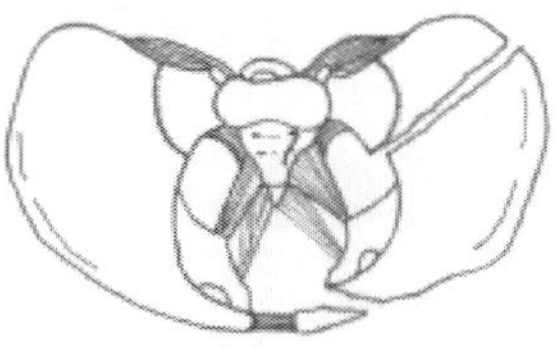
III	Complete SI joint disruption with lateral displacement, disrupted anterior SI, sacrotuberous, and sacrospinous ligaments; disrupted posterior SI ligaments	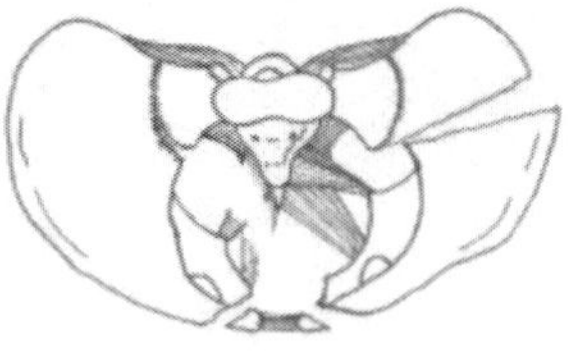
Lateral Compression	Horizontally oriented pubic rami fractures anteriorly and varying degrees of injury severity posteriorly	
I	Internal rotation of pelvis causes ipsilateral sacral compression fracture	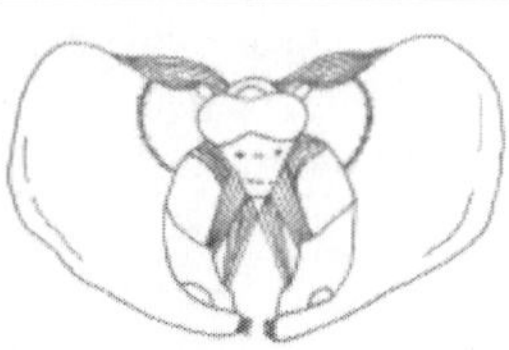

Category	Description	
II	Ipsilateral cresent fracture of iliac wing	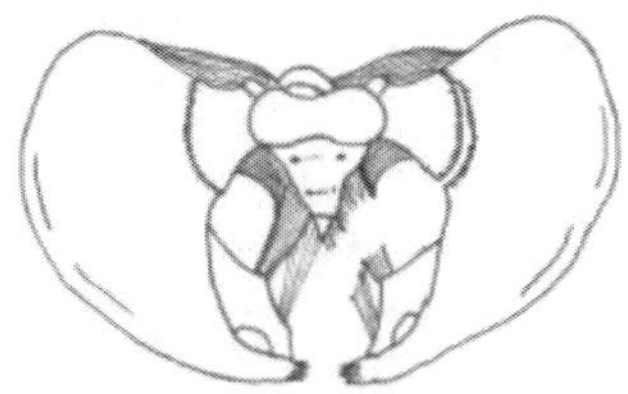
III	Ipsilateral LC I or LC II injury with contralateral open-book (APC) injury	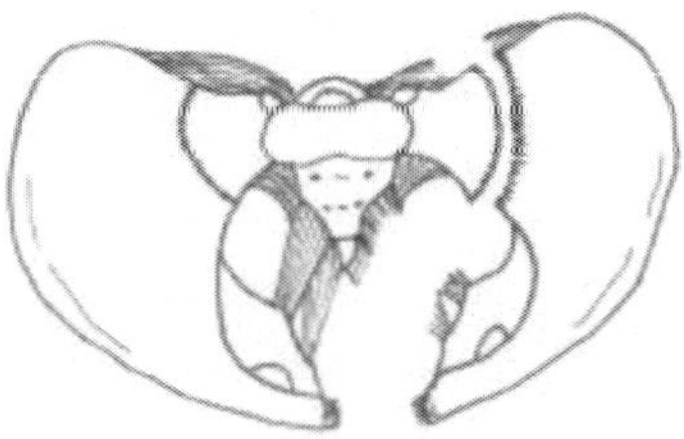
Vertical Shear	Most unstable injury. Vertical displacement of the hemipelvis following symphyseal diastasis or rami fractures anteriorly and iliac wing fractures, sacral fractures, or SI joint dislocations posteriorly	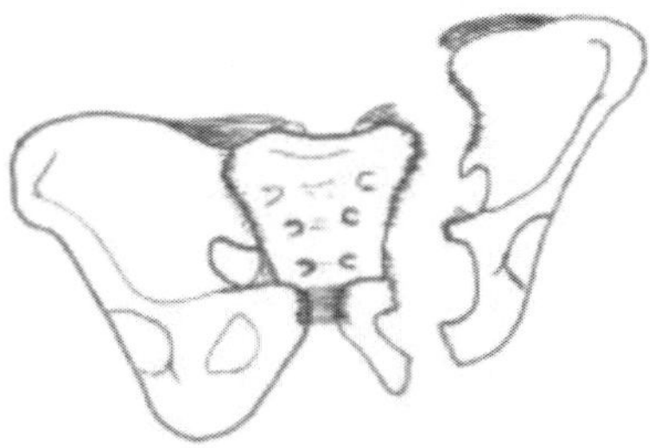
Combination Injury	Combination of injury patterns. Most commonly LC/VS	

This is currently the most commonly used classification system for describing pelvic fractures as it clearly relates the mechanism of injury to the severity of fracture.

Orthopaedic Trauma Association of Pelvic (Six) Ring (One) Fractures

The A-B-C system was described by Müller, Isler and Ganz in which they combine Pennal's work on pure mechanism of injury with Tiles classification, relating to instability of the pelvic girdle. This comprehensive system is designed to standardize fracture patterns in a more detailed and accurate way by categorizing a complete alphanumeric graduation of all injuries by separated reflection of the anterior, posterior, left and right pelvic segments.

Table 5. Describes the Orthopaedic Trauma Association (OTA) Classification for pelvic fractures [6, 12]

Type 61	Description
A	Lesion sparing (no displacement of the posterior arch)
1	Avulsion fracture of the innominate bone
2	Direct fractures of the innominate bone
3	Transverse fractures of the sacrum and coccyx
B	Lesion of anterior pelvic girdle, partial disruption of the posterior arch; partially stable
1	Unilateral external rotation (open-book) injury, partial disruption of the posterior arch
2	Unilateral internal rotation (LC injury) injury, partial disruption of the posterior arch
3	Bilateral injury, partial disruption of the posterior arch
C	Complete disruption of the posterior arch; unstable
1	Unilateral injury, complete disruption of the posterior arch
2	Bilateral injury, ipsilateral complete disruption of the posterior arch but incomplete disruption contralaterally
3	Bilateral injury, complete disruption of the posterior arch

This classification system is more useful for research purposes as opposed to application in routine clinical settings.

Sacral Fractures

Although sacral fractures appear with type A 3, type B and type C fractures on the AO/OTA classification system, for routine clinical use, it is best to use the tried and tested Dennis classification. This system is based on three zones in relation to the sacral foramina and also enables estimation of the expected rate of neurological damage of the sacral neural plexus.

Abdominal Trauma

Unrecognised abdominal and pelvic injury remains a cause of preventable death.

Table 6. Describes the Dennis Classification for Sacral fractures [6, 13]

Zone	Description	Risk of neurological damage
I	Fracture located laterally across the sacral ala 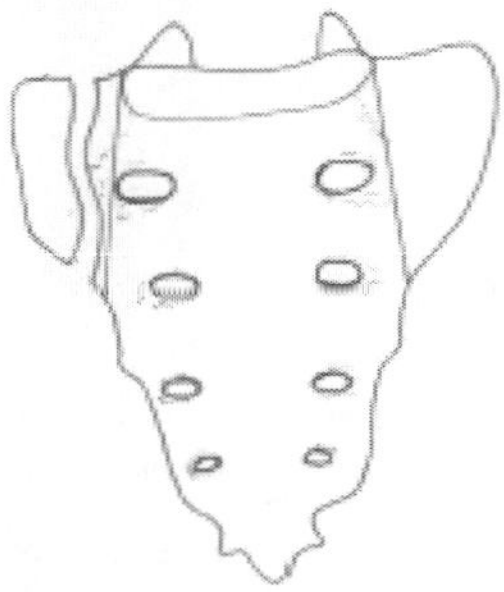	6% risk of L5 root impingement
II	Fracture bordered by the sacral foramina. Injuries may involve the neuroforamina but not the spinal canal 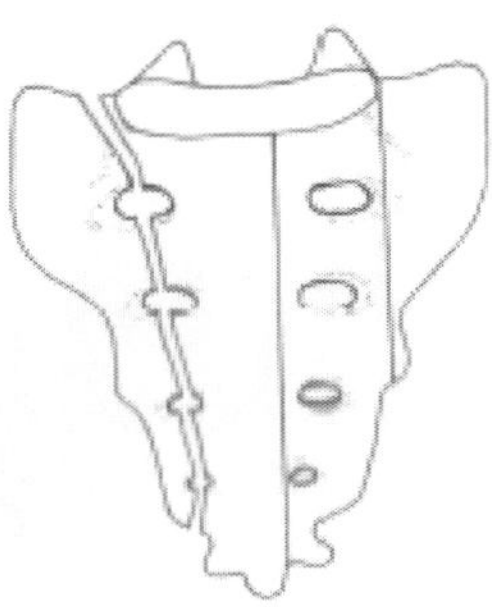	28% risk of L5, S1, or S2 root impingement
III	Fracture located medially to the sacral foramina and involve the spinal canal 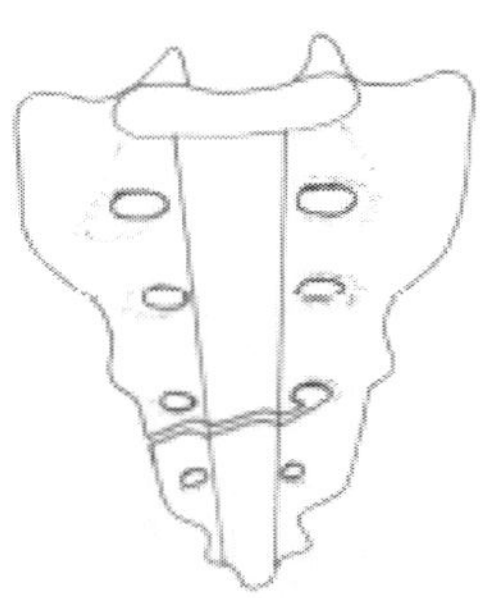 Sub-classified by Roy-Camille et al.: 1. simple flexion deformity of sacrum 2. partial translation and hyperkyphotic 3. complete translation with no fracture overlap	57% risk of neurological injury

Although this chapter focuses mainly on pelvic trauma, it is important not to ignore the structures contained within the pelvis and understand how they can be damaged. Gaining an understanding of the mechanism of injury is imperative for enabling early identification and treatment of potential injuries:

Blunt Trauma

Blunt trauma caused by a direct blow can cause compression or crush injuries to abdominal viscera and to the pelvis. Due to the mechanism of energy transfer, solid and hollow viscera are deformed in such a way that causes rupture. Indeed, patients involved in road traffic collisions (RTCs) are prone to deceleration injuries in which the fixed parts of viscera slow down and non-fixed parts continue at a comparatively greater speed. Restraint devices such as seat belts, when worn incorrectly, cause shearing injuries, which is another type of compression injury. Shearing and deceleration injuries will tend to cause visceral lacerations at the site of their ligamentous support or vascular pedicles. Secondary injuries such as haemorrhage and contamination of the abdominal cavity with associated peritonitis then ensues [4]. Table 7 shows the organs most frequently injured following blunt trauma.

Penetrating Trauma

The important differentiation to make is between stab wounds and low velocity gunshot wounds; which both cause damage to tissue by lacerating it, and high velocity gunshot wounds; which cause a greater amount of damage due to higher kinetic energy transfer to tissue, and cause cavitation and bullet fragmentation [4].

Combination Injuries

Explosive devices can inflict blunt and penetrating trauma. Patients in close proximity to an explosion will suffer primary blast injury in which a sudden increase in air pressure can cause lung injury as well as injury to the other hollow viscera such as the gastrointestinal tract. Penetrating trauma usually results from secondary blast injury in which bomb fragments and debris are picked up by the blast and energised.

Table 7. Demonstrates the organs commonly affected following penetrating trauma, this will also be dependant upon trajectory [4]

Organ affected	Incidence of organ damage with blunt trauma	Incidence of organ damage with penetrating trauma	
		Stab wound	Gun shot
Liver	35%-45%	40%	30%
Small bowel	5%-10%	30%	50%
Colon	-	15%	40%
Diaphragm	-	20%	-
Abdominal vessels	-	-	25%
Spleen	40%-55%	-	-
Retroperitoneal haematoma	15%	-	-

Blunt trauma results from tertiary blast injury in which the blast wind displaces the body and propels it through the air causing collision and contusion [4].

Concomitant Injury Following Pelvic Fracture

Pelvic fractures associated with visceral injury indicate a high-energy mechanism and are associated with increased mortality. Genitourinary injury is seen in 15% to 20% of pelvic fractures and commonly includes urethral, corpus cavernosa, bladder and bladder neck injury. Genitourinary injury tends to result from either shearing forces, or as a result of direct laceration by a bony spicule. These injuries tend to greatly impact long-term morbidity; in a review by Basta et al. of 119 patients with anterior pelvic fractures, they concluded that patients with inferomeidal pubic rami fractures or pubic symphysis diastasis of greater than 1cm had a strong association with urethral injury. They also found that for every millimetre of pubic symphysis diastasis, there was a 10% increased risk of urethral injury [14]. Metze and Tiemann et al. report that 61% of men complain of sexual dysfunction following pelvic fracture but that 19% had persistent erectile dysfunction. These injuries were usually associated with disruptions of the posterior ring [15].

Gastrointestinal injury associated with pelvic fracture occurs in 3.3% of adults and 5.3% of children, with solid organ injuries occurring in 17% and 14% of those cases respectively [16].

Current literature reports that in 5% to 18% of cases, patients will experience an ileus that usually resolves after 3 days. Patients complaining of ileus persisting for longer than 3 days should undergo CT imaging with enteric contrast to rule out an occult bowel injury such as entrapment at the pelvic fracture site, which can present with persistent or intermittent ileus [12].

Haemorrhage

The American College of Surgeons, state that the overall mortality for patients with a pelvic fracture of any type is around 1 in 6 (5%-30%), but that this increases to 1 in 4 (10%-42%) for patients with closed pelvic fractures with hypotension and is as high as 50% of patients with open pelvic fractures. This is predominantly caused by haemorrhage and is the most significant potentially reversible cause of death associated with pelvic injury [4].

Common sources of blood loss include laceration of the retroperitoneal veins of the pelvis or branches of the internal iliac artery or from cancellous bone at the fracture site, and accounts for haemodynamic instability in as many as 1 in 4 cases [12].

Blackmore et al. performed a retrospective cohort study of 627 patients with pelvic fractures, in which 20% had major pelvic haemorrhage. They sought to identify any reliable predictors of major haemorrhage following pelvic fracture. Four predictors were found and include: a haematocrit <30 in resus, a heart rate >130bpm, a displaced obturator ring fracture, and pubic symphysis diastasis >1cm. Patients without any predictors had a 1.6% chance of major haemorrhage, but those with three or more predictors more than a 66% chance of major haemorrhage [17].

A retrospective review of 289 patients by Magneussen et al., attempted to quantify blood transfusion requirements following pelvic fracture within the first 24 hours of admission. They found that patients with isolated pelvic fractures with major ligament disruption (APC II or III, LC III, vertical shear, or combined mechanisms) were 44% more likely than other fracture types to receive a blood transfusion compared to other pelvic fracture types.

Acetabular fractures classified as both column, anterior column, anterior column posterior hemi-transverse, or T type were 56% more likely to receive a blood transfusion compared to other acetabular fracture types [18].

Diagnosis/Investigation

History

Due to the potential for extensive loss of blood volume and concomitant intra-abdominal injury associated with pelvic fracture, it is important to distinguish the life-threatening clinical scenarios associated with polytrauma or complex injury from the haemodynamically stable situation of a solitary pelvic ring fracture. As such, initial management must proceed according to ATLS® principles [4].

Evaluation of the abdomen and pelvis is included in the initial assessment of circulation during primary survey but can provide diagnostic challenges in determining the source of occult bleeding. Taking a history may provide the key to understanding the location and mechanism of injury including the direction and magnitude of forces involved. The ability to gain such information in the acute setting may be challenging, the patient may be compromised following intoxication by alcohol or illicit drugs, indeed injury to the brain, spinal cord or chest wall will limit patient responsiveness [4].

Clinical Examination

Inspection must be carried out with the patient fully exposed enabling one to comprehensively examine the inferior aspect of the chest, the anterior and posterior abdomen and the perineum. These areas should be inspected for signs of abrasions, contusions, lacerations, penetrating wounds or impaled foreign bodies, haematomas, and eviscerated organs such as small bowel or omentum. We know that hypothermia contributes to coagulopathy, therefore a well rehearsed and rapid examination is required [4].

Guidance from ATLS® advocates that in the context of suspected pelvic fracture, patients should be cautiously log rolled. This enables examination of the flanks, perianal and scrotal area. Signs not miss include blood at the urethral meatus as well as swelling, ecchymosis, or laceration of the perineum, vagina, rectum or buttocks. Following blunt trauma, a rectal examination is useful in assessing the integrity of rectal mucosa, as well as sphincter tone and to determine whether the patient has a high-riding prostate indicative of urethral disruption resulting from significant pelvic fracture. Following penetrating trauma, gross blood from bowel perforation may be apparent on rectal examination [4].

Palpating the abdomen may be useful in eliciting signs of peritoneal irritation and can be used to distinguish between superficial and deep tenderness. Involuntary guarding is a reliable sign of peritoneal irritation. Rebound tenderness can also be sought to confirm peritonism. Whilst palpating the abdomen, it is important to ensure that a gravid uterus is also not missed. Clinical skills such as percussion and auscultation of the abdomen are an unreliable means of identifying pathology at the best of times and prove even more difficult to elicit in a noisy resus bay [4].

Mechanical instability of the pelvic ring should be assumed in patients with pelvic fractures who are hypotensive and have no other obvious source of blood loss. Indeed any of the physical signs mentioned above indicate major haemorrhage originating from the pelvis. For patients with an obvious pelvic fracture who are in shock, it is deemed detrimental to manually manipulate the pelvis to assess for instability as the risk of dislodging an organised haemtoma, which has a role in preventing further blood loss, is too high. Only if the patient is haemodynamically stable and a solitary pelvic ring fracture is suspected, should one consider testing the mechanical stability of the pelvic ring. In this case, gentle but firm compression over the iliac wings, with distractive movements applied downwards and internally and then outwards, referred to as the compression distraction maneuver, may reveal laxity or instability. Translational motion of the pelvis, indicative of posterior ligament disruption, can be assessed by palpating the posterior iliac spine and tubercle while pushing and pulling the unstable hemipelvis. To limit the risk of haemorrhage, these maneuvers should only be attempted once, if at all [4].

Diagnostic Tools

The mainstay of diagnostic imaging in the resus setting is focused assessment with sonography for trauma (FAST) and X-ray.

The use of more sophisticated imaging tools such as CT scanning and angiography are only utilised once the patient has been stabilised and so do not constitute first line imaging.

Focused Assessment with Sonography for Trauna (FAST)

FAST scanning has an undisputed role in screening for sources of haemorrhage in the resus environment.

Within minutes, the entire abdomen can be examined for signs of free fluid, lacerations to parenchymal organs including the kidney, liver and spleen. Within the pelvis, signs of a retroperitoneal haematoma can also be found as well as signs of a peri- or intra-vesical bleed [4, 19].

It is important to note that for patients with pelvic fractures, a negative examination does not rule out intraperitoneal haemorrhage. A retrospective review by Friese et al. of 146 patients with pelvic fracture exhibiting clinical signs of haemorrhage, indicated by a systolic blood pressure of less than 100 mmHg or an unstable pelvic fracture pattern was performed to assess the sensitivity and specificity of FAST scanning for detecting intraperitoneal bleeding. A total of 126 patients underwent a FAST scan and 104 of those patients underwent confirmatory evaluation of their abdomen with either operative exploration or CT scan. The sensitivity and specificity of FAST scanning to detect intraperitoneal bleeding as a result of pelvic fracture was 26% and 96% respectively, the positive and negative predictive values were 85% and 63% respectively [19].

X-Rays

An A.P. chest x-ray is always recommended for patients with multisystem blunt trauma as potentially life threatening conditions such as a tension pneumothorax, haemothorax, haemopneumothorax, pericardial haematoma or aortic disruption may be found. Free air under the diaphragm indicates a ruptured hollow viscus in the abdominal cavity. The ATLS® manual insists that an A.P. chest film is not necessarily indicated for haemodynamically abnormal patients with penetrating abdominal trauma as this would be an indication for emergency laparotomy. Instead, a haemodynamically normal patient with penetrating trauma above the umbilicus or a suspected junctional injury of the thoracoabdominal region would indicate a need for an erect chest x-ray [4]. For patients who are haemodynamically abnormal in whom the source of haemorrhage is unclear, an A.P. view of the pelvis may be helpful in establishing the source of blood loss. Indeed a pelvic x-ray may be performed if the mechanism of injury indicates some form of pelvic trauma or if the patient complains of pelvic pain or tenderness. If involvement of the posterior ring pelvic is suspected, views of the pelvic inlet can demonstrate horizontal dislocation, whereas outlet views can show vertical dislocations and can be sought by tilting the x-ray tube 45° in the frontal plane cranially and caudally, respectively.

Although this technique has to a large extent, been replaced by CT scanning, a number of pelvic surgeons find these initial images a useful comparison intra-operatively when trying to reduce vertical shear type injuries [4, 6].

CT Scanning

CT scans can provide information about the extent of organ injury within the abdomen and pelvis and can be helpful in diagnosing retroperitoneal injury that is challenging to assess on physical examination or FAST scanning. They are also useful in enabling visualization of the entire dimension of the osseous and ligamentous lesions of the posterior pelvic girdle, which is useful for the purposes of classification. Indeed three-dimensional reconstructions can be created to help with orientation of dislocated fracture lines [4, 20].

There are however some important limitations to CT scanning in the context of abdominal and pelvic trauma. It is important to remember that it is a time consuming investigation and so should only be performed in haemodynamically normal patients or patients who have responded to fluid resuscitation who do not have an indication for an emergency laparotomy [4].

A review of the diagnosis and management of pelvic fractures by McCormack et al. claims it is often difficult to determine whether the source of haemorrhage is arterial or venous. They believed that CT scans of the pelvis are sensitive in revealing the presence of a haematoma but not specific in locating the source of the bleed. In a more recent study by Romano et al., they aimed to determine the role of Helical CT scans in identifying vascular injuries in patients with blunt pelvic trauma.

Accurate differentiation between high flow haemorrhage indicating arterial injury and low flow haemorrhage, indicating venous haemorrhage, was achieved enabling appropriate management [20]. Of course angiography and venography are utilised to further delineate and treat the source of arterial and venous haemorrhage respectively.

Angiography

In cases of pelvic trauma presenting with persistent haemodynamic instability, digital subtraction agiography (DSA) is indicated so that the internal iliac artery can be visualised and embolised for bleeds greater than 3 mls/minute using coils or gelofoam paritcles. However, the majority of bleeds are venous in origin and so more often than not, angiography seems not to be indicated. A 5 year study by Agolini et al. of 806 patients with pelvic fracture showed that only 35 patients (4.3%) required angiography.

The most commonly injured arteries were the internal pudendal, lateral sacral, and superior gluteal vessels. Of the patients requiring angiography, only 15 patients (1.9%) required embolisation, which was performed with a successs rate of 100%. No patient required subsequent re-embolisation [21].

Treatment

Differentiating between pelvic fractures with or without life-threatening haemorrhage is vital in the initial management of these injuries.

Treatment for Major Pelvic Disruption

Major pelvic disruption requires haemorrhage control and fluid resuscitation. Life saving treatment can be implemented in both the pre-hospital and the resus setting.

Major pelvic disruption is typically caused by either open book or vertical shear injuries, and is associated with massive haemorrhage. Large volumes of crystalloid should be avoided in favour of O negative packed red cells initially, followed by cross matched blood once it can be obtained, clotting factors are also integral to the major haemorrhage protocol. Instead, small crystalloid boluses of 250-500mls are given to assess haemodynamic stability. A haemodynamically unstable patient is defined as a non-responder or transient responder to intravenous fluids.

Despite adequate attempts with fluid resuscitation, if only temporary improvement or even no improvement is seen in cardiovascular status, the patient must be actively bleeding. In such cases, permissive hypotension is adopted until haemorrhage control can be achieved [4].

Mechanical compression of the pelvic space is key and can be achieved temporarily by using a pelvic binder or improvised using a sheet applied at the level of the greater trochanters of the femur.

The necessity for a pelvic binder to remain in situ must be reviewed once the patient is resuscitated and the coagulopathy is corrected, as they are known to cause pressure sores over bony prominences.

If an unstable pelvic fracture pattern has been identified, permission to remove a pelvic binder should only be granted once a semi-permanent or permanent form of pelvic fixation has been achieved [4].

Applying a C-clamp can be a useful means of external fixation for Type C injuries in which the posterior sacral or anterior prevesical venous plexus may be damaged. The C-clamp is placed at the intersection of the line between the anterior and posterior iliac spine and the posterior border of the femur.

If the clamp is applied too distally, it may enter the sciatic notch, damaging the sciatic nerve. If the clamp is positioned too ventrally, the iliac wing is at risk of perforation. The threaded tube is then tightened which compresses the posterior pelvic ring [6].

An external fixator can also be used for emergency pelvic stabilisation and is particularly useful for open book type injuries. However, permanent stabilisation, especially of the posterior pelvic ring, cannot be substituted for by this means unless surrounding soft tissue coverage is so poor that external fixation is the only option. Reduction is performed by inserting a pair of Schanz screws cranially at each side of the pelvis into the iliac crest, as well as a pair of caudal screws in the supraacetabular region, close to the anterior inferior iliac spine. The screws are drilled at an angle of 45-60°, which corresponds to the inclination of the iliac wings.

Once the pins on either side of the pelvis have been connected, the entire assembly can be used as a lever for reduction of rotational displacement before adding the longitudinal rods. There is a risk of pin site infection with every external fixation device, in the case of pelvic fixation this may result in loosening and osteomyelitis of the iliac wing. A careful risk: benefit analysis must be undertaken before deciding to proceed [6].

It is worth noting that pelvic binders enable clots to form at sites of venous haemorrhage but will not control arterial haemorrhage and so the haemodynamic response to the binder can be helpful in determining the source of vascular injury.

These patients will require some form of endovascular control. Those patients who become haemodynamically stable following application of a pelvic binder will can proceed to a CT scanner to further delineate the source of bleeding as well as the pelvic fracture pattern. If an arterial blush is seen on the on CT, patients should proceed for angio-embolisation [4, 6].

Resuscitative Endovascular Balloon Occlusion of the Aorta (REBOA)

REBOA was first reported as early as the Korean War as a means of improving haemorrhage control and temporarily increasing proximal or central perfusion to the heart and brain. The technology involved is not new, but has received a resurgence following the military's need to improve their management of haemorrhagic shock whilst in Afghanistan [22, 23].

Stannard et al. described a practical guide for performing REBOA. Arterial access is gained through the femoral artery and can be achieved with either an open cut down, or more commonly an ultrasound guided percutaneous approach. A sheath is then inserted over a wire to form a working port. To ensure the balloon is inflated in the most clinically important area, three distinct occlusion zones have been defined to help refine the technique. Zone I comprises the descending thoracic aorta between the origins of the left subclavian and coeliac arteries. Zone II is the paravisceral area and, due to the risk of occluding the renal arteries, has been proposed as a non-occlusion zone. Zone III is the infrarenal area from the most inferiorly located renal artery to the aortic bifurcation and is useful in stopping haemorrhage following major pelvic and lower limb trauma. See figure 1. The average distance from the femoral artery access point to each zone have been measured, therefore to target a specific occlusion zone, it is a case of selecting the correctly sized balloon catheter for that zone [22].

Although REBOA's principle advantage over thoracotomy and aortic clamping is its less invasive manner, sparing an already compromised patient from further morbidity, its use in civilian trauma has not yet been widely adopted. Possible explanations for the lag in application of this procedure include latent technology as well as this being a poorly understood skill with minimal clinical evidence to support its widespread use [22].

In a recent series by Brenner et al., REBOA was performed on 4 patients with blunt trauma and 2 with penetrating injury. REBOA was accomplished quickly and enabled an average increase in blood pressure of 55mmHg with an average occlusion time of only 18 minutes. Three patients underwent zone I occlusion and three patients had zone III occlusion. In all six cases, there were no complications associated with the use of REBOA and none of the patients in this cohort died as a result of haemorrhage. This study supports REBOAs use as a feasible and highly effective means of haemorrhage control for patients in end-stage shock but may take some time before it becomes common place in both pre-hospital and resus settings [23].

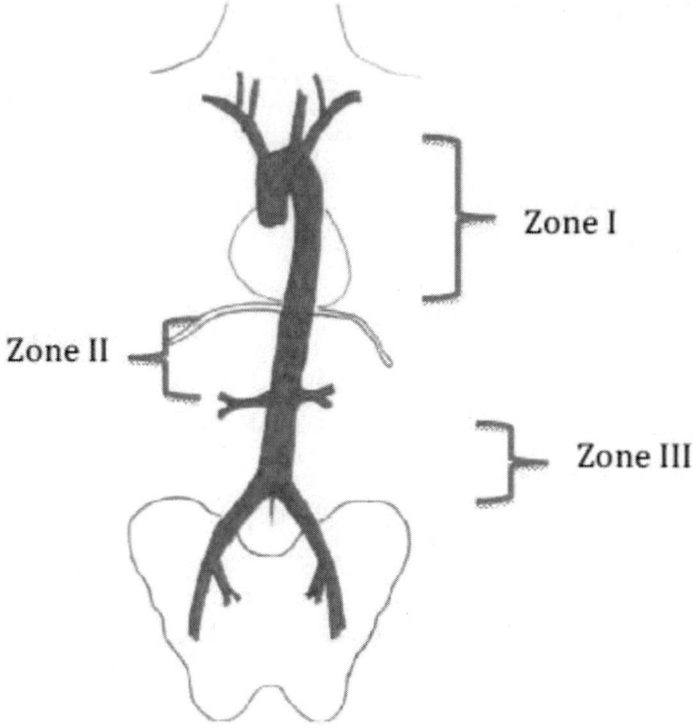

Figure 1. The REBOA 'Zones of Aortic Occlusion'.

Damage Control Orthopaedics

In the case of continuous haemodynamic instability that has failed to resolve within 15-30 minutes of adequate fluid resuscitation as well as application of a pelvic binder, the patient should be transferred to the operating theatre for an emergency laparotomy and pelvic packing. The extraperitoneal space is inspected and any massive haematomas removed.

The true pelvis is packed including both sides of the bladder to tamponade the posterior presacral region. This is only useful with counterpressure established by temporary external stabilisation of the pelvic ring [4].

In the past, the temptation for polytraumatised patients was to perform Early Total Care (ETC), in which definitive fracture fixation would be performed within the first 24-48 hours of injury.

We now know much more about the pathophysiological and immunological mechanisms regulating the host response to injury.

Following traumatic injury, a systemic inflammatory response (SIRS) occurs, followed by a period of recovery mediated by the counter-regulatory anti-inflammatory response (CARS). Following major polytrauma, the corresponding inflammatory response is significant and may lead to multi-organ dysfunction (MODS) followed by multi-organ failure and even death.

If the initial inflammatory response following trauma constitutes a "first hit" to the body, then surgery can be responsible for a "second hit". Indeed the impact of surgery is dependent on the patients own biological reserve, as well as the nature and timing of surgical intervention.

Damage control surgery is about softening the impact of the "second hit". Damage control orthopaedics (DCO) is achieved by setting modest goals for initial operative intervention which include: obtaining sufficient fracture stabilisation that also prevents further tissue damage; reducing the risk of compartment syndrome; enable the patient to be mobilised for tests and pulmonary care. This is why external fixation is the treatment of choice for DCO. It can be rapidly applied, is less invasive than definitive fixation and limits the amount of blood loss [24].

Pape et al. described four classes of patients, based on their clinical status: stable, borderline, unstable, and in extremis. A patient is classified into one of these four classes, if he or she meets the criteria in at least three of the four pathophysiological parameters, as reported in table 8. The indication for DCO is reserved for "unstable" and "in extremis" patients, as the risk of a "second hit" is deemed too high [25].

Definitive fixation and reconstruction should be performed during a second-look procedure 5-10 days after injury. Any sooner than this and the immunological changes and fluid shifts will not have normalised. Any later than 2 weeks and the risk of external fixator pin site infection increases substantially. See figure 2 for a definitive protocol [24, 25].

Post-operatively, patients should be transferred to intensive care for aggressive resuscitation with blood and blood products. Every effort must be made to correct coagulopathy as well as clear persistent signs of tissue hypoperfusion. Warming to normothermia is also a key aspect for managing the damage control patient. Until definitive fixation has occurred, the patient will still require a pelvic binder. Log rolling and other manoeuvres should be kept to an absolute minimum [25].

Table 8. Describes the assessment of a trauma patient in to four grades based on a number of clinical parameters. This can be utilised to identify which patients require damage control surgery [25]

	Parameter	Stable (grade I)	Borderline (grade II)	Unstable (grade III)	In extremis (grade IV)
Shock	BP (mmHg)	≥ 100	80 - 100	60 - 90	< 50 - 60
	Blood units (2h)	0 - 2	2 - 8	5 - 15	> 15
	Lactate levels	Normal range	Approx. 2.5	> 2.5	Severe acidosis
	Base deficit (mmol/L)	Normal range	No data	No data	> 6 - 18
	ATLS classification	I	II - III	III - IV	IV
	UO (mL/h)	> 150	50 - 150	< 100	< 50
Coagulation	Platelet count (μg/mL)	> 110000	90000 - 110000	< 70000 - 90000	< 70000
	Factor II and V (%)	90 - 100	70 - 80	50 - 70	< 50
	Fibrinogen (g/dL)	> 1	Approx. 1	< 1	DIC
	D-Dimer	Normal range	Abnormal	Abnormal	DIC
Temperature		> 35°C	33 - 35°C	30 - 32°C	30°C or less
Soft tissue injuries	Lung function, PaO2/FiO2	> 350	300	200 - 300	< 200
	Chest trauma score, AIS	AIS I or II	AIS ≥ 2	AIS ≥ 2	AIS ≥ 3
	TTS	0	I - II	II - III	IV
	Abdominal trauma score (moore)	≤ II	≤ III	III	≥ III
	Pelvic Trauma (AO classification)	A	B or C	C	C (crush, added abdo trauma)
	Extremities	AIS I or II	AIS II - III	AIS III - IV	Crush, extremities

Abbreviations: BP: Blood pressure, ATLS: Advnaced Trauma Life Support, UO: Urine Output, AIS: Abbreviated Injury Score, TTS: Thoracic Trauma Score, DIC: Disseminated Intravascular Coagulation.

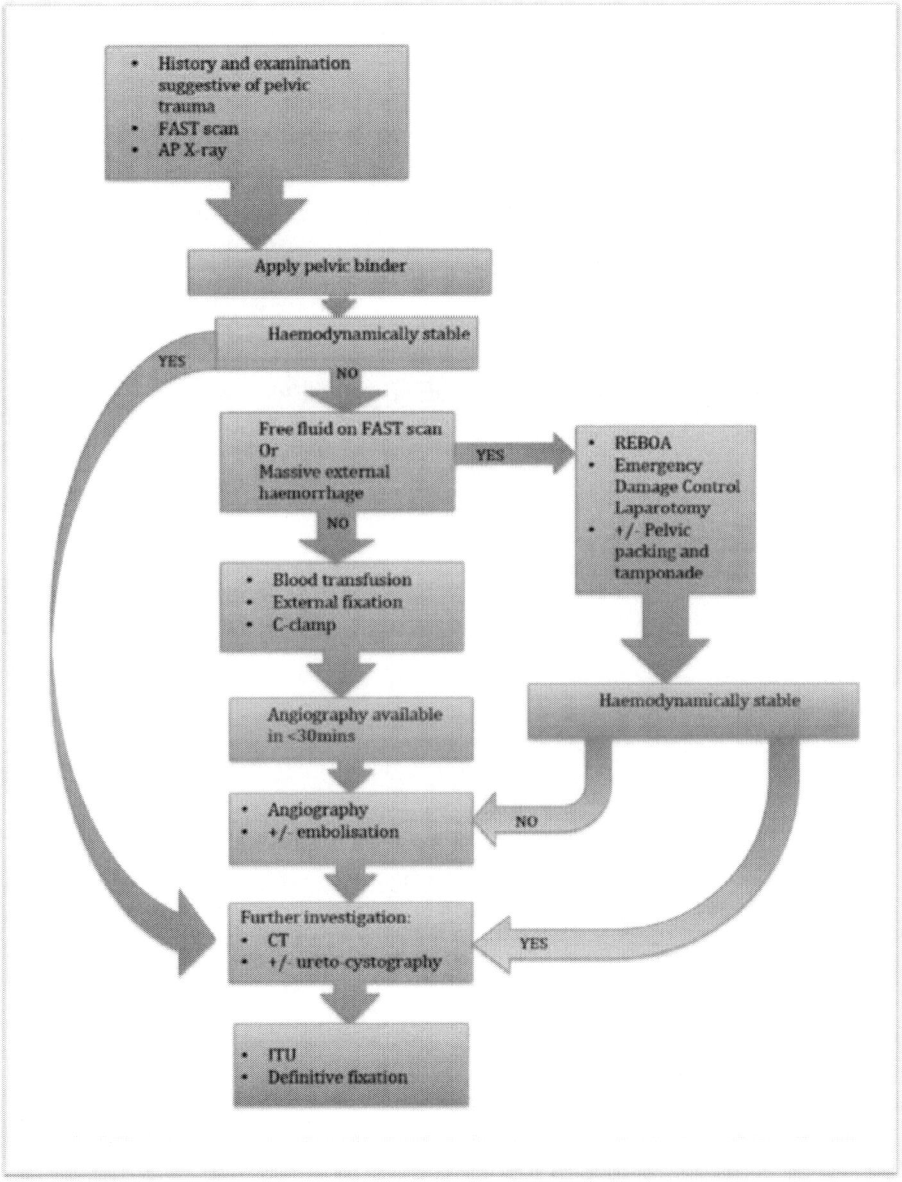

Figure 2. An example of definitive protocol for the management of pelvic trauma patients.

Treatment of Pelvic Injuries without Haemodynamic Instability

Stable pelvic ring fractures such as type A injuries, which include fractures of the pubic rim, undisplaced iliac wing fractures as well as transverse fractures of the sacrum below the linea terminalis, only require a short amount of bed rest until the patient gains relief from fracture pain [6].

Avulsion fractures of the iliac spine or of the ischial tuberosity can be treated non-operatively by nonweightbearing for 1 to 2 weeks. Healing occurs because alteration to the length of muscle that occurs following avulsion fractures of the inferior anterior iliac spine or ischial tuberosity for example, is compensated for when the hip joint is carried in extension as this relaxes the hamstrings [6].

Definitive Pelvic Fixation

Non-operative treatment of type B and C fractures will often cause painful instability due to ligamentous disruption and will result in deformities of the pelvic ring. Internal fixation is therefore vital for enabling weight bearing and reducing the time required for immoblisation [6].

Fixation Tactics

The key principle for fixing type B fractures is to close the anterior pelvic ring. The most common indication is rupture of the symphysis, which always requires open reduction and internal fixation with a plate. Unstable transpubic fractures can be fixed using an external fixator or by using transpubic screws. Stabilisation of the posterior ring may be necessary in the case of severe type B fractures in which there is additional external instability. Due to the rotational and vertical instability caused by type C fractures, it is necessary to reconstruct and stabilize both the anterior and posterior pelvic ring. The approach to operative fixation is determined by the site of injury, surrounding soft tissue damage, as well as concomitant injury. Patients with sacral fractures who have neurological deficits will need a laminectomy or foraminotomy to decompress the sacral roots. This can be performed using a posterior approach as described below [6].

Table 9. Describes the approach and operative techniques that can be used to definitively treat fractures of the anterior and posterior pelvic ring [6]

Region of Pelvic Ring	Indication	Approach	Operative Technique
Anterior Pelvic Ring	Transsymphyseal instability	Pfannenstiel approach Or Median longitudinal laparotomy	• Sharp reduction into obturator foramen • Flush closure of symphysis attempted • Four hole 4.5mm DC plate placed over the cranial area of the pubic rim • cortical screws drilled 30° to the vertical plane dorsally and caudally
Transymphyseal stabilisation with DC plate 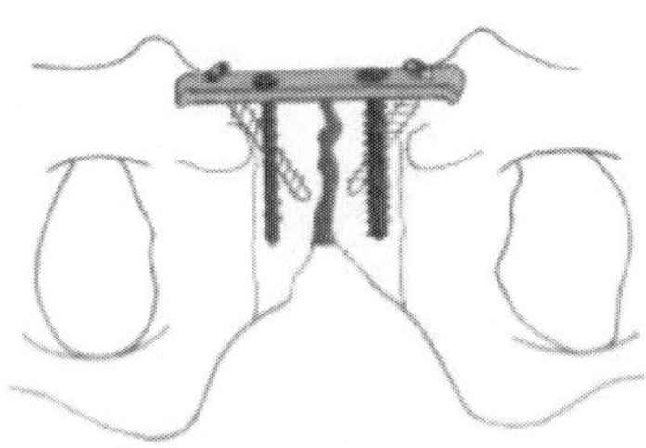			
Anterior Pelvic Ring	Unstable pubic rim fracture	Small medial incisions	• medial cortex of pubic rim drilled • creeping intramedullary cortical screws inserted • lag the fracture line
Posterior Pelvic Ring	• Transiliac instability • Transacral instability • Small anterior fracture of the sacrum	Antero-lateral approach • Supine position • Incision medial to the iliac crest • Psoas retracted medially by subperiosteal preparation • 1st radix of the sacral plexus can be found below the transverse process of the 5th lumbar vertebrae	• Reduce fracture using traction, abduction/adduction or rotation of the leg • Tension band wiring can also be used over two screws inserted either side of the fracture line • 2x short 3 or 4 hole small fragment plates • Plates to form an angle of 70-80° from the cranial plate on the upper iliac crest and the caudal plate on the linea terminalis • Avoid the "parallelogram effect"

Table 9. (Continued)

Region of Pelvic Ring	Indication	Approach	Operative Technique
Iliac stabilisation with DC plate and screws: 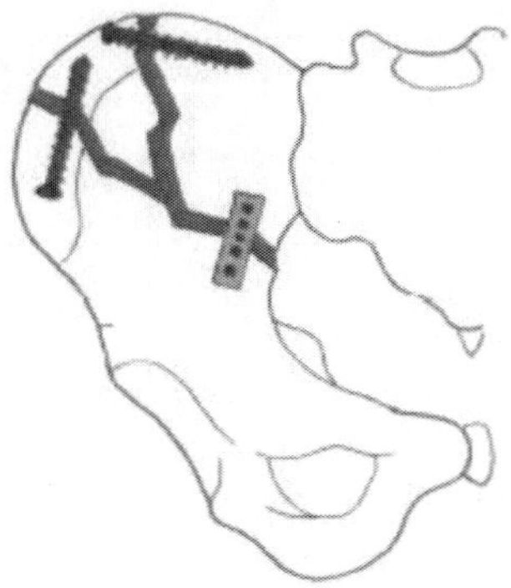			
Posterior Pelvic Ring	• Sacral fractures • Bilateral sacroiliac dislocations	Posterior approach • Prone position • Incision is made 1.5cm lateral to the posterior iliac spine along the posterior iliac crest • Cut gluteal fascia and retract laterally • Continue distally to the sciatic notch • Protect gluteal vessels	• Reduce sacroiliac dislocation using a sharp reduction clamp or Jungbluth clamp fixed at two screws inserted into the sacroiliac joint (use image intensifier with inlet/outlet views to ensure controlled reduction/ palpate finger into the sciatic notch) • For fixation use two 7.0- or 7.3-mm cannulated screws anchored into the body of the 1st vertebral body of the sacrum (entry point is 3-4cm lateral to the posterior iliac crest) • Screws are inserted at a 10° angle in the frontal plane, vertically to the plane of the iliac wing Trans-sacroiliac screwing: • Controlled reduction with image intensifier (II) • Entry point defined by II in the lateral view • Outlet view shows the exact level of entry • Inlet view controls the angle to the frontal plane Transsacral lesions: • angle <10°, parallel to the frontal plane into 1st vertebral body of the sacrum

Region of Pelvic Ring	Indication	Approach	Operative Technique
			Posterior Transiliac fractures with small iliac fragments: • Fix SIJ with shaped reconstruction plate anchored into the sacrum caudally Bilateral SIJ dislocations: • fix with posterior transverse plates (two 4.5-mm DC plates) shaped at the 1st and 3rd level of the sacrum in the posterior iliac spine or ala laterals of the sacrum Transforaminal sacral fractures (S1 and S1): • H shaped plates used for local internal fixation • Performed via the pedicles and ala laterals of the sacrum • Stabilisation of the anterior pelvic ring to achieve a tension band effect. Sacral bursting fractures: • Vertebro-pelvic fixation using an internal fixator • Pedicular screws are anchored into the 5th lumbar body and posterior iliac spines • Reduce the fracture by applying traction via the longitudinal support • Trans-sacroiliac screwing will increase rotational stability

Trans-sacroiliac stabilisation with screws

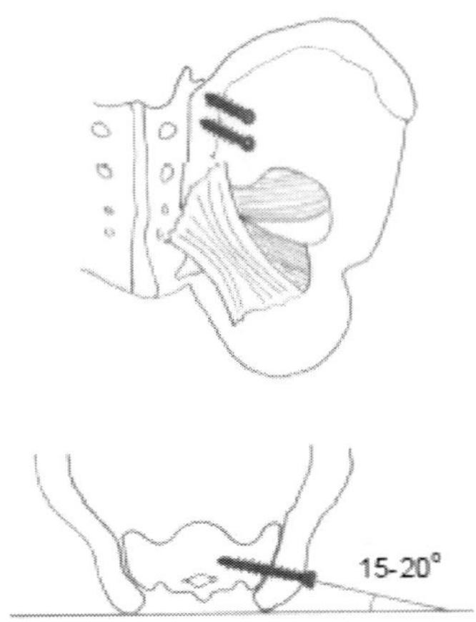

Internal fixation via vertebro-pelvic stabilisation

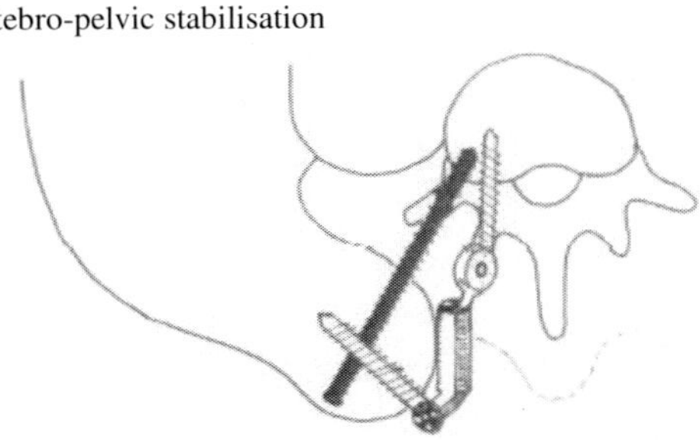

Post Operative Management

The risk of deep vein thrombosis (DVT) for patients who have sustained major pelvic trauma stands between 35% and 61%. Steele et al. performed a prospective study of 103 consecutive patients undergoing surgical stabilisation of pelvic and acetabular fractures who were on DVT prophylaxis. Patients were administered low-molecular-weight heparin (LMWH) within 24 hours of injury or on achieving haemodynamic stability and were screened for DVT using duplex ultrasonography 10-14 days post operatively. There was a 10% incidence of proximal DVT and a 5% incidence of pulmonary embolus. Only 3% of patients with a proximal DVT received LMWH within 24 hours of injury, 22% received LMWH more than 24 hours post operatively ($p<0.01$). This lead to a conclusion that LMWH administered without delay is a safe and effective method of thromboprohylaxis in patients with major pelvic and acetabular fractures [26].

Post-operative infection following major pelvic trauma and pelvic fracture fixation can cause considerable morbidity. Risk factors are dependant on the extent of soft tissue damage. Torbert et al. performed a retrospective audit of 211 patients who underwent surgery for postoperative infection in an attempt to determine speciation and drug resistance profiles associated with fracture fixation cases. Stapphylococcus Aureus was present in 56% of infections, with 58% of those (32% of all cases) being methicillin-resistant S. aureus. Gram-negative rods (GNR) were found in 32% of cases, with 4% being multidrug resistant. The rate of GNR infection in the pelvis, acetabulum and proximal femur was found to increase to 63%, which was statistically significant ($P=0.0002$) compared to a rate of 23% in other locations. As a result, this centre considered the use of aminoglycosides in the treatment of pelvic, acetabular and proximal femoral fractures [27].

A review by Hauser et al. of the prophylactic use of antibiotics in open fractures acknowledges that prolonged use of broad-spectrum antibiotics is commonly cited as the standard for best practice in preventing infection. They go on to warn clinicians that multi-drug-resistant systemic infections are attributable to antibiotic overuse and can commonly cause life-threatening problems in the intensive care setting. Their review supports the conclusion that a short course of first-generation cephalosporin, initiated as soon as possible after injury, significantly reduces the risk of infection provided prompt orthopaedic fracture wound management is also carried out [28].

Post-operative mobilisation is another important consideration. Generally, this is at the surgeon's discretion.

For patients who have undergone stable internal fixation, it is feasible to be partially weightbearing 15-20kg on the affected side immediately after surgery. Indeed partial weightbearing can also be permitted following anterior stabilisation of type B injuries, as well as posteriorly fixed type C injuries. Full weightbearing is permitted following fixation of symphyseal disruptions. Weight bearing following external fixation remains a contentious issue. The consensus remains however, that full weightbearing is permitted immediately post-operatively provided the posterior ring is stable. Radiographs of the a.p, inlet and outlet views should be taken 6 and 12 weeks post-operatively to monitor fracture union [6].

In the case of complex trauma, in which there may be a lack of soft tissue coverage caused by crush injuries, contusions or lacerations, multiple second-look procedures may be required. This may call for collaboration with plastic surgical services, as further debridement and grafting is often necessary.

As with most orthopaedic surgery, removal of implants and metal work is generally considered once they start to cause pain.

In pelvic surgery, there are a number of implants for which removal is recommended as a matter of course. Symphyseal rupture takes around 4 months to heal, but after time physiologic movement will loosen the screws and so they should be removed between 6 and 12 months post-operatively. Indeed, trans-sacroiliac screws should also be removed within same time period [6].

Complications

The table below describes the early general and early local complications as well as late complications associated with pelvic fractures. This highlights the need for a multidisciplinary approach towards patients suffering pelvic trauma.

Patients with pelvic fractures that result in nonunion or malunion may complain of instability, leg length discrepancy and painful weightbearing. Fractures of the sacrum can cause persistant neurological pain and deficit, where as fractures of the pubic rim can cause a misalignment resulting in bladder dysfunction [6].

Details of reconstructive methods for correction of nonunion, malunion and instability will not be covered in this chapter.

Table 10. Lists the early general, early local and late complications pelvic trauma and surgical fixation [1, 6, 26-28]

Type of Complication	Complication	Incidence
Early general	Deep Vein Thrombosis	35% - 61%
	Pulmonary Embolus	2% - 3%
Early local	Haematoma	6% - 7%
	Infection	6% - 7%
	Nerve damage (predominantly sciatic nerve)	8% - 10%
Late	Painful sacroiliac joint	27%
	Painful non-unions	3%
	Fractures malalignment	5% - 8%
	Leg length discrepancy >2cm	3% – 6%
	Sexual dysfunction (males)	10%
	Sexual dysfunction (females)	2%
	Impotence	50% - 60%

Prognosis

Following a large multicenter study by the AO foundation, they state that anatomical healing of pelvic ring fractures is achieved in 80% of cases. They go on to reveal that a good or excellent clinical outcome is only achieved in 66% of cases, and that this discrepancy may due to concomitant neurological, urological or ligamentous injuries.

Naturally, complaints such as persistent pain are more common following a more severe injury pattern with 10-30% occurring with Type A injuries, 15-40% after type B injuries and 30-45% after Type C injuries [6].

Lefaivre et al. performed a systematic review to evaluate the use and interpretation of functional outcome tools following the surgical treatment of pelvic ring fractures. A total of 28 papers were included. The Short-Form 36 (SF-36) was by far the most commonly used generic outcome instrument, used in 12 papers. The pelvis-specific outcome instruments were used in 19 studies; the Majeed score in ten, Iowa pelvic score in six, Hannover pelvic score in two and the Orlando pelvic score in one. Four authors tested construct validity based on correlation with the SF-36, and performed psychometric testing on patients who used the Majeed, IPS and Orlando pelvis-specific outcome measures.

No testing of responsiveness, content validity or reproducibility was performed. They concluded that the existing literature in this area is inadequate to inform surgeons or patients about the functional outcomes of these fractures after fixation [29].

In a later publication, Lefaivre et al. went on to test the validity of 3 previously published pelvic outcome questionnaires. A total of 38 patients were recruited to their study after a mean time of 57 months post-operatively. Of these patients, 15 had an OTA C fracture and 23 patients had an OTA B fracture. Patients cited difficulty with recreational mobility, emotional stress and family strain, employment and financial difficulty, sleep disturbance and anxiety, as well as sexual dysfunction as the most important consequences of their injuries. Each of the 3 pelvic outcome questionnaires showed a high correlation with the Physical Component Score of the SF-36, and both indices of the Short Musculoskeletal Function Assessment questionnaire (SMFA). None of the outcome measures had a high correlation with the Mental Component Score of the SF-36, indicating that these scores do not capture psychological distress and wellbeing, social functioning, and overall vitality. Therefore no outcome tool is able to capture every important consequence following pelvic fracture and operative fixation [30].

Acetabular Fractures

The acetabulum is a loadbearing area and therefore restoration of the congruence of the hip joint is key. Failure to correct any remaining steps or gaps in the articular surface, especially the main weighbearing area of the acetabular dome, can result in premature osteoarthritis of the hip joint [6].

Epidemiology

Only 10% of pelvic disruptions involve the acetabulum and although they often occur in conjunction with other fractures, in the context of pelvic injury, acetabular fractures are considered as an independent entity [1, 6].

Acetabular fractures have an overall incidence of 3 per 100,000/year and demonstrate a bimodal distribution of incidence relating to mechanism of injury and age. High-energy blunt trauma occurs in the young and is most commonly caused by Road Traffic Collisions (RTCs), a fall from height greater than 10ft and pedestrians hit by cars.

Posterior wall fractures are the most common, comprising of 24% of acetabular fractures. Around 15% of acetabular fractures are associated with a pelvic ring injury, 50% will have a concomitant injury to another organ system and 36% of patients will also have an associated lower limb injury.

Elderly patients will present following low energy mechanisms of injury such as a fall from height less than 10ft, and will usually present with an isolated injury [1, 6, 31].

When considering options for surgical fixation of acetabular fractures, it is important to take in to account the patient's pre-morbid status. Elderly patients will often have reduced bone stock and a number of significant co-morbidities and so this may influence decision making in definitive management. For fracture patterns that are easily reconstructable in elderly patients with good pre-morbid status, acetabular stabilisation should be performed. Patients with complex fracture patterns, requiring extensive bone grafting, or with complex co-morbidities should undergo primary endoprosthetic replacement. This may require a two-step process in which the acetabulum is reconstructed with cancellous bone graft from the femoral head. Paediatric acetabular fractures are incredibly rare, with an incidence of 0.01% of all reported paediatric fractures. An incredibly high-energy mechanism of injury is required to cause such fractures and there is a risk of disrupting the epiphyseal growth plates. Except for the need of smaller plates and screws, reconstruction and stabilisation is achieved in much the same way as with adults.

For children younger than 10 years of age, partial weightbearing is recommended for 4-6 weeks post-operatively followed by removal of K-wires within 6-8 weeks, and removal of plates within 5-6 months to avoid premature closure of the epiphyseal plates. Follow-up radiographs should be taken biannually to ensure this has not occurred [6].

Classifying Acetabular Injuries

A number of classification systems for acetabular fractures exist and are primarily based on the 'two column' theory. The most robust classification for acetabular fractures was established by Judet and Letournel, in which there are a total of 10 different fracture types; 5 with elementary fracture types caused by 1 major fracture line, and 5 different combined fracture types composed of at least 2 fracture types. Simple fracture types account for only 20% of acetabular fractures, the most commonly occurring fractures are therefore combined types [6, 32].

Table 11. Describes the Judet and Letournel classification for acetabular fractures [6, 32]

Fracture Type	Description	
Simple	Elementary fracture type caused by one fracture line	
Posterior wall	Involves the posterior articular surface, often with the retroacetabular surface.	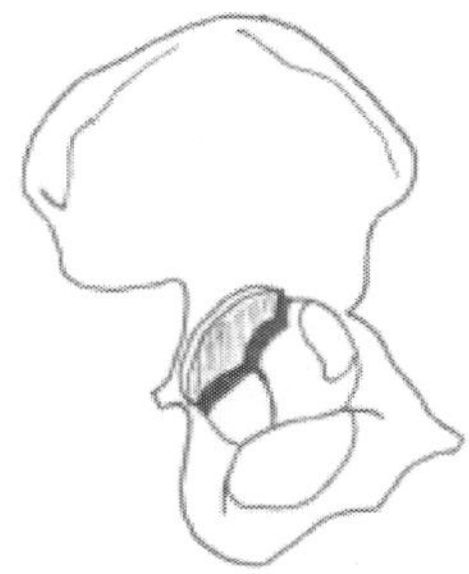
Posterior column	The posterior column is completely disconnected from the acetabulum. Fracture line crosses the obturator foramen toward the inferior pubic rim. The femoral head is often dislocated inwards.	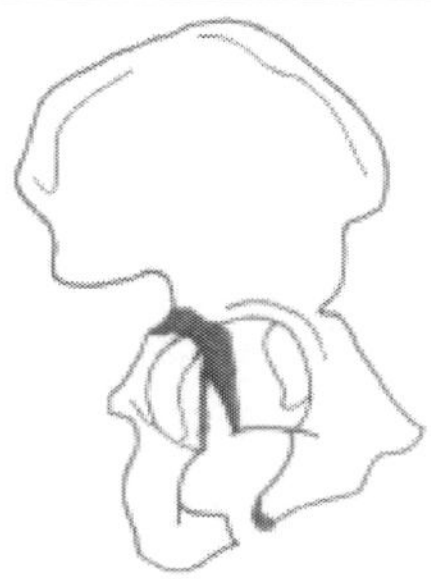
Anterior wall	Fractures occur along the iliopectineal line.	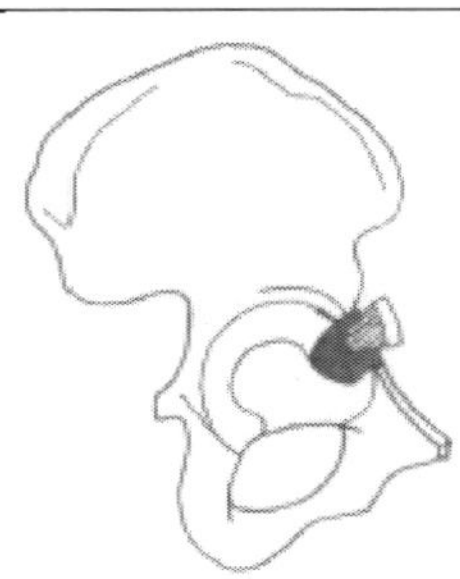
Anterior column	Fractures initiate above the anterior iliac spine and pass through the obturator foramen.	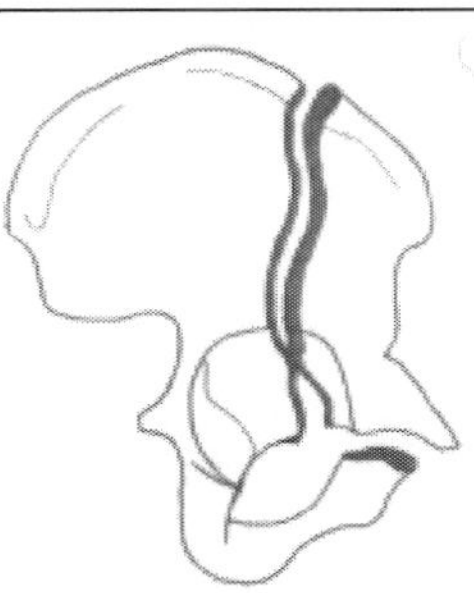

Table 11. (Continued)

Fracture Type	Description	
Simple	Elementary fracture type caused by one fracture line	
Transverse fracture	Fracture line crosses the acetabulum horizontally. Both columns are involved.	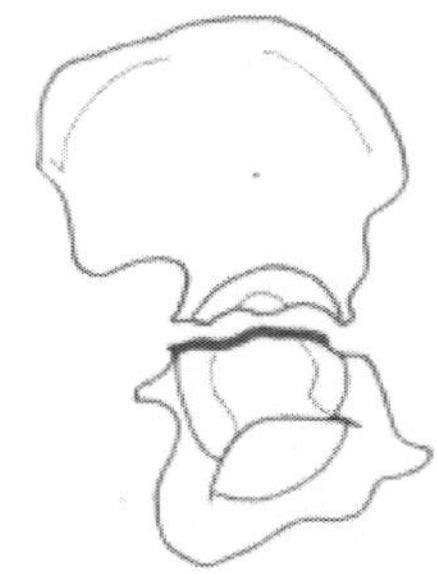
Combined	Combined fracture type caused by at least two fracture lines	
Posterior column and posterior wall	The posterior wall is mostly displaced cranially.	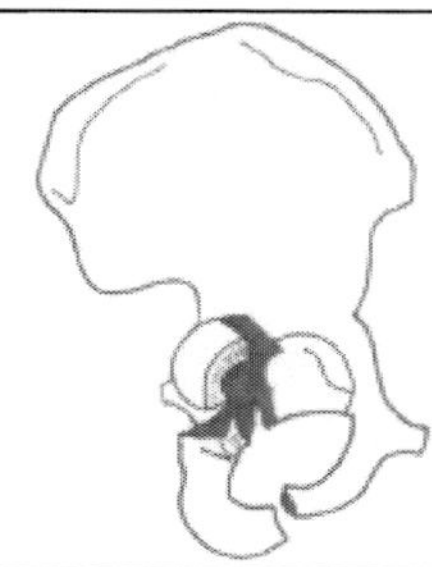
Transverse and posterior wall	The posterior wall fragment tends to be dislocated posteriorly.	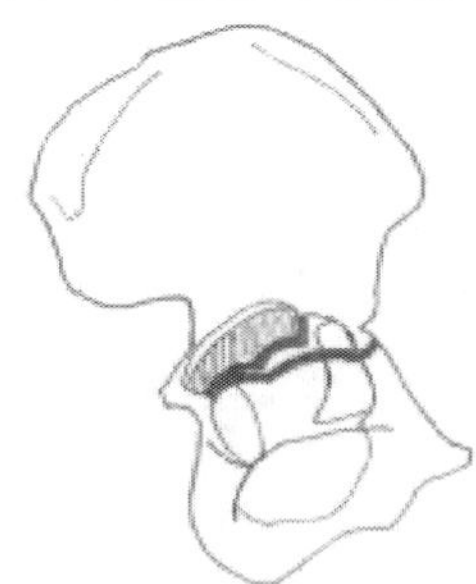
T-Shaped	This is a transverse fracture with an additional vertical fracture that crosses the obturator foramen.	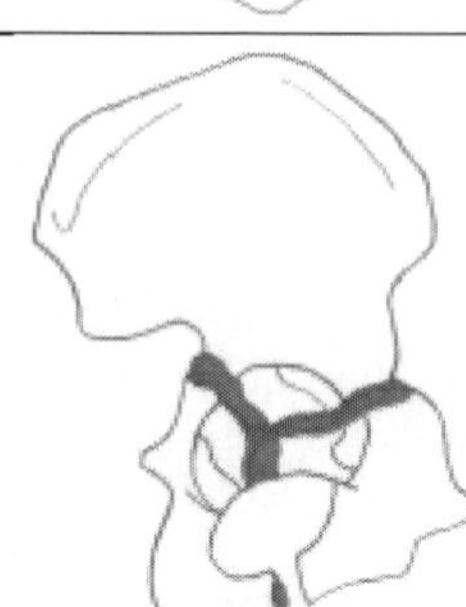

Fracture Type	Description	
Simple	Elementary fracture type caused by one fracture line	
Anterior column and hemitransverse	Two separate fracture lines; a concave fracture of the anterior column running cranio-caudally and a transverse fracture line separating the posterior column at the level of the acetabulum.	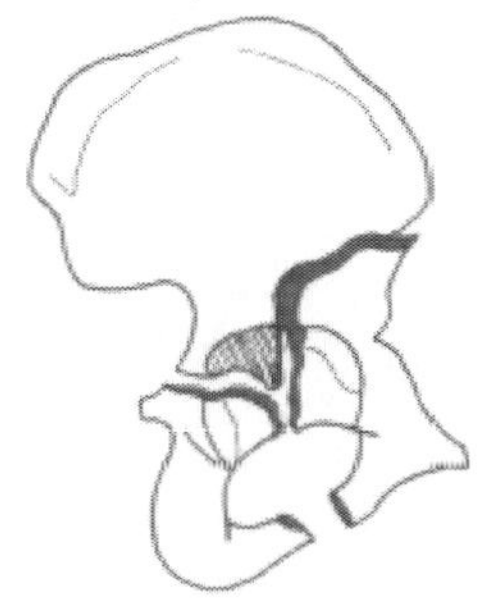
Both column	All parts of the acetabulum are separated from the stable iliac segment – results in several fracture lines of the iliac wing. The acetabulum loses all stability.	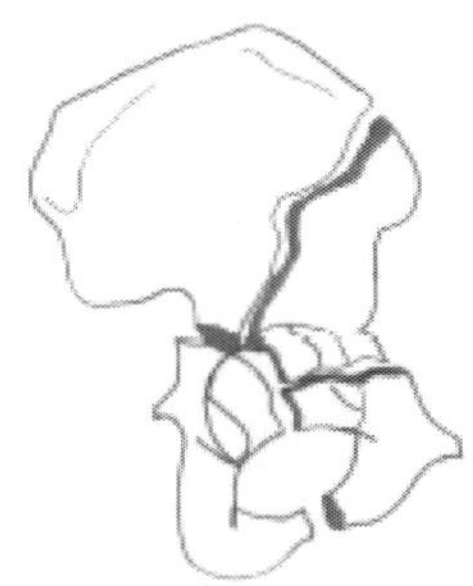

The column theory presents the notion that the acetabulum is supported by two columns of bone to form an “inverted Y”, which is connected to the sacrum through the sciatic buttress. The anterior column is comprised of the anterior ilium, the anterior wall and dome of the acetabulum, the iliopectineal eminence and the lateral superior pubic ramus. The posterior column is comprised of the quadrilateral surface, the posterior wall and dome of the acetabulum, the ischial tuberosity and the greater/lesser sciatic notches [6, 32].

Diagnosis/Investigation

History

As with pelvic fractures, gaining a clear idea of the mechanism of injury is the key to identifying patients at risk of sustaining an acetabular fracture. For example, a high index of suspicion should be afforded to patients who fall from a height greater than 10ft or sustain a dashboard injury following a road traffic collision (RTC).

Clinical Examination

Important findings on clinical examination include a painful restriction of motion of the hip joint, as well as shortening and/or a rotational deformity of the leg. As there is a 10% associated risk of sciatic nerve injury with acetabular fractures, particularly following posterior column involvement, a thorough neurological examination should be undertaken and carefully documented [6, 32].

Diagnostic Tools

X-Ray

Initial radiographs in the a.p, ala, and obturator views are essential for operative planning. The ala view is obtained by raising the intact hemipelvis by 45°, and provides a good view of the iliac wing, the posterior column, and the anterior acetabular border. The obturator view is obtained by raising the injured hemipelvis by 45° and enables one to see the obturator foramen, the anterior column and the posterior acetabular boarder [6].

Various landmarks exist that may help with discerning the fracture pattern and enabling accurate classification. The iliopectineal line demonstrates the anterior column, whereas the ilioischial line marks the posterior column. Disruptions in those lines can therefore help with identification of fractures to the corresponding walls of the acetabulum. There are a number of important assumptions that can also be made with regards to x-ray findings and fracture classification. A column fracture or T-fracture must be assumed if the obturator foramen is involved. Fracture lines crossing the iliac wing are indicative of an anterior column or two-column fracture. The spur sign is pathognomonic for a two columns fracture type and arises following internal rotation of caudal fracture fragments and the iliac bone attached to the sacroiliac joint [6, 32].

CT Scanning

Although the x-ray views described above provides an accurate picture and are helpful with fracture classification, CT scanning is necessary for precise operative planning as well as post-operative comparison following fracture reduction. Impressions of the articular surface and of the femoral head can be sought through three-dimensional reconstructions, which are helpful in gaining spatial orientation of the course of fracture lines.

Axial views are particularly useful as they enable column fractures to be characterized by a transverse course, transversal fractures by a vertical course, and wall fractures by a typical angular fracture course [6, 32].

Treatment

Instability of the femoral head as well as congruency of the articular surface of the acetabulum are important factors influencing the need for surgical intervention. This is assessed using the acetabular roof arc angle, a measurement made using the a.p, obturator and iliac views. A line is drawn to the geometric center of the acetabulum and another is drawn through the point where the fracture line intersects the acetabulum and again to the geometric center of the acetabulum.

The angle drawn in this way represents the medial, anterior, or posterior roof arc as seen on the a.p., obturator or iliac views respectively. The medial roof arc angle applies to transverse acetabular fractures and is deemed unstable requiring surgical stabilisation if less than 45°. The anterior roof arc applies to anterior column fractures and is deemed unstable requiring surgical fixation if less than 25°.

The posterior roof arc applies to posterior column fractures and is deemed unstable requiring surgical fixation is less than 70°. Fracture gaps greater than 2mm increase the risk of developing post-traumatic arthritis [6, 32, 33].

Undiscplaced fractures; small, minimally displaced posterior wall fragments; minimally displaced anterior column fractures lying outside the roof arc; and undisplaced low transverse fractures can all be treated non-operatively. Patients should be encouraged to partially weightbear 15-20kg on the affected leg for 6-12 weeks once analgesic control has been established. The progression of fracture healing should be monitored and weightbearing status adjusted accordingly [6, 32, 33].

Operative Fixation

Acetabular surgery demands careful operative planning. Operative fixation is best performed 5-8 days following injury once haemodynamic stability has been achieved and other, more life threatening injuries treated. Performing surgery any later than 2-3 weeks after injury increases the risk of callus formation hindering an optimum clinical outcome.

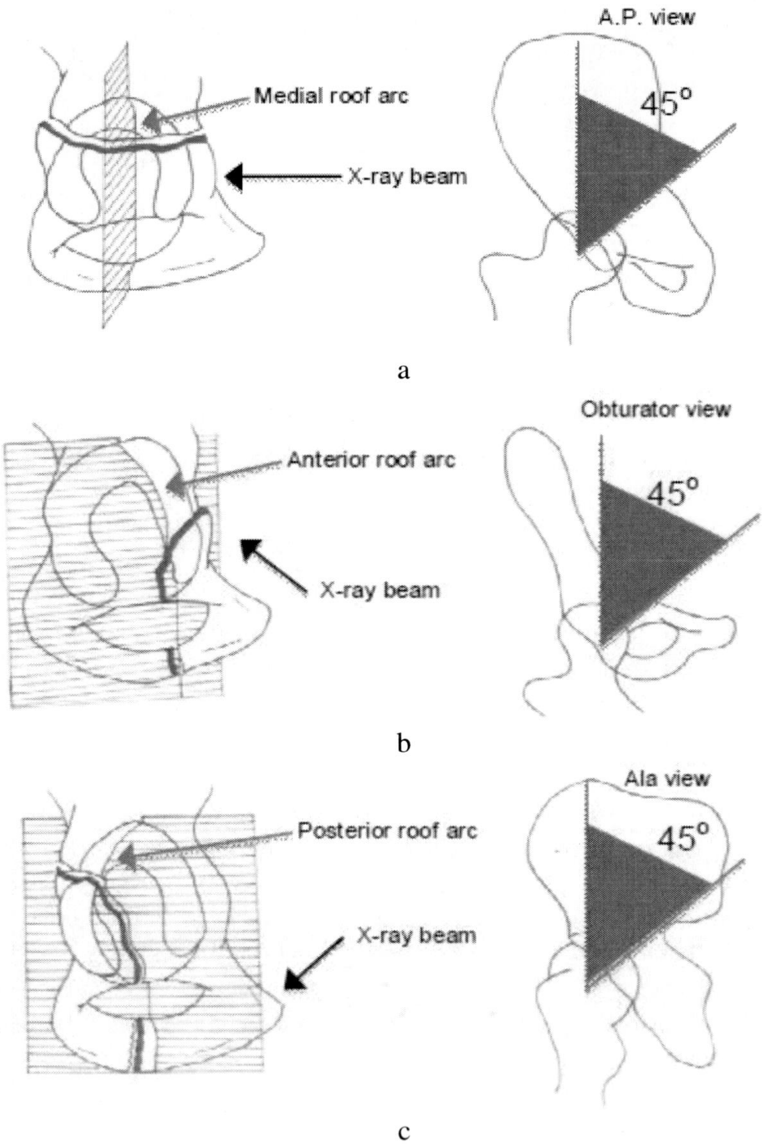

Figure 3. The Matta Roof arcs.

Emergency acetbaular surgery is only required following open injuries with vascular damage or in the case of posterior dislocations in which closed reduction is not possible [6, 32].

Below is a table of the different approaches and fixation methods for different fracture types. Satisfactory fracture reduction is a vital first step in acetabular reconstruction and often requires considerable force. Schanz screws inserted into the femoral neck are useful for applying traction. If inserted into the ishcial tuberosity, they can also be used to achieve de-rotation of the posterior column.

Table 12. Describes the approach and operative techniques that can be used to definitively treat acetabular fractures [6, 32]

Fracture Location	Approach	Method of Fixation
• Posterior wall • Posterior column • Transverse • T-type	Kocher-Langenbeck • Lateral position • Incision from proximal lateral thigh crossing greater tuberosity dorsally • Gluteus maximus dissected • Small external rotators detached close to the femur and retracted dorsally • Sciatic nerve and superior gluteal vessels identified • Trochanteric flip osteotomy + Z-shaped incision of posterior capsule to expose anterior acetabulum	• Combination of small fragment 3.5-mm cortical screws to achieve a lag effect and 3.5-mm reconstruction plates • Two plates are usually required
Anterior Column fixation using lag screws 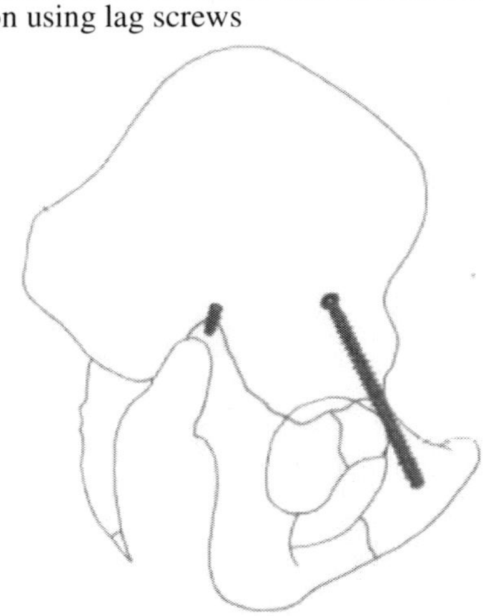		

Table 12. (Continued)

Fracture Location	Approach	Method of Fixation
Fixation of combined posterior column and wall fractures 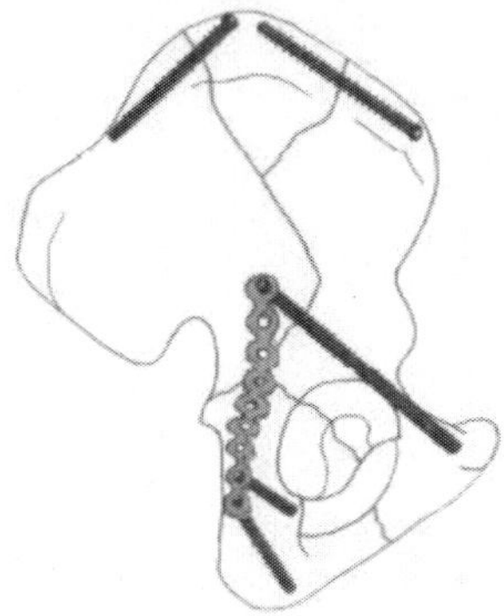		
Plate fixation of the posterior column 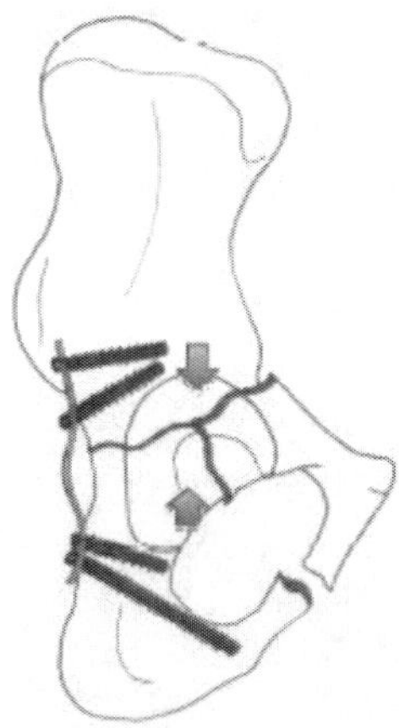		
• Anterior wall • Anterior column • Anterior column and posterior hemitransverse • T-type • Both columns	Ilioinguinal • Supine position • Incision from the posterior iliac crest to the anterior superior iliac spine along the inguinal ligament • External oblique aponeurosis incised • Iliopsoas detached subperiostally	• Combination of small fragment 3.5-mm cortical screws to achieve a lag effect and 3.5-mm reconstruction plates • Lag screw to the anterior column increases stability • Further stabilisation of the anterior column achieved by applying a reconstruction plate to the linea terminalis

Fracture Location	Approach	Method of Fixation
	• Posterior wall of the inguinal canal dissected • Psoas and femoral nerve identified and looped • Lateral femoral cutaneous nerve preserved • Femoral vessels and spermatic cord identified and looped • Musculature of iliac wing retracted • 1st window lateral to iliopsoas – exposes iliac wing and SIJ • 2nd window between psoas and femoral vessels – exposes SIJ/acetabular roof • 3rd window medial to inguinal canal – exposes superior pubic rim + pubic symphysis	
Alternative of anterior column fixation using a plate via the ilioinguinal approach 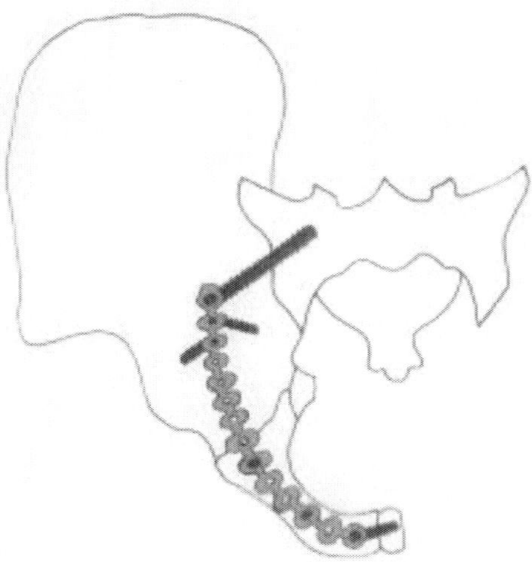		
Both column fracture	Extended Iliofemoral • Lateral position, knee flexed • Incision starts at the PSIS continues along the iliac crest to the anterior border of the iliotibial tract • Extension of sub-periosteal preparation medially or laterally of the iliac wing • Osteotomy of the greater femoral tuberosity	

Clamps such as the Jungbluth, Matta or Frabeuf have been designed to gain leverage from temporary screws or tangenital bore holes. K-wires are another useful adjunct for attempting to reconstruct multi-fragment fractures.

Any attempts to reduce acetabular fractures should be attempted in a controlled fashion using an image intensifier. Satisfactory reduction is said to be achieved with gaps of less than 2mm [6, 32].

Post Operative Management

Provided pain has been adequately controlled, partial weightbearing of 15-20kg through the affected leg should be permitted. Full weightbearing should commence 8-12 weeks postoperatively.

Postoperative x-rays of standard acetabular views should be taken at 6 and 12 weeks. Due to the risk of periarticular ossification and infection, removal of hardware is seldom performed in adult cases [6, 32].

Complications

Many of the complications of acetabular fracture fixation are shared with those following pelvic fracture fixation. Bleeding and nerve damage are the most significant intraoperative complications.

Commonly, bleeding arises from the superior gluteal artery, although the femoral vessels can also be damaged iatrogenically with anteromedial dissection during the Kocher-Langenbeck approach. The most common nerve injury associated with acetabular surgery is to the sciatic nerve, which often occurs following extensive traction with hooks during the Kocher-Langenbeck approach for posterior fractures. Curved retractors and knee flexion can go some way to avoiding this complication.

Less commonly, damage to the superior gluteal nerve can occur whilst attempting to control bleeding from the superior gluteal artery. The ilioinguinal approach also has an inherent risk to the lateral femoral cutaneous and femoral nerves [6, 32].

A useful outcome measure following acetabular fracture fixation is the Harris Hip Score (HHS), a clinician-based outcome measure with ten items assessing pain, function, absence of deformity, and range of motion. The pain domain measures pain severity and its effect on activities as well as the need for analgesia. Pooled HHS outcome scores and complication rates published by the AO foundation found that satisfactory reduction and stabilisation of acetabular fractures was achieved in 94% of cases and that 77-85% have good to excellent outcomes [6, 32].

Predictably, poor outcomes following acetabular fracture are associated with an older age at injury, fracture patterns with a high degree of comminution as well as complete loss of joint space, suboptimal fracture reduction and delays in definitive fixation [1, 6, 32].

Heteroptopic ossification (HO) appears to occur most commonly with the extended iliofemoral approach and is very uncommon with the ilioinguinal approach. It is also more common in males, patients with concomitant head or chest trauma, a high Injury Severity Score, and T-shaped fractures. Historically it was thought that the rate of HO could be reduced by taking a course of indomethacin 25mg TDS for 6 weeks postoperatively or by using 800 Gy of radiation within 72 hours postoperatively.

Matta et al. studied 107 patients prospectively who were randomly selected to either receive a 6-week course of indomethacin as treatment against HO following acetabular reconstruction, or a placebo. Nearly 8 months after surgery, HO was shown in 47.4% of the 57 patients who received indomethacin and in 56.8% of the 44 patients who received the placebo. The difference was not statistically significant. Indomethacin was therefore not effective in preventing HO postoperatively for acetabular fractures. A number of other studies have shown that radiation is as effective as indomethacin at reducing HO and a lot more expensive, which leads to the conclusion that neither are an effective means of reducing this phenomenon [34, 35].

Prognosis

Matta et al. performed a two to twenty-year survivorship study of 816 patients who underwent open reduction and internal fixation for displaced acetabular fractures. They performed a Kaplan-Meir survivorship analysis of the hip in which the worst-case scenario was either a total hip arthoplasty or hip arthrodesis as the end point. The cumulative survivorship over a twenty-year period was 79% [37]. Briffa et al. reported the outcome of 257 patients who underwent surgical fixation of acetbaular fractures over a 10-year period. They used the Merle D'Aubigné score, a validated outcome assessment tool that assess pain, range of movement of the hip joint and mobility. Simple fractures were observed in 108 patients (42%) and associated fractures in 149 patients (58%).

A total of 75 patients (47%) reported excellent results, 41 patients (25%) reported good results, fair results by 12 patients (7%) and poor results were reported by 33 patients (20%) [38].

Table 13. Shows a summary of the complications that can arise following acetabular surgery as well as their associated incidences [1, 26, 34-36]

Type of Complication	Complication	Incidence
General	Deep Vein Thrombosis	10% - 20%
	Pulmonary Embolus	4% - 10%
Local	Bleeding (extended iliofemoral approach)	1.6L
	Bleeding (Kocher-Langenbeck approach)	900mls
	Infection	3% - 9%
	Nerve palsy traumatic	16%
	Nerve palsy iatrogenic	7.8%
Late	Heterotopic ossification	30% (23.6% following extended iliofemoral approach)
	Severe osteoarthritis	19.1%
	Avascular necrosis of the femoral head	3%

A large study by Letournel and Judt of 492 patients who underwent operative fixation of acetabular fractures found excellent to good results in 80-90% of cases in which patients had acquired simple fracture types. The worst outcome was seen in patients with combined posterior column and posterior wall fractures, in which only 47% of patients reported good and excellent functional results.

Non-anatomical fracture reduction, age greater than 40 years, anterior hip dislocation, post-operative incongruence of the acetabular roof, involvement of the posterior acetabular wall, acetabular impaction, a femoral head cartilage lesion, initial displacement of the articular surface of ≥20 mm, and utilization of the extended iliofemoral approach were all significant negative independent predictors of hip survival [37].

Depending on the fracture type as well as the surgeons experience, anatomical healing without signs of post-traumatic arthritis can be expected in 70-80% of cases. The development of arthritis usually depends on un-modifiable factors such as patient age and bone quality. The majority of post-traumatic femoral head necrosis occurs within the first 2 years of injury. Ranawat et al. analysed the outcomes for post –traumatic arthritis following acetabular fracture.

The average time from fracture to total hip arthroplasty (THA) was 36 months. A total of 32 patients underwent THA for post-traumatic arthritis, 24 (75%) were initially treated with open reduction and internal fixation, 8 managed conservatively. This increased their Harris Hip score from 28 (range 0-56) to 82 (range 20-100) [39].

The high rate of hip survivorship at twenty-years as well as the excellent functional outcome scores following open reduction and internal fixation of acetabular fractures, leads to the conclusion that current surgical methods of fixation are effective but do not leave much room for error. Acetabular facture fixation requires careful pre-operative planning as well as skilled operative technique.

References

[1] Pynsent, P. B., Fairbank, J. C. T., Carr, A. J. 1994. The Pelvis and Acetabulum. In: *Outcome Measures in Trauma*. Oxford: Reed Elsevier Group. Pg. 216-236.

[2] O'Sulivan, R. E. M., White, T. O., Keating, J. F. 2005. Major Pelvic Fractures; Identification of Patients at High Risk. *Journal of Bone and Joint Surgery*. [Online]. 87-B(4), pg. 530-533. [Accessed 9th October 2014]. Available from: http://www.bjj.boneandjoint.org.uk/content/87-B/4/530.full.

[3] Guthrie, H. C., Owens, R. W., Birhcher, M. D. 2010. Fractures of the pelvis. *Journal of Bone and Joint Surgery*. 92(11), pg. 481-8.

[4] ACS Committee on Trauma. Abdominal and Pelvic Trauma. In: *Advanced Trauma Life Support*. 9th Edition. US: Hearthside Publishing. Pg. 123-147.

[5] Lee, D. *The Pelvic Girdle*. 4th Edition. 2011. Toronto: Elsevier.

[6] Wirbel, R. and Pohlemann, T. Pelvic and Acetabular Fractures. In: Arnold, W. and Ganzer, U. 2014. *Bone and Joint Injuries: Trauma Surgery III*. Berlin: Springer. Pg. 197-225.

[7] Balogh, Z., King, K. L., Mackay, P., et al. The epidemiology of pelvic ring fractures: a population-based study. *J. Trauma*. 2007 Nov;63(5): 1066-73.

[8] Demetriades, D., Karaiskakis, Toutouzas, K., et al. Pelvic fractures: epidemiology and predictors of associated abdominal injuries and outcomes. *J. Am. Coll. Surg*. 2002 Jul; 195(1): 1-10.

[9] Demetriades, D., Karaiskakis, Velmahos, G. C., et al. Pelvic fractures in paediatric and adult trauma patients: are they different injuries? *J. Trauma*. 2003 Jun; 54(6): 1146-51.

[10] Pohlemann, T., Gänsslen, A., Schellwald, O., et al. Outcome evaluation after unstable injuries of the pelvic ring. *Unfallchirurg*. 1996 Apr; 99(4): 249-59.

[11] Siegmeth, A., Müllner, T., Kukla, C., et al. Associated injuries in severe pelvic trauma. *Unfallchirurg*. 2000 Jul; 103(7): 572-81.

[12] McCormack, R., Strauss, E. J., Alwattar, B J., et al. Diagnosis and Management of Pelvic Fractures. *Bulletin of the NYU Hospital for Joint Diseases* 2010;68(4):281-91.

[13] Van Rensburg, L. *Sacral Fractures [Online]*. 2009 [2015/01/26]. Available from: URL: http://www.rcsed.ac.uk/fellows/lvanrensburg/classification/pelvis/sacrum.htm.

[14] Basta, A. M., Blackmore, C. C., Wessells, H. Predicting urethral injury from pelvic fracture patterns in male patients with blunt trauma. *J. Urol.* 2007;177(2):571-5.

[15] Metze, M., Tiemann, A H., Josten, C. Male sexual dysfunction after pelvic fracture. *J. Trauma*. 2007; 63:394-401.

[16] Demetriades, D., Karaiskakis, M., Velmahos, G. C., et al. Pelvic fractures in paediatric and adult trauma patients: are they different injuries? *J. Trauma*. 2003 Jun;54(6):1146-51.

[17] Blackmore, C. C., Cummings, P., Jurkovich, G. J., et al. Predicting major haemorrhage in patients with pelvic fracture. *J. Trauma*. 2006 Aug;61(2):346-52.

[18] Magnussen, R. A., Tressler, M. A., Obremskey, W. T., et al. Predicting blood loss in isolated pelvic and acetabular high-energy trauma. *J. Orthop. Trauma*. 2007 Oct;21(9): 603-7.

[19] Friese, R. S., Malekzadeh, S., Shafi, S., et al. Abdominal ultrasound is an unreliable modality for the detection of hemoperitoneum in patients with pelvic trauma. *J. Trauma*. 2007 Jul;63(1):97-102.

[20] Romano, L., Pinto, A., De Lutio Di Castelguidone, E., et al. Spiral computed tomography in the assessment of vascular lesion of the pelvis due to blunt trauma. *Radiol. Med.* 2000 Jul-Aug;100(1-2):29-32.

[21] Agolini, S. F., Shah, K., Jaffe, J., et al. Arterial embolization is a rapid and effective technique for controlling pelvic fracture haemorrhage. *J. Trauma*. 1997 Sep;43(3):395-9.

[22] Stannard, A., Eliason, J. L., Rasmussen, T. E. Resuscitative endovascular ballon occlusion of the aorta (REBOA) as an adjunct for the hemorrhagic shock. *J. Trauma*. 2011 Dec;71(6):1869-72.

[23] Brenner, M. L., Moore, L. J., DuBose, J. J., et al. A clinical series of resuscitative endovascular balloon occlusion of the aorta for hemorrhage control and resuscitation. *J. Trauma Acute Care Surg*. 2013 Sep; 75(3): 506-11.

[24] Nicola, R. *Early Total Care versus Damage Control: Current Concepts in the Orthopedic Care of Polytrauma Patients [Online]*. 2013 [2015/01/26]. Available from: URL: http://www.ncbi.nlm.nih.gov/pmc/articles/PMC4045290/.

[25] Pape, H. C., Giannoudis, P. V., Krettek, C., et al. Timing of fixation of major fractures in blunt polytrauma: role of conventional indicators in clinical decision making. *Journal of Orthopaedic Trauma*. 2005;19(8): 551-562.

[26] Steele, N., Dodenhoff, R. M., Ward, A. J., et al. Thromboprophylaxis in pelvic and acetabular trauma surgery. The role of early treatment with low-molecular-weight heparin. *J. Bone Joint Surg. Br*. 2005 Feb;87(2): 209-12.

[27] Torbert, J. T., Joshi, M., Moraff, A., et al. Current bacterial speciation and antbiotic resistance in deep infections after operative fixation of fractures. *J. Orthop. Trauma*. 2015 Jan;29(1):7-17.

[28] Hauser, C. J., Adams, C. A. Jr, Eachempatic, S. R. Surgical Infection Society guideline: prophylactic antibiotic use in open fractures: an evidence-based guideline. *Surg. Infect*. (Larchmt). 2006 Aug;7(4):379-405.

[29] Lefaivre, K. A., Slobogean, G. P., Valeriote, J., et al. Reporting and interpretation of the functional outcomes after surgical treatment of disuptions of the pelvic ring: a systematic review. *J. Bone Joint Surg. Br.* 2012 Apr;94(4):549-55.

[30] Lefaivre, K. A., Slobogean, G. P., Ngai, J. T., et al. What outcomes are important for patients after pelvic trauma? Subjective responses and psychometric analysis of three published pelvic-specific outcome instruments. *J. Orthop. Trauma*. 2014 Jan;28(1):23-7.

[31] Laird, A. and Keating, J. F. Acetabular fractures: 16-year prospective epidemiological study. *J. Bone Joint Surg. Br*. 2005 Jul;87(7):969-73.

[32] Weatherford, B. *Acetabular Fractures [Online]*. 2014 [2015/01/26]. Available from: URL: http://www.orthobullets.com/trauma/1034/acetabular-fractures.

[33] Clifford, R. *Roof arc measurements for roof arc angles for acetabular fractures [Online]*. 2014 [2015/01/26]. Available from: URL: http://www.wheelessonline.com/ortho/roof_arc_measurements_for_acetabular_frx.

[34] Matta, J. M. and Siebenrock, K. A. Does indomethacin reduce heterotopic bone formation after operations for acetabular fractures? A prospective randomised study. *J. Bone Joint Surg. Br*. 1997 Nov;79(6): 959-63.

[35] Moore, K. D., Goss, K., Anglen, J. O. Indomethacin versus radiation therapy for prophylaxis against heterotopic ossification in acetabular fractures: a randomised, prospective study. *J. Bone Joint Surg. Br*. 1998 Mar;80(2):259-63.

[36] Trafton, P. *AO Foundation; Acetabulum [Online]*. 2007 [2015/01/26]. Available from: URL: https://www2.aofoundation.org/wps/portal/!ut/p/a0/04_Sj9CPykssy0xPLMnMz0vMAfGjzOKN_A0M3D2DDbz9_UMMDRyDXQ3dw9wMDAx8jfULsh0VAdAsNSU!/?BackMode=trueandbone=PelvisandcontentUrl=%2Fsrg%2Fpopup%2Fevidence_sum%2F62%2F62-Evidence-Summ.jspandpopupStyle=diagnosisandsegment=AcetabulumandsoloState=true#JumpLabelNr5.

[37] Tannast, M., Najibi, S., Matta, J. M. Two to twenty-year survivorship of the hip in 810 patients with operatively treated acetabular fractures. *J. Bone Joint Surg. Am*. 2012 Sep. 5;94(17):1559-67.

[38] Briffa, N., Pearce, R., Hill, A. M., et al. Outcomes of acetabular fracture fixation with ten years' follow-up. *J. Bone Joint Surg. Br*. 2011 Feb;93 (2):229-36.

[39] Ranawat, A., Zelken, J., Helfet, D. Total hip arthroplasty for posttraumatic arthritis after acetabular fracture. *J. Arthroplasty*. 2009 Aug; 24(5):759-67.

In: Abdominal Injuries
Editor: Chad L. Barrett

ISBN: 978-1-63482-590-0

Chapter 4

Endoscopic Stent Placement for the Treatment of Traumatic Pancreatic Duct Ruptures in Children

Johannes Mayr[1,*], Frank-Martin Häcker[1] and Lukas Degen[2]

[1]Department of Pediatric Surgery, University Children's Hospital Basel, Switzerland, Basel, Switzerland

[2]Division of Gastroenterology and Hepatology, University of Basel, Switzerland, Basel, Switzerland

Abstract

Pancreatic duct ruptures in children are predominantly caused by bicycle handlebar injuries. Acute onset of abdominal symptoms and subsequent pancreatic pseudocyst formation occur within hours or days after the injury. Pancreatic duct ruptures are diagnosed by contrast-enhanced computer tomography (CT), magnetic resonance pancreaticography (MRP), or endoscopic retrograde pancreaticography

* Corresponding author: Johannes M. Mayr, M.D., Department of Pediatric Surgery, University Children's Hospital Basel, Spitalstrasse 33, 4031 Basel, Switzerland. Tel: 0041 61 704 2811; Fax: 0041 61 704 12 47; E-mail: johannes.mayr@ukbb.ch.

(ERP). Pancreatic duct ruptures usually require surgery or other interventional therapy and carry a significant risk of morbidity. ERP-guided stent placement of the proximal pancreatic duct, with or without stenting of the rupture site, has been reported recently.

Case Report

Two boys, aged 6 and 6.5 years, sustained pancreatic duct ruptures in handlebar injuries when riding their bicycles. In both cases, free abdominal fluid was noted using ultrasonographic imaging, and levels of serum amylase on admission were 251 U/L and 398 U/L (normal range: <100 U/L), respectively. Octreotide (2 x 0.025 mg/day) was administered intravenously starting on day 1 and day 7, respectively. Both pancreatic duct ruptures (American Association for the Surgery of Trauma [AAST] grade 3) were confirmed with abdominal contrast-enhanced CT scans on the day of admission and 8 days after the injury. Both children underwent ERP-guided stent placement (5.0 French, 8.0 and 7.0 cm in length, respectively) of the major pancreatic duct. In both boys, oral nutrition was started 1 day after the endoscopic intervention and was well tolerated thereafter. The two boys returned home 2 days and 7 days after the intervention. In both patients, peripancreatic fluid accumulation resolved after 2 days and 4 weeks, respectively. Stents were removed by endoscopy after 4 and 9 weeks. Follow-up for 87 and 82 months was uneventful.

Conclusion

ERP-guided stent placement represents a safe and efficient treatment option for pancreatic duct injuries AAST grade 3 in children and may replace more complex surgical treatment in selected cases. Further studies are required to confirm our findings.

Keywords: pancreatic duct, injury, pediatric, ERP, stent

Introduction

Pancreatic injury in childhood is rare, constituting 0.3% to 0.7% of all trauma admissions at large pediatric trauma centers [1, 2, 3]. Most blunt pancreatic injuries occur if the border region of the pancreatic head and corpus are forcefully compressed against the vertebral column. Injury to the neck of the pancreas is usually the result of a blunt impact on the tube-shaped end of a bicycle handlebar, or deceleration injury in motor vehicle collision with seat belts running across the belly of the child [4, 5, 6, 7, 8]. A low body mass index may predispose to pancreatic duct injuries in children because of insufficient soft tissue [4].

Pancreatic injuries are graded according to the guidelines of the American Association for the Surgery of Trauma (AAST) into 5 categories, i.e., grade 1: minor contusion; grade 2: major contusion; grade 3: distal transection or parenchyma and duct injury (to the left of the superior mesenteric vein [SMV]); grade 4: proximal transection or parenchyma and duct injury (to the right of the SMV); grade 5: massive disruption of pancreatic head [9].

Most pancreatic injuries in children are benign parenchymal contusions grade 1 or grade 2, which are amenable to nonoperative treatment [2]. Lesions of the major pancreatic duct (grade 3 and grade 4) are very rare in children and are sometimes diagnosed after an interval of several days when pseudocyst formation results in obstructive symptoms of the alimentary tract, or if signs of chemical peritonitis develop. Lesions of the major pancreatic duct cause prolonged hospitalization and give rise to significant morbidity. Diagnosis of major pancreatic duct injuries is sometimes delayed because of the exclusive use of ultrasonography or plain X-ray imaging instead of contrast-enhanced CT or even better magnetic resonance pancreaticography (MRP). However, in injured children aged less than 7 years, MRP intervention may be unduly traumatizing if no sedation or anesthesia is provided.

For primary investigation, some authors advocate endoscopic retrograde pancreaticography (ERP) as the gold standard if major pancreatic duct injury is suspected [10]. Use of endoscopic retrograde cholangiopancreaticography (ERCP) in children has become more common in recent years, despite a complication rate of 13.5% [10]. ERP also allows for simultaneous insertion of an endoscopically placed transpapillary stent to secure the low pressure outflow of pancreatic duct secretions into the duodenum, or to insert a nasopancreatic drain [4, 11, 12]. However, endoscopically inserted pancreatic duct stents to treat pancreatic major duct lesions in children are discussed controversially, with some authors advocating nonoperative management and others recommending operative interventions such as spleen-preserving pancreatic resection within the first 72 h after injury [1, 2, 13, 14, 15]. Thus, experience with pancreatic duct stenting is limited [13].

This case report describes the management of lacerations of the major pancreatic duct (grade 3) in two boys, using endoscopically placed pancreatic duct stents.

Case Report

Case 1

A 6-year old boy hit the end of the handlebar of his bicycle during a fall injury in the afternoon. He initially complained of abdominal pain, but the pain subsided and he was subsequently able to eat normally. Due to increasing abdominal pain, he was admitted to the accident and emergency ward thereafter, where a circular bruise mark in the epigastrium was noted. Guarding and massive abdominal pain were present. Initial laboratory tests yielded the following values: hemoglobin 12.1 g/L, leucocyte count 14.9 x 10^9/L, ASAT 166 U/L, ALAT 128 U/L, serum amylase 251 U/L (normal range: <100 U/L), and serum lipase 335 U/L (normal range: <40 U/L).

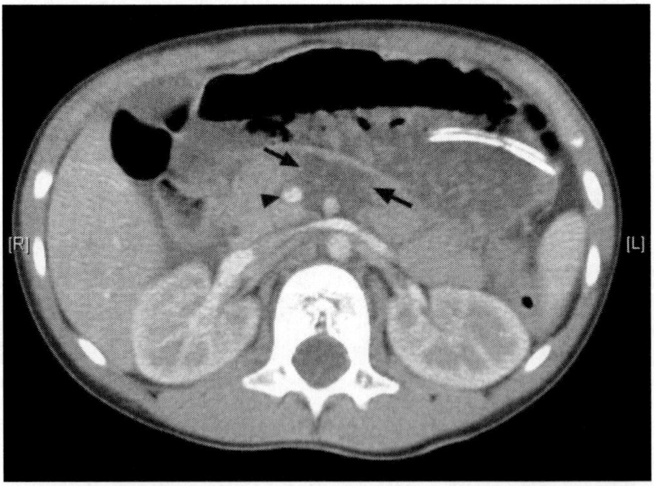

Figure 1a. Contrast-enhanced CT scan of the abdomen obtained on the day of injury. Rupture of the pancreas (arrows) and the major pancreatic duct anterior and to the left of the superior mesenteric vein (SMV; marked by arrowhead) and to the right of the superior mesenteric artery (SMA). The transection zone is visualized by a low attitude line across the pancreas.

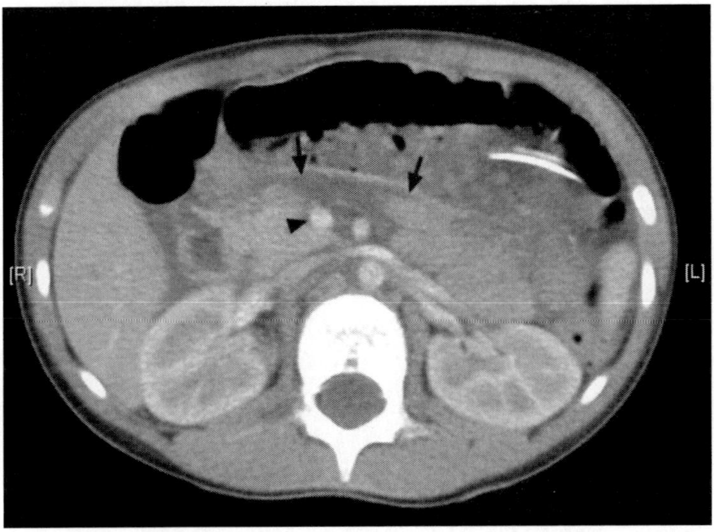

Figure 1b. Minimal amount of fluid visible between the pancreas and stomach (marked by arrows). SMV marked by arrowhead.

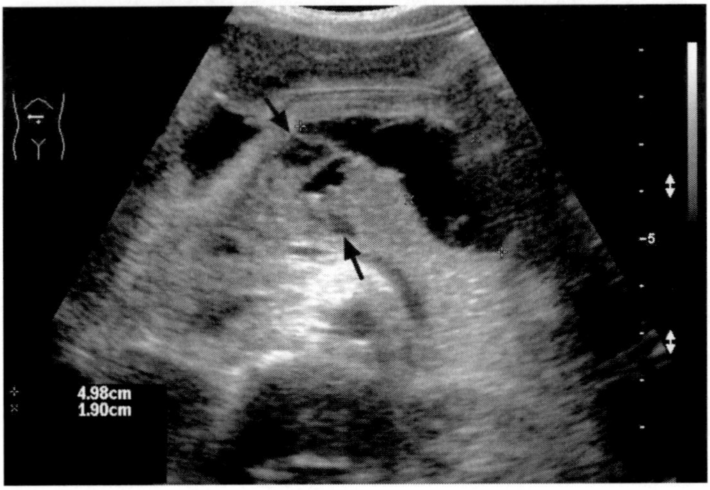

Figure 2. Transverse ultrasonographic scan of the upper abdomen obtained 5 days after the injury. Pseudocyst of 5.0 x 1.9 cm in size, in close vicinity to the rupture zone (arrows) across the neck of the pancreas.

Ultrasonographic scanning of the abdomen showed a swollen pancreatic head region, with blurred margins of the pancreas, a contusion zone within the liver, and moderate amounts of free intraperitoneal fluid. Contrast-enhanced CT of the abdomen performed on the day of admission showed edema of the pancreatic head and a small laceration of the pancreatic corpus (Figure 1a and 1b). A small amount of free intraperitoneal fluid behind the urinary bladder was noted. The boy was admitted to the pediatric intensive care unit for observation. Total parenteral nutrition was initiated, and octreotide (Sandostatin®, Novartis Pharmaceuticals, Basel, Switzerland) was administered intravenously (0.025 mg twice daily). A nasogastric tube was inserted. Hypocalcemia was corrected by intravenous calcium administration. On day 3, a central intravenous line was placed as the child tolerated no fluid by mouth. During the first days after the injury, abdominal symptoms gradually improved and the pain subsided, but further ultrasonic scanning showed a pseudocyst of 5.0 x 1.9 cm in size (Figure 2) causing small bowel paralysis.

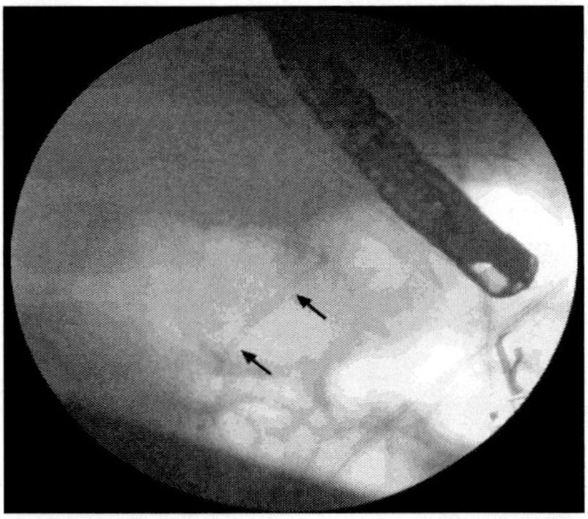

Figure 3a. ERP with insertion of a pigtail catheter (size 5 French, length 8.0 cm; arrows) into the major pancreatic duct.

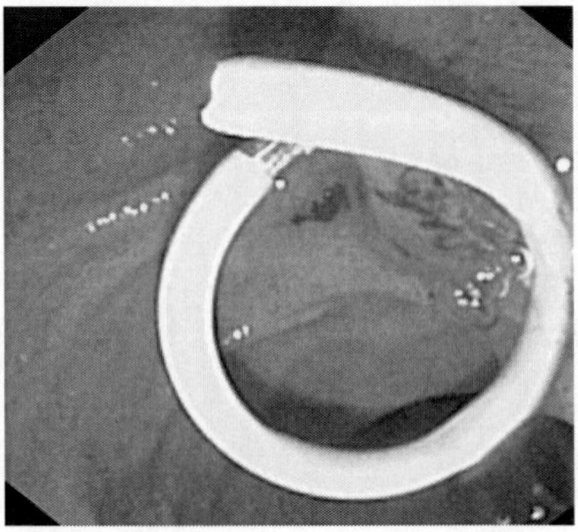

Figure 3b. Endoscopic image of the proximal end of the pancreatic pigtail stent.

ERP, performed by an experienced gastroenterologist (L.D.) one week after the injury, revealed partial disruption of the major pancreatic duct to the left of the SMV, indicative of grade 3 pancreatic injury [9]. A 5.0 French pancreatic stent (Wilson-Cook Medical Inc., Winston Salem, NC, USA) with a length of 8.0 cm was inserted as described by Canty and Weinman and Lin et al. [12, 16] (Figure 3a and 3b). One day after the intervention, serum levels of amylase and lipase declined, and a reduced amount of peripancreatic fluid was noted on ultrasonographic examination. Oral nutrition was initiated and remained well tolerated. Three days after stent insertion, ultrasonographic imaging confirmed the reduction of peripancreatic fluid accumulation (Figure 4a and 4b). One week after ERP intervention, the boy left hospital; overall length of stay (LOS) at the hospital was 14 days. Three weeks after stent insertion, an episode of acute pancreatitis occurred, with a maximum level of serum amylase of 1010 U/L and serum lipase of 387 U/L. Pancreatitis resolved upon intravenous fluid administration, antibiotic therapy, and pain treatment without further intervention. Ultrasonographic scanning obtained 3 weeks after endoscopic stent placement showed a residual pancreatic pseudocyst of 1.0 cm x 1.5 cm in size (Figure 5) and consolidation of the pancreas at the site of rupture. Four weeks after insertion, the stent was removed by endoscopy (Figure 6). Three weeks after stent removal, ultrasonographic scanning revealed a residual 3.3 mm dilatation of the pancreatic main duct at the site of injury (Figure 7).

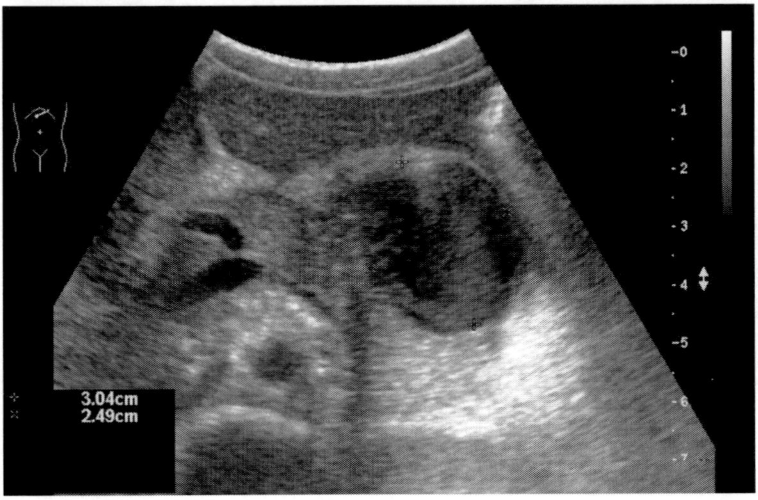

Figure 4a. Ultrasonographic transverse upper abdominal scan of the pancreatic rupture site obtained on day 3 after endoscopic stent insertion. The pseudocyst measures 3.0 x 2.5 cm, and the content of the cyst consists of hypoechogenic fluid.

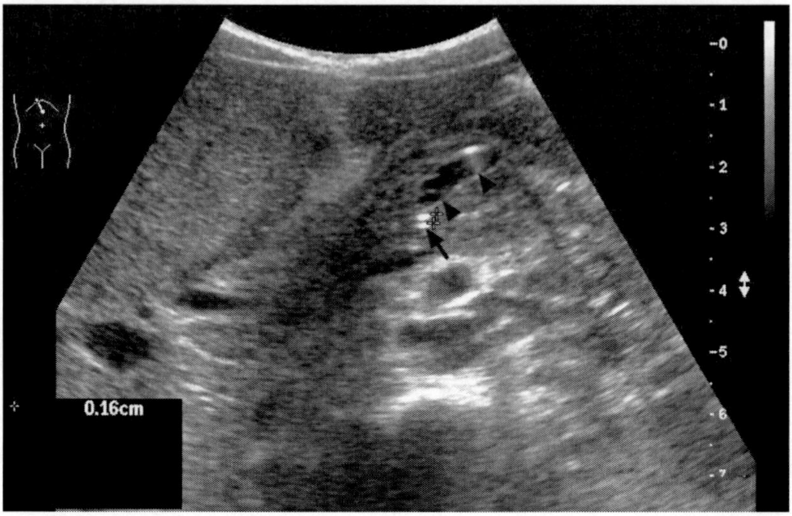

Figure 4b. Ultrasonographic sagittal scan of the pancreatic body. The endoscopically placed stent (arrow) is located dorsally to the hypoechogenic area of the pancreatic rupture (arrowhead).

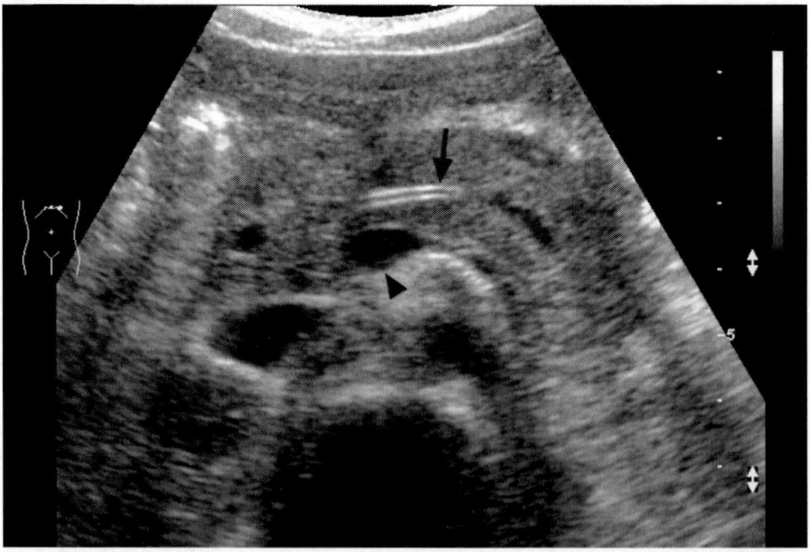

Figure 5. Transverse upper abdominal ultrasonographic scan of the pancreas obtained 3 weeks after endoscopic stent placement. The rupture site is marked by arrowhead. The pancreatic main duct is splinted by the stent (arrow). Minimal dilatation of the distal pancreatic major duct. A small residual pseudocyst (1.5 x 1.0 cm; arrowhead) dorsally to the healing pancreatic rupture is discernable.

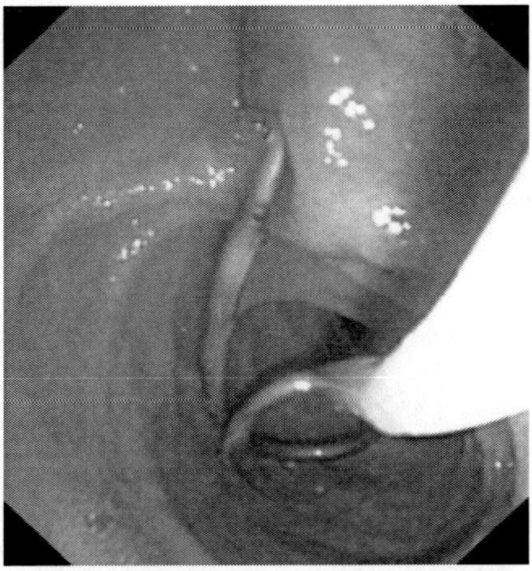

Figure 6. Endoscopic image obtained 4 weeks after endoscopic stent insertion. The pigtail stent is removed using a sling.

Sonographic follow-up obtained 16 months after stent removal confirmed a normal diameter of the major pancreatic duct, and there was no atrophy of the pancreas parenchyma (Figure 8). The pseudocyst was no longer discernable. Serum lipase levels had returned to normal. The child no longer complained of abdominal pain, and he tolerated all types of food.

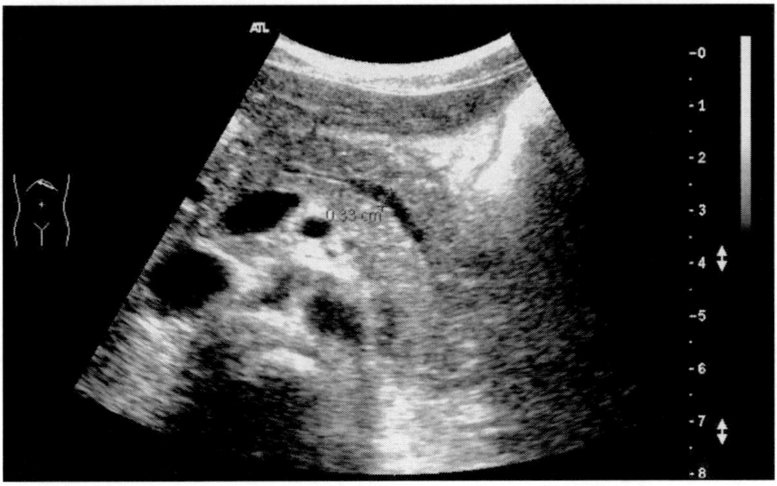

Figure 7. Transverse upper abdominal ultrasonographic scan showing the major pancreatic duct distally to the site of injury. Diameter of the major pancreatic duct measures 3.3 mm.

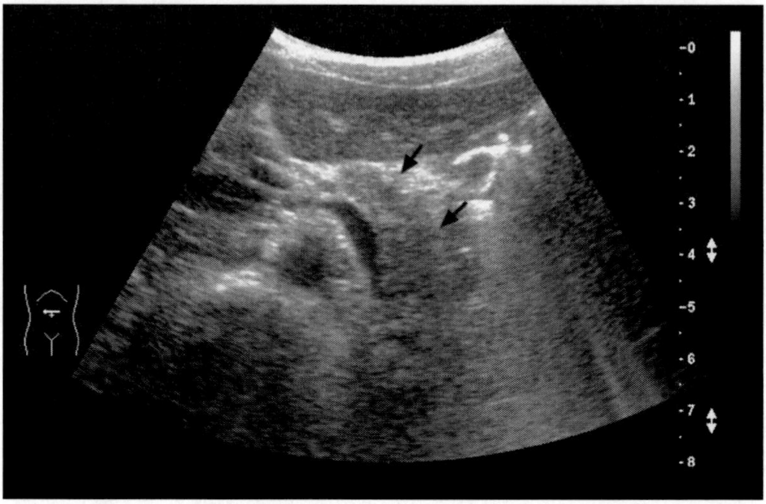

Figure 8. Transverse upper abdominal ultrasonographic scan showing normal width of the pancreatic body (anterior margin of the pancreas marked by arrows).

Seven years after the injury, the boy reported no sequelae of the pancreatic duct rupture.

Case 2

A 6.5-year old boy fell onto the tube-shaped open end of his bicycle handlebar. He complained about increasing epigastric pain within the following hours. At the local hospital, ultrasonic scanning of the abdomen revealed free intra-abdominal fluid, and the child was referred to our level I pediatric trauma center for further management. A small bruise was noted above the left iliac crest, and periumbilical pain was recorded on admission to our trauma center.

At initial investigation, clinical chemistry values were as follows: hemoglobin 11.6 g/L, leucocyte count 13.3 x 10^9/L, ASAT 82 U/L, ALAT 61 U/L, and serum amylase 398 U/L. Ultrasonographic scanning of the abdomen showed a minimal amount of free intraperitoneal fluid, and the pancreas was not visualized due to distended, air-filled bowel loops.

Small amounts of liquid were given orally, and parenteral nutrition was initiated. Serum amylase levels increased steadily, peaking 5 days after the injury (1450 U/L), whereas serum lipase levels peaked 8 days after the injury (389 U/L). Periumbilical pain persisted, and the child was unable to tolerate adequate oral nutritional intake. Octreotide (Sandostatin(R), Novartis Pharmaceuticals, Basel, Switzerland) was administered at a dose of 0.025 mg twice a day. A contrast-enhanced CT scan of the abdomen, performed 5 days after the injury, confirmed rupture of the pancreatic major duct in the region between the pancreatic head and corpus, anterior and to the left of the SMV (grade 3 pancreatic injury) [9]; (Figure 9a and 9b). Due to persisting upper abdominal pain and high levels of urine amylase (16,620 U/L; normal range: <270 U/L) on day 17 after the injury, ERP was undertaken by an experienced gastroenterologist (L.D.) 18 days after the injury. ERP confirmed partial disruption of the major pancreatic duct. A 5.0 French, 7.0 cm pancreatic stent was inserted endoscopically.

One day after the intervention, octreotide administration was stopped. Serum and urine levels of amylase declined, and oral nutrition was increasingly tolerated. Two days after the ERP intervention, the boy left hospital, and subsequent ultrasonographic scanning confirmed the absence of peripancreatic fluid 2 days thereafter (Figure 10). Overall LOS was 21 days.

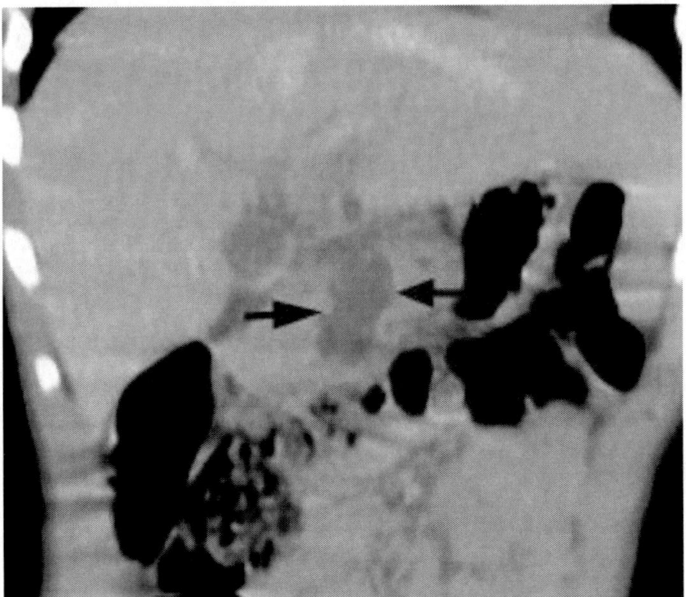

Figure 9a. Contrast-enhanced CT scan of the abdomen. In the coronal plane reconstruction, the area of pancreatic laceration is characterized by a hypodense zone (marked by arrows).

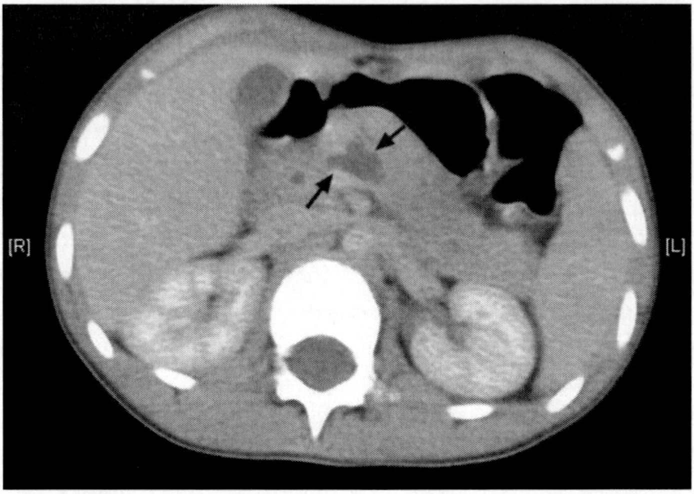

Figure 9b. Contrast-enhanced transverse CT scan of the upper abdomen. The pancreatic rupture (arrows) is anterior to the SMA and SMV.

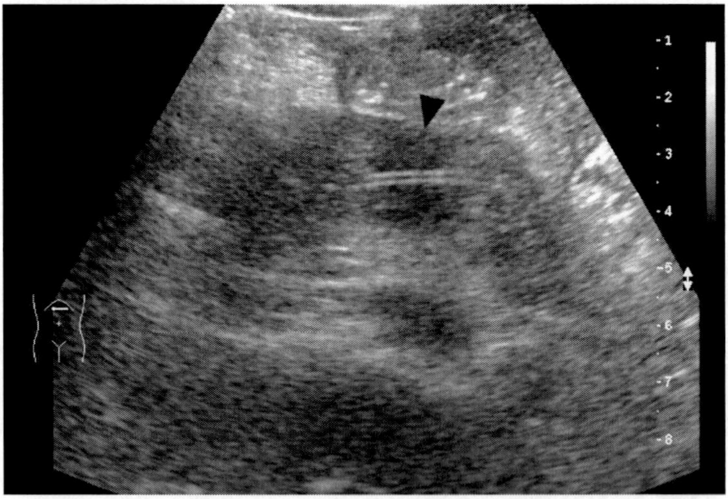

Figure 10. Transverse upper abdominal ultrasonographic scan obtained 2 days after endoscopic stent placement showing the stent within the major pancreatic duct. The stent was progressed across the rupture site (arrowhead) of the major pancreatic duct.

Because removal of the stent was not possible 4 weeks after the injury for family reasons, the stent was removed by endoscopy after 9 weeks. At follow-up 32 months after the injury, ultrasonographic scanning of the abdomen showed a normal shape of the pancreas. Serum amylase level was 63 U/L, and serum glucose level was 7.1 mmol/L.

At follow-up after almost 7 years, the boy reported to be free of complaints. In the meantime, he had gained adequate body weight and height.

Discussion

Both our patients had elevated serum amylase and/or lipase levels at the time of hospital admission. This is in agreement with de Blaauw et al. and Haugaard et al., who reported that 50% to 90% of their patients had elevated serum levels of amylase on admission [8, 17]. In line with Houben et al. and Abbo et al., our patients were assessed by initial ultrasonographic scanning, and diagnosis of pancreatic major duct injury was confirmed by contrast-enhanced CT scanning [4, 7]. Delayed detection of injuries of the major pancreatic duct in children is a well-known phenomenon [4]. A significant diagnostic time delay occurred in our second patient, in whom we obtained the contrast-enhanced CT scan that confirmed major duct injury 5 days after the accident. This time delay compares well with findings of other authors, who reported a median time delay until diagnosis of pancreatic duct injury up to 11 days [4, 6] or a range of 0.75 h to 216 h [1]. In our second patient, we had initially based our diagnostic work-up solely on clinical examination, serial ultrasonographic scans, and laboratory tests. This underlines the fact that ultrasonographic examination is not sufficient to rule out major duct injuries of the pancreas [4]. Condition of the major pancreatic duct is the most relevant prognostic factor for treating pancreatic injuries [16]. The most important factors to diagnose major pancreatic duct injury are confirmation of a 50% laceration of the pancreas, complete transection of the pancreas, and visualization of early pancreatic fluid accumulation [4].

Therefore, many authors advocate contrast-enhanced CT scans on admission to diagnose major duct injuries [1, 2, 5, 18]. Contrast-enhanced high-resolution CT scanning is superior to routine abdominal CT [2]. The CT scan might be repeated after one day if suspicion of pancreatic injury persists despite a negative finding in the initial CT scan [19]. Other authors recommend MRP or even ERP imaging [13, 20, 21]. However, MRP and ERP imaging in children less than 7 years of age usually requires conscious sedation or even anesthesia.

ERP represents the most accurate method to diagnose pancreatic trauma [22]. Rescorla et al. described the use of early ERP in children [20]. However,

ERP is invasive and is associated with potential complications. In addition, the method is not widely available at pediatric trauma centers, and its application in children requires expertise [22]. MRP and secretin-enhanced magnetic resonance cholangiopancreatography (MRCP) are probably of equal value to ERP in diagnosing pancreatic duct injuries [22, 23, 24].

The proponents of ERP argue that this technique is not only a diagnostic tool but also allows for therapeutic pancreatic stent insertion within the same anesthetic procedure [4, 11, 12, 16]. When performed by well-trained endoscopists, ERCP is useful and safe in children [10, 25, 26]. Canty and Weinman described early stent placement in children suffering from pancreatic duct ruptures [12]. An overview of studies evaluating the role of endoscopic transpapillary pancreatic duct drainage in children and adults was published by Bhasin et al. [22]. Houben et al. reported on a series of 9 children who suffered pancreatic major duct injuries treated with ERP and pancreatic stent insertion [4]. In all of these children, pancreatic resection was avoided [4]. A stent was placed across the injured duct site in 3 children [4]. However, clinical improvement was most pronounced in the children in whom the tip of the stent was placed within the accumulated fluid at the site of the lesion of the major pancreatic duct [4].

Endoscopic insertion of pancreatic stents to drain the site of injury of the major pancreatic duct or to splint the site of duct lesion by advancement of the stent over the pancreatic duct laceration zone has been described by several authors [4, 12, 16]. However, it remains debatable whether the distal end of the stent should by progressed over the rupture site of the pancreatic main duct, thus providing a splinting effect for the healing duct, and possibly preventing post-traumatic pancreatic duct stenosis [4, 11]. Other authors recommend placing the distal end of the pancreatic duct splint in the region of the major duct laceration to optimize drainage of secretions at the site of pancreatic injury, thus avoiding pancreatic pseudocyst formation or treating a developing pseudocyst [4]. There is a risk of post-traumatic pancreatic major duct strictures at the site of the ruptured duct, and some authors recommend repeated ERP and endoscopic dilatation of the duct stricture immediately after removal of the pancreatic stent [16].

However, the ideal time period between insertion and removal of the pancreatic stent in grade 3 and grade 4 injuries of the pancreas in children needs to be determined. In children, a stenting interval of 3 months was described [11]. Lin et al. reported that the duration of stent treatment was shortened from 2 months to 3 weeks in adult patients who had sustained injuries to the pancreatic duct, in order to prevent ductal stricture [16]. In our patients, we monitored peripancreatic fluid regression by serial ultrasonic scanning as suggested by Houben et al. [4].

Optimal treatment of an injured major pancreatic duct (grade 3 and grade 4) in children is discussed controversially [1]. In line with our treatment strategy, Abbo et al. described treatment of pancreatic duct lesions with total parenteral nutrition and administration of octreotide (Sandostatin(R), Novartis Pharmaceuticals, Basel, Switzerland) [7].

Wood et al. undertook pancreatic resection in all patients suffering from pancreatic transections detected by ERP and used a nonoperative approach for all minor pancreatic duct lesions [6]. However, Kawahara et al. suggested that distal pancreatectomy should not be routinely performed in patients with isolated pancreatic duct injury [27]. While many authors opt for spleen-preserving pancreatic resection [1, 6, 14], others advocate nonoperative management of pancreatic injuries in children [15, 18, 28, 29] with or without administration of octreotide [1, 8]. However, the usefulness of somatostatin treatment remains controversial [29].

The nonoperative failure rate in children suffering from pancreatic injuries is as high as 26% [1]. Furthermore, 35% to 40% of children with grade 2 or grade 3 injuries develop pancreatic pseudocysts [1, 7, 8, 30], but 50% of pseudocysts regress spontaneously [5]. Persisting pseudocysts were drained percutaneously under ultrasonographic or CT-assisted guidance [29], or were drained after maturation into the stomach under endoscopic guidance [30] or surgically by creating a cyst-gastrostomy or cyst-jejunostomy using a Roux-en-Y loop [5, 30]. Lin et al. suggested treating post-traumatic pseudocysts with grade 1 to grade 3 pancreatic injuries with percutaneous drainage, and grade 4 injuries with endoscopic stent placement [16]. In children, more than 70% of pancreatic pseudocysts can be managed nonoperatively, regardless of the diameter of the pseudocyst [31]. However, the number of days to full oral feeding in children suffering from pseudocysts is 30 days [31].

In a multicenter review, the LOS for children with grade 2 and grade 3 pancreatic injuries who underwent surgery was comparable to that for children who were managed nonoperatively [5]. In high-grade pancreatic injuries (grade 3 and grade 4), nonoperative management was associated with more days on total parenteral nutrition, and more complications than in children managed operatively [18, 32].

Both the median LOS (13 days) after early resection for complete main duct transection and median LOS for nonoperative treatment (17 days) reported by Wood et al. [6] are slightly shorter than our total LOS (14 days and 21 days). However, the postoperative LOS after endoscopic stent insertion in our patients amounted to 2 and 7 days, which is shorter than the postoperative LOS reported by Wood et al. [6].

De Blaauw et al. argue that nonoperative management of pancreatic injuries in children has a good outcome, despite the mean duration of treatment of 24 days [8]. They also state that there is little to gain with ERP and stenting [8].

Regardless of the type of nonsurgical treatment, some children will suffer atrophy of the distal part of the pancreas [18]. This usually does not result in diabetes or exocrine insufficiency of the pancreas in the majority of children [18], a fact that is well known from the follow-up of children who underwent partial pancreatic resection [33, 34].

Conclusion

Endoscopic management of pancreatic major duct injuries represents a minimally invasive option to treat these severe injuries. However, prospective multicenter studies are necessary to confirm the efficiency and safety of this endoscopic treatment strategy in children.

References

[1] Mattix KD, Tataria M, Holmes J, Kristoffersen K, Brown R, Groner J, Scaife E, Mooney D, Nance M, Scherer L. Pediatric pancreatic trauma: predictors of nonoperative management failure and associated outcomes. *J Pediatr Surg.* 2007 Feb;42(2):340-4.

[2] Meier DE, Coln CD, Hicks BA, Guzzetta PC. Early operation in children with pancreas transection. *J Pediatr Surg.* 2001 Feb;36(2):341-4.

[3] Jobst MA, Canty TG Sr, Lynch FP. Management of pancreatic injury in pediatric blunt abdominal trauma. *J Pediatr Surg.* 1999 May;34(5):818-23; discussion 823-4.

[4] Houben CH, Ade-Ajayi N, Patel S, Kane P, Karani J, Devlin J, Harrison P, Davenport M. Traumatic pancreatic duct injury in children: minimally invasive approach to management. *J Pediatr Surg.* 2007 Apr;42(4):629-35.

[5] Paul MD, Mooney DP. The management of pancreatic injuries in children: operate or observe. *J Pediatr Surg*. 2011 Jun;46(6):1140-3.

[6] Wood JH, Partrick DA, Bruny JL, Sauaia A, Moulton SL. Operative vs nonoperative management of blunt pancreatic trauma in children. *J Pediatr Surg*. 2010 Feb;45(2):401-6.

[7] Abbo O, Lemandat A, Reina N, Bouali O, Ballouhey Q, Carfagna L, Lemasson F, Harper L, Sauvat F, Galinier P. Conservative management of blunt pancreatic trauma in children: a single center experience. *Eur J Pediatr Surg*. 2013;23:470-3.

[8] de Blaauw I, Winkelhorst JT, Rieu PN, van der Staak FH, Wijnen MH, Severijnen RS, van Vugt AB, Wijnen RM. Pancreatic injury in children: good outcome of nonoperative treatment. *J Pediatr Surg*. 2008 Sep;43(9):1640-3.

[9] Moore EE, Cogbill TH, Malangoni MA et al. Organ injury scaling, II: Pancreas, duodenum, small bowel, colon and rectum. *J Trauma* 1990; 30:1427-9.

[10] Paris C, Bejjani J, Beaunoyer M, Ouimet A. Endoscopic retrograde cholangiopancreatography is useful and safe in children. *J Pediatr Surg*. 2010 May;45(5):938-42.

[11] Cay A, Imamoglu M, Bektas O, Ozdemir O, Arslan M, Sarihan H. Nonoperative treatment of traumatic pancreatic duct disruption in children with an endoscopically placed stent. *J Pediatr Surg*.2005 Dec;40(12):e9-12.

[12] Canty TG Sr, Weinman D. Treatment of pancreatic duct disruption in children by an endoscopically placed stent. *J Pediatr Surg*. 2001 Feb;36(2):345-8.

[13] Hall RI, Lavelle MI, Venables CW. Use of ERCP to identify the site of traumatic injuries of the main pancreatic duct in children. *Br J Surg*. 1986 May;73(5):411-2.

[14] Smith SD, Nakayama DK, Gantt N, Lloyd D, Rowe MI. Pancreatic injuries in childhood due to blunt trauma. *J Pediatr Surg*.1988 Jul;23(7):610-4.

[15] Keller MS, Stafford PW, Vane DW. Conservative management of pancreatic trauma in children. *J Trauma*. 1997 Jun;42(6):1097-100.

[16] Lin BC, Liu NJ, Fang JF, Kao YC. Long-term results of endoscopic stent in the management of blunt major pancreatic duct injury. *Surg Endosc*. 2006 Oct;20(10):1551-5.

[17] Haugaard MV, Wettergren A, Hillingsø JG, Gluud C, Penninga L. Non-operative versus operative treatment for blunt pancreatic trauma in children. *Cochrane Database Syst Rev.* 2014 Feb 12;2:CD009746.

[18] Wales PW, Shuckett B, Kim PC. Long-term outcome after nonoperative management of complete traumatic pancreatic transection in children. *J Pediatr Surg.* 2001 May;36(5):823-7.

[19] Bosboom D, Braam AW, Blickman JG, Wijnen RM. The role of imaging studies in pancreatic injury due to blunt abdominal trauma in children. *Eur J Radiol.* 2006 Jul;59(1):3-7.

[20] Rescorla FJ, Plumley DA, Sherman S, Scherer LR 3rd, West KW, Grosfeld JL. The efficacy of early ERCP in pediatric pancreatic trauma. *J Pediatr Surg.* 1995 Feb;30(2):336-40.

[21] Chandler C, Waxman K. Demonstration of pancreatic ductal integrity by endoscopic retrograde pancreatography allows conservative surgical management. *J Trauma.* 1996 Mar;40(3):466-8.

[22] Bhasin DK, Rana SS, Rawal P. Endoscopic retrograde pancreatography in pancreatic trauma: need to break the mental barrier. *J Gastroenterol Hepatol.* 2009 May;24(5):720-8.

[23] Soto JA, Alvarez O, Múnera F, Yepes NL, Sepúlveda ME, Pérez JM. Traumatic disruption of the pancreatic duct: diagnosis with MR pancreatography. *AJR Am J Roentgenol.* 2001 Jan;176(1):175-8.

[24] Gillams AR, Kurzawinski T, Lees WR. Diagnosis of duct disruption and assessment of pancreatic leak with dynamic secretin-stimulated MR cholangiopancreatography. *AJR Am J Roentgenol.* 2006 Feb;186(2): 499-506.

[25] Vegting IL, Tabbers MM, Taminiau JA, Aronson DC, Benninga MA, Rauws EA. Is endoscopic retrograde cholangiopancreatography valuable and safe in children of all ages? *J Pediatr Gastroenterol Nutr.* 2009 Jan;48(1):66-71.

[26] Hsu RK, Draganov P, Leung JW, Tarnasky PR, Yu AS, Hawes RH, Cunningham JT, Cotton PB. Therapeutic ERCP in the management of pancreatitis in children. *Gastrointest Endosc.* 2000 Apr;51(4 Pt 1):396-400.

[27] Kawahara I, Maeda K, Ono S, Kawashima H, Deie R, Yanagisawa S, Baba K, Usui Y, Tsuji Y, Fukuta A, Sekine S. Surgical reconstruction and endoscopic pancreatic stent for traumatic pancreatic duct disruption. *Pediatr Surg Int.* 2014 Sep;30(9):951-6.

[28] Kertai MA, Boehner C, Maiss J, Huemmer HP, Reingruber B. Nonoperative management of the child with severe pancreatic and splenic injury: should this become our preferred approach? *J Trauma.* 2010 Feb;68(2):E44-8.

[29] Shilyansky J, Sena LM, Kreller M, Chait P, Babyn PS, Filler RM, Pearl RH. Nonoperative management of pancreatic injuries in children. *J Pediatr Surg.* 1998 Feb;33(2):343-9.

[30] Sharma SS, Maharshi S. Endoscopic management of pancreatic pseudocyst in children –a long-term follow-up. *J Pediatr Surg.* 2008 Sep;43(9):1636-9.

[31] Russell KW, Barnhart DC, Madden J, Leeflang E, Jackson WD, Feola GP, Meyers RL, Scaife ER, Rollins MD. Non-operative treatment versus percutaneous drainage of pancreatic pseudocysts in children. *Pediatr Surg Int.* 2013 Mar;29(3):305-10.

[32] Beres AL, Wales PW, Christison-Lagay ER, McClure ME, Fallat ME, Brindle ME. Non-operative management of high-grade pancreatic trauma: is it worth the wait? *J Pediatr Surg.* 2013 May;48(5):1060-4.

[33] Lovvorn HN 3rd, Nance ML, Ferry RJ Jr, Stolte L, Baker L, O'Neill JA Jr, Schnaufer L, Stanley CA, Adzick NS. Congenital hyperinsulinism and the surgeon: lessons learned over 35 years. *J Pediatr Surg.* 1999 May;34(5):786-92; discussion 792-3.

[34] Al-Shanafey S, HabibZ, Al-Nassar S. Laparoscopic pancreatectomy for persistent hyperinsulinemic hypoglycemia of infancy. *J Pediatr Surg.* 2009 Jan;44(1):134-8; discussion 138.

Index

#

A

B

G

H

I

J

K

L

M

Q

R

S

T

NATURAL DISASTER RESEARCH, PREDICTION AND MITIGATION

NATURAL CATASTROPHES

RISK FINANCING AND INSURANCE ISSUES

NATURAL DISASTER RESEARCH, PREDICTION AND MITIGATION

Additional books in this series can be found on Nova's website under the Series tab.

Additional E-books in this series can be found on Nova's website under the E-book tab.

NATURAL DISASTER RESEARCH, PREDICTION AND MITIGATION

NATURAL CATASTROPHES

RISK FINANCING AND INSURANCE ISSUES

OLIVER H. ROHDE
EDITOR

nova publishers
New York

For permission to use material from this book please contact us:
Telephone 631-231-7269; Fax 631-231-8175
Web Site: http://www.novapublishers.com

Library of Congress Cataloging-in-Publication Data

ISBN: 978-1-62948-449-5

Published by Nova Science Publishers, Inc. † New York

CONTENTS

PREFACE

The four major types of natural environmental hazards that can result in property damages or lost lives are (1) geophysical events, such as earthquakes, tsunamis, and volcanic eruptions; (2) meteorological events, such as hurricanes and tropical storms, typically generated in the Caribbean Sea and Atlantic Ocean; (3) hydrological events, such as floods; and (4) climatological events, such as extreme temperature, drought, and wildfires. Economic losses (both insured and uninsured) from natural environmental hazards, especially from meteorological and climatological events, have increased in recent decades and have occurred with large spatial and interannual variability. For example, 8 of the 10 most costly catastrophes in the United States have occurred since 2000, including Hurricane Katrina (2005), which caused more than $80 billion in economic losses (both insured and uninsured) to private property and infrastructure and, more recently, Hurricane Sandy (2012), which caused more than $65 billion in economic losses. Most observers agree that it is highly likely that the United States will continue to experience increasing losses from natural catastrophes and that those losses will place increasing fiscal pressure on federal, state, and local governments as well as private risk transfer markets, which are currently responsible for a sizable share of the total cost of financing recovery and reconstruction. This book examines the rising cost of financing the recovery and reconstruction following natural disasters; reports of the nation's increasing vulnerability (and resilience) to coastal hazards; questions concerning the capacity of state and local government officials and private insurers to deal with the rising costs; and disagreements concerning the appropriate role for the federal government in dealing with these costs which have all become major topics of congressional debate.

Chapter 1 - The federal government has an established institutional framework for disaster preparedness, reduction, prevention, and response—mainly disaster assistance. However, concerns have been expressed about the nation's increasing exposure and vulnerability to natural hazards. The rising cost of financing recovery and reconstruction following natural disasters, reports of the nation's increasing vulnerability to coastal hazards, questions concerning the capacity of state and local governments and private insurers to deal with the rising costs, and disagreements concerning the appropriate role of the federal government in dealing with these costs have all become major topics of congressional debate.

The financial consequences of catastrophic natural disasters, such as Hurricanes Katrina (2005) and Sandy (2012), are largely a result of increasing population growth and the rising concentration of property assets in vulnerable disaster-prone areas. According to the National Oceanic and Atmospheric Administration (NOAA), Hurricane Katrina caused more than $80 billion in economic losses (both insured and uninsured) to private property and infrastructure and, more recently, Hurricane Sandy caused more than $65 billion in economic losses. New York and New Jersey—two of the nation's most populous states—were especially affected by Hurricane Sandy-induced storm surge and coastal flooding. Sandy also triggered a sustained and heightened policy interest in the potential effects of climate change and population growth on the National Flood Insurance Program (NFIP), the feasibility of innovative public-private sector catastrophe risk management and financing initiatives, and consideration of cost-effective and practical adaptation strategies to make society more financially resilient.

In the wake of Hurricane Sandy, a key policy question for Congress is whether the federal government should intervene in U.S. risk transfer markets to ensure the continued availability and affordability of homeowners' insurance for all residents. Advocates of federal intervention in property catastrophe insurance markets argue that an inevitable mega-catastrophe event will exceed the financial capacity of private insurers and reinsurers, as well as state insurance programs. Thus, they argue, the federal government should consider establishing a national catastrophe risk-financing program to transfer diversified pools of risk to the capital markets to help states achieve better terms with regard to the cost of insurance protection.

In essence, advocates argue that state residual property insurance pools would benefit from global diversification by transferring government's catastrophe risk to capital market partners through catastrophe swap or directly to capital market investors through (catastrophe) bond issuance, or the purchase options on their exposure to extreme weather events (weather hedge). These options would presumably reduce pressure on public budgets and help improve insurers' access to capital to ensure adequate capacity and solvency of the insurance industry to meet consumer needs.

Opponents of federal intervention argue that the insurance and reinsurance industry—with access to existing innovation for risk-financing transactions—has withstood unprecedented recent extreme natural disaster events with minimal disruption.

As will be discussed, several catastrophic risk-financing legislative options are before the 113th Congress. For example, H.R. 737, the Homeowners' Defense Act of 2013, would establish a National Catastrophe Risk Consortium to facilitate multistate pooling of catastrophe exposures (covering a variety of event probabilities and types) and transferring such risk through catastrophe-linked securities and insurance derivatives directly to investors in the capital markets.

H.R. 240, the Homeowners Insurance Protection Act of 2013, would create the National Commission on Catastrophe Preparation and Protection to provide for reinsurance of state disaster insurance programs. Under this proposal, the Treasury would auction excess-of-loss reinsurance contracts to public and private catastrophe risk-bearers, insurers, and state funds to improve the availability and affordability of coverage for homes. H.R. 549, the Homeowner Catastrophe Protection Act of 2013, would amend the Internal Revenue Code to allow insurers to establish pre-tax reserves by creating disaster protection funds for claims arising from future catastrophic events. Income allocated to the catastrophe reserves would be taxable as income only when withdrawn for the payment of losses.

Chapter 2 - On August 23, 2011, a rare, powerful magnitude 5.8 earthquake and aftershocks hit Mineral, VA, shutting down two North Anna Power Plants located about 7 miles from the earthquake's epicenter. The earthquake was felt from Georgia to southeast Canada. Other earthquakes have also occurred in the area, as well as in surrounding areas. For example, on July 16, 2010, a 3.6 magnitude earthquake occurred in Gaithersburg, MD, about 110 miles from the epicenter. Seismologists report that although Virginia is classified as a "moderate" seismic risk zone, since 1977, the state has experienced 160 earthquakes, of which just 16% were felt. According to the U.S. Geological Survey (USGS), this earthquake was the strongest earthquake to hit the entire states since the 5.8 magnitude tremor in 1897.

Separately, on March 11, 2011, a massive 9.0 magnitude earthquake struck off the coast of Honshu, Japan. It was the most severe and likely the costliest earthquake to hit Japan in the 130 years of recorded history. The Japan earthquake and tsunami caused more than 10,000 casualties, widespread property and infrastructure damage, blackouts, fire, and nuclear meltdowns. The nuclear crisis has compounded the challenges faced by a nation struggling to clean up and recover from the earthquake and tsunami. Two weeks later, the disaster triggered a crisis at the nuclear power facility; Japan's government said there was a leaking reactor core at the Fukushima Dai- ichi nuclear reactor complex, releasing radioactive contamination into the atmosphere and groundwater.

In the aftermath of the recent East Coast earthquake (and shut down of the North Anna nuclear power plants) and Japan's technological and natural disaster, U.S. policymakers are asking if it could happen here and, if so, how associated costs would be financed. In the event of a major natural disaster, several catastrophe risk financing and insurance issues could arise, including (1) the need to revisit the nature, extent, and timing of potential earthquake and tsunami hazards in the United States; (2) the adequacy of nuclear third-party liability insurance capacity; and (3) the challenges of financing recovery from natural disasters and making earthquake insurance more affordable. The latter challenge is largely a function of the national financial markets' capacity to absorb the cost and economic burden of a devastating mega-earthquake.

Given the economic devastation in Japan, there is heightened congressional interest in finding ways to reduce disaster risk for homeowners, insurance companies, financial firms, and both federal and state governments. This report examines earthquake catastrophe risk and insurance in the United States in light of recent developments. It examines both traditional and non-traditional approaches for financing recovery from earthquake losses as well as challenges in financing catastrophe losses with insurance. The report also explores the feasibility of a federal residential earthquake insurance mechanism and assesses policy implications of such a program. Finally, the report examines legislation introduced in the 112th Congress that addresses issues related to earthquakes, including S. 637, the Earthquake Insurance Affordability Act. S. 637 would authorize the U.S. Treasury to guarantee up to $5 billion in bonds available to certified public entities, like the California Earthquake Authority (CEA), following a catastrophic seismic event. The entity would have to exhaust its claims-paying ability before the federal guarantee becomes available. The measure is designed to reduce earthquake insurance rates by reducing the need to purchase reinsurance. The bonds would be repaid with premiums.

This report examines catastrophic earthquake risk and insurance issues facing the United States in light of the recent devastating Japan earthquake and tsunami. It examines both traditional and non-traditional approaches for financing recovery from earthquake losses as well as challenges in financing catastrophe losses with insurance. Much of earthquake disaster and nuclear-accident liability is currently borne by taxpayers. This report explores the feasibility of a federal residential earthquake insurance mechanism and concludes with policy implications of such a program.

Chapter 3 - In late October 2012, Hurricane Sandy caused widespread flood-related property damage in coastal areas of states throughout the Northeast and the mid-Atlantic region. The storm exposed vulnerabilities in the region's public transportation and infrastructure and underscored the nation's growing exposure to extreme weather events, sea-level rise, and coastal flooding. Although the full economic cost of Sandy will not be known for years, the storm has resulted in substantial federal disaster recovery assistance, including tens of billions for flood and hurricane protection and coastal restoration, and the rebuilding of mass transit systems and housing.

Government payouts under the National Flood Insurance Program (NFIP) are estimated to be between $12 billion and $15 billion in flood insurance claims. In the immediate aftermath of Sandy, this amount quickly exceeded the $4 billion in cash and remaining borrowing authority from the Treasury Department. By January 2013, the NFIP had processed more than 140,000 claims for Sandy-related damages totaling about $1.7 billion. To protect the financial integrity of the NFIP and ensure that the NFIP has the financial resources to cover its existing commitments following the devastation caused by Sandy, the Obama Administration requested that Congress pass legislation to increase the NFIP's borrowing authority. On January 4, 2013, Congress passed, and the President two days later signed into law, H.R. 41 to provide a $9.7 billion increase in the NFIP's borrowing authority, from $20.725 billion to $30.425 billion, to pay flood claims related to Hurricane Sandy.

Policymakers have expressed views on several flood management challenges facing the NFIP. These challenges include finding ways to (1) improve the accuracy of flood risk assessment and mapping of hurricane and coastal storm hazard areas; (2) strengthen the financial sustainability of the NFIP in the face of expected future extreme weather events (climate change), sea-level rise, and coastal flooding; (3) address potential affordability challenges associated with mandatory purchase requirements and implementation of full actuarial premium rates, beginning in 2014; (4) reduce the likelihood of future emergency supplemental spending to finance recurring recovery expenditures by making communities stronger and more resilient; (5) address uncertainty surrounding human settlement patterns and the NFIP's ability to contain the nation's growing exposure to floods; and (6) explore the creation of effective hazard-reduction strategies—linked to land use planning techniques (and construction standards)—to direct development and people out of, and away from, flood-prone areas.

Early in 2012, Congress passed and President Barack Obama signed into law the Biggert-Waters Flood Insurance Reform Act of 2012, P.L. 112-141. The law reauthorized the NFIP through September 30, 2017, and made a number of reforms to strengthen the future financial solvency and administrative efficiency of the NFIP. In the wake of Sandy, Congress might choose to consider policy options to achieve greater sustainability and cost savings by addressing long-term flood management challenges. Options include the use of flood policies (10-20 years, rather than 1 year), privatization of flood risk, issuance of community based flood insurance contracts, and regulatory and tax changes to encourage financial innovation in financing recovery from large- scale natural disasters.

This report provides an analysis of flood risk management, summarizes major challenges facing the NFIP, and outlines key reforms enacted in the Flood Insurance Reform Act of 2012. The report identifies and presents some key remaining flood management issues for congressional consideration, and concludes with a discussion of policy options for the future financial management of flood hazards in the United States.

On October 29, 2012, Hurricane Sandy hit the East Coast, flooding some coastal areas and causing massive economic disruptions in states throughout the Northeast and the mid-Atlantic region. Communities in New York, New Jersey, and Connecticut were particularly hard hit. In the wake of disaster recovery from Hurricane Sandy, policymaker attention has refocused on the effectiveness of the existing unified national program for floodplain management in reducing the loss of life and property from weather-related coastal hazards (hurricanes, storm surges, and tornadoes), aging coastal protection infrastructure and increasing vulnerability to storm impacts, persistently low insurance participation in the National Flood Insurance Program (NFIP), and the escalating cost of flooding to taxpayers.

Despite billions spent on preparedness and structural and non-structural mitigation measures to reduce disaster-related losses, the nation faces growing exposure to flood-related losses. Some argue that storms of Sandy's strength and intensity will occur more frequently, resulting in increasing incidents of major flooding and damage. This situation raises at least five policy concerns and questions. First, is federal flood insurance that complements land use management still a workable method of managing flood risk, reducing the costs and human suffering from floods, and distributing burdens equitably among those protected by flood insurance and the general public? Second, is flood risk possible for private insurers to underwrite? Third, could flood risk be effectively transferred to the private sector through reinsurance or to capital markets through catastrophe bonds? Fourth, should the NFIP debt to the Treasury be forgiven? Fifth, are the consequences of flood risks and the level of protection offered by hurricane protection systems communicated effectively to the public? These are some of the issues of contention that remain after recently passed NFIP-reform legislation in Congress.

This report provides an analysis of U.S. flood risk management policy, summarizes major challenges facing the NFIP, and outlines key insurance reform provisions in the Biggert-Waters Flood Insurance Reform Act of 2012 (Flood Insurance Reform Act of 2012). The report also identifies and presents some key remaining flood management issues of contention for congressional consideration, and it concludes with a discussion of policy options for the future financial management of flood hazard costs.

In: Natural Catastrophes
Editor: Oliver H. Rohde

ISBN: 978-1-62948-449-5

Chapter 1

FINANCING NATURAL CATASTROPHE EXPOSURE: ISSUES AND OPTIONS FOR IMPROVING RISK TRANSFER MARKETS*

Rawle O. King

SUMMARY

The federal government has an established institutional framework for disaster preparedness, reduction, prevention, and response—mainly disaster assistance. However, concerns have been expressed about the nation's increasing exposure and vulnerability to natural hazards. The rising cost of financing recovery and reconstruction following natural disasters, reports of the nation's increasing vulnerability to coastal hazards, questions concerning the capacity of state and local governments and private insurers to deal with the rising costs, and disagreements concerning the appropriate role of the federal government in dealing with these costs have all become major topics of congressional debate.

The financial consequences of catastrophic natural disasters, such as Hurricanes Katrina (2005) and Sandy (2012), are largely a result of increasing population growth and the rising concentration of property assets in vulnerable disaster-prone areas. According to the National Oceanic and Atmospheric

---

* This is an edited, reformatted and augmented version of the Congressional Research Service publication, CRS Report for Congress R43182, dated August 15, 2013.

Administration (NOAA), Hurricane Katrina caused more than $80 billion in economic losses (both insured and uninsured) to private property and infrastructure and, more recently, Hurricane Sandy caused more than $65 billion in economic losses. New York and New Jersey—two of the nation's most populous states—were especially affected by Hurricane Sandy-induced storm surge and coastal flooding. Sandy also triggered a sustained and heightened policy interest in the potential effects of climate change and population growth on the National Flood Insurance Program (NFIP), the feasibility of innovative public-private sector catastrophe risk management and financing initiatives, and consideration of cost-effective and practical adaptation strategies to make society more financially resilient.

In the wake of Hurricane Sandy, a key policy question for Congress is whether the federal government should intervene in U.S. risk transfer markets to ensure the continued availability and affordability of homeowners' insurance for all residents. Advocates of federal intervention in property catastrophe insurance markets argue that an inevitable mega-catastrophe event will exceed the financial capacity of private insurers and reinsurers, as well as state insurance programs. Thus, they argue, the federal government should consider establishing a national catastrophe risk-financing program to transfer diversified pools of risk to the capital markets to help states achieve better terms with regard to the cost of insurance protection.

In essence, advocates argue that state residual property insurance pools would benefit from global diversification by transferring government's catastrophe risk to capital market partners through catastrophe swap or directly to capital market investors through (catastrophe) bond issuance, or the purchase options on their exposure to extreme weather events (weather hedge). These options would presumably reduce pressure on public budgets and help improve insurers' access to capital to ensure adequate capacity and solvency of the insurance industry to meet consumer needs.

Opponents of federal intervention argue that the insurance and reinsurance industry—with access to existing innovation for risk-financing transactions—has withstood unprecedented recent extreme natural disaster events with minimal disruption.

As will be discussed, several catastrophic risk-financing legislative options are before the 113th Congress. For example, H.R. 737, the Homeowners' Defense Act of 2013, would establish a National Catastrophe Risk Consortium to facilitate multistate pooling of catastrophe exposures (covering a variety of event probabilities and types) and transferring such risk through catastrophe-linked securities and insurance derivatives directly to investors in the capital markets.

H.R. 240, the Homeowners Insurance Protection Act of 2013, would create the National Commission on Catastrophe Preparation and Protection to provide for reinsurance of state disaster insurance programs. Under this proposal, the Treasury would auction excess-of-loss reinsurance contracts to public and private catastrophe risk-bearers, insurers, and state funds to improve the availability and affordability of coverage for homes. H.R. 549, the Homeowner Catastrophe Protection Act of 2013, would amend the Internal Revenue Code to allow insurers to establish pre-tax reserves by creating disaster protection funds for claims arising from future catastrophic events. Income allocated to the catastrophe reserves would be taxable as income only when withdrawn for the payment of losses.

INTRODUCTION: DEFINING THE PROBLEM AND CURRENT CHALLENGES

The four major types of natural environmental hazards[1] that can result in property damages or lost lives are (1) *geophysical events*, such as earthquakes, tsunamis, and volcanic eruptions; (2) *meteorological events*, such as hurricanes and tropical storms, typically generated in the Caribbean Sea and Atlantic Ocean; (3) *hydrological events*, such as floods; and (4) *climatological events*, such as extreme temperature, drought, and wildfires.[2] Economic losses (both insured and uninsured) from natural environmental hazards, especially from meteorological and climatological events, have increased in recent decades and have occurred with large spatial and interannual variability. For example, 8 of the 10 most costly catastrophes[3] in the United States have occurred since 2000, including Hurricane Katrina (2005), which caused more than $80 billion in economic losses (both insured and uninsured) to private property and infrastructure and, more recently, Hurricane Sandy (2012), which caused more than $65 billion in economic losses.[4]

Most observers agree that it is highly likely that the United States will continue to experience increasing losses from natural catastrophes and that those losses will place increasing fiscal pressure on federal, state, and local governments as well as private risk transfer markets, which are currently responsible for a sizeable share of the total cost of financing recovery and reconstruction.

The rising cost of financing recovery and reconstruction following natural disasters, reports of the nation's increasing vulnerability (and resilience) to coastal hazards, questions concerning the capacity of state and local government officials and private insurers to deal with the rising costs, and disagreements concerning the appropriate role for the federal government in dealing with these costs have all become major topics of congressional debate.

The financial consequences of severe natural disasters, such as Hurricanes Katrina (2005) and Sandy (2012), are largely a result of increasing population growth and the rising concentration of property assets in vulnerable disaster-prone areas, such as coastal regions exposed to windstorms, river basins exposed to floods, and urban areas exposed to earthquakes. Climate change may also play a role. Moreover, the hazards posed by extreme weather-induced coastal hazards—namely sea level rise, storm surge, coastal flooding, and erosion—could prove challenging, not only for individuals and businesses, but also for affected state and local governments, especially given concerns about private insurers' ability and willingness to manage and finance low-probability, high-consequence events. For example, New York and New Jersey—two of the nation's most populous states—were especially affected by Hurricane Sandy-induced storm surge and coastal flooding. Sandy triggered a sustained and heightened policy interest in the potential effects of climate change and population growth in coastal areas for the National Flood Insurance Program (NFIP), the feasibility of innovative public-private sector initiatives for managing and financing catastrophic risks, and consideration of cost-effective and practical adaptation strategies to make society more resilient to damages from natural environmental hazards.[5]

This report opens with an examination of the current role of private insurers in managing disaster risk and their capacity and willingness to deal with the rising cost of financing recovery and reconstruction following natural disasters. This discussion focuses on the traditional mechanisms insurers use to hedge risk (e.g., reinsurance and retrocession) by arranging for the right to receive some level of reimbursement or indemnification when losses actually occur.

The report then examines the current role of federal, state, and local governments in managing disaster risk and dealing with the rising cost of financing recovery and reconstruction following natural disasters. This discussion focuses on the federal disaster recovery framework, which includes policies concerning disaster relief, insurance, and mitigation.

The report also examines various alternative risk (ART) financing options in light of the current level of uncertainty concerning the probability of catastrophic losses and the increased exposure and vulnerability of coastal areas to natural disaster damages. Some of these risk-financing options include state-sponsored loss-sharing financing mechanisms and private ART methods, such as insurance-linked securities (e.g., catastrophic bonds and contingent capital securities).

The report concludes with an examination of the rationale for and against government intervention in risk transfer markets and other legislative options currently under congressional consideration. For example, H.R. 737, the Homeowners' Defense Act of 2013, would establish a National Catastrophe Risk Consortium to facilitate both multistate pooling of catastrophic risks (covering a variety of event probabilities and types) and natural disaster-linked securitization, thereby strengthening the financial capacity of these programs. H.R. 240, the Homeowners Insurance Protection Act of 2013, would create the National Commission on Catastrophe Preparation and Protection with the authority to establish a federal reinsurance program to make reinsurance coverage available to eligible state natural catastrophe insurance programs to improve the availability and affordability of coverage for homes and the solvency and capacity of homeowners' insurance markets. H.R. 549, the Homeowner Catastrophe Protection Act of 2013, would allow insurers to make tax-deductible contributions to a tax-exempt policyholder disaster protection fund established for the payment of policyholders' claims arising from certain catastrophic events.

Advocates of federal intervention in catastrophe insurance markets argue that an inevitable mega- catastrophe event will exceed the financial capacity of private insurers and reinsurers, as well as state insurance programs. Thus, they argue, the federal government should consider proposals for improving insurers' access to capital in the reinsurance, banking, and securities markets to ensure adequate capacity and solvency of the industry to meet consumer needs. Opponents of federal intervention, on the other hand, argue that the insurance industry has withstood unprecedented recent natural disaster events with minimal disruption and insurers have the financial engineering tools and instruments to transfer insurance risk to investors in capital markets.

The Role of Private Insurers

There is general agreement that disaster risk and uncertainties must be cost-effectively managed and financed to ensure economic growth and maximize social welfare. People and organizations typically purchase an ordinary insurance policy, the most common risk management technique, to reduce uncertainty and worry from their inability to predict individual future outcomes. The insured pays a fee in exchange for the insurer's promise to pay a certain sum of money provided a stipulated event occurs. The insurer is able to offer protection against financial loss by pooling the risks from a large group of independent and identically distributed risks. In many cases, however, the risks to different individuals are not independent. For example, in a major hurricane, earthquake, or flood, many people may suffer at the same time. Economists refer to this situation as correlated losses. Insurers spread such risks not only across individuals (geographically or spatially) but also across time (intertemporal) through reinsurance contracts placed with separately capitalized reinsurers or loss reserves (surplus) built up in good years to offset unusually high losses in catastrophic loss years.

An understanding of the role of private insurers in the economy must begin, therefore, with the concepts of *risk* (or the variation in possible outcomes of a situation) and *uncertainty*, which is one of the decisive determinants of individual behavior. Economists observe that the goal of individuals is to maximize expected utility, and this has meant mitigating uncertainty with the purchase of an insurance policy.

Under a typical insurance transaction, individuals transfer risk to an independent pool and, via the law of large numbers,[6] insurers convert risky contracts into almost sure things. This pooling process permits the systematic accumulation of funds that provide for payment of losses in accordance with the terms of the ordinary insurance contract. Individuals in the group pay a specific premium rate instead of risking the uncertainty of a (potentially large) loss. The premium rate is equal to the actuarial value of the loss plus an amount to compensate the insurer for assuming the risk.

Economists observe that when risk transfer occurs in an uncertain environment, two basic problems arise: *moral hazard*[7] and *adverse selection*.[8] Both are founded on imperfect information. Moral hazards in insurance, for example, occur because the insurer does not have costless access to information possessed by the insured and therefore does not know whether the loss is caused by the insured's carelessness or by chance. The insurer typically will reduce moral hazard by requiring the insured to bear some of the costs of the contingency, for example, by requiring a deductible. Insurers have addressed the adverse selection problem with proper risk identification and assessment, risk segmentation, risk-based premiums, and effective underwriting.

The traditional insurance mechanism is not sufficient for diversifying the risk of loss arising from large-scale natural disasters—a problem that became increasingly apparent to policymakers following Hurricane Hugo (1989), Hurricane Andrew (1992), and the Northridge earthquake (1994). The problem is that catastrophic natural disaster losses tend to be correlated, unpredictable, and costly when the events occur. Insurers traditionally protect themselves against catastrophic losses through reinsurance agreements with separately capitalized reinsurers. Reinsurers, like insurers, pool risk and diversify (spread) risk by writing many unrelated policies, and sometimes purchase reinsurance themselves, called "retrocession," or enter into reciprocal loss-sharing agreements with other reinsurers to manage their risk portfolios.

Given the relatively small capital and surplus of the reinsurance industry—compared with probable maximum losses from a potential mega-catastrophic event—insurers recognized during the 1990s that the global reinsurance industry might not have been capable of funding large-scale catastrophic losses in the United States. Concerns expressed by policymakers ranged from the adequacy of insurance capital to the liquidity and transparency in the U.S. risk transfer market. By the mid-1990s, insurers and reinsurers began issuing insurance-linked securities, namely catastrophe bonds, to augment underwriting capacity and effectively hedge against potential catastrophic losses.

During the 1990s and 2000s, Congress held relatively frequent oversight and investigation hearings into the competitive nature and solvency of the insurance industry and possible causes for market dislocation, especially pertaining to the availability and affordability of property insurance (and reinsurance) in high-risk areas following a major catastrophic event. More recently, Congress has held relatively few hearings on the subject, perhaps because of the increased use and availability of competitively priced (property) catastrophe bond issuance (i.e., insurance linked securities) that complement traditional catastrophe reinsurance. The main factor contributing to these relatively recent developments—with implications for reinsurance pricing, availability, and structure—is sustained capital growth in 2012 and 2013, and downward pressure on rates in the traditional reinsurance market to remain competitive, driven by an influx of capacity from alternative or "convergence" capital sources.[9] As will be discussed later, institutional asset managers (primarily pensions) and sophisticated institutional investors (e.g., endowments and multi-strategy hedge funds) have increasingly shown an interest in accessing catastrophe risk on a liquid basis and stable, modest returns on investments that are non-correlated to the balance of their portfolios.[10] The result is that—for the first time—insurance linked securities (ILS) pricing is delivering a more cost effective risk transfer solution than traditional (reinsurance) vehicles.

Separately, a new potential catastrophic risk financing challenge appears to be emerging. Even if there is a sufficiently large and growing catastrophe risk transfer market—as most observers would argue appears to be the case—property insurers exposed to hurricane-driven, storm-surge damage to residential property risk along the Atlantic and Gulf coasts might still choose to restrict supply in favor of other, potentially more profitable, investments.[11]

In summary, with respect to the role of private insurers in financing natural catastrophic risks, Congress faces several policy issues and questions, including

1. **Uncertainty concerning the probability of catastrophic losses.** Uncertainty about how often catastrophic natural disasters occur (frequency), the geographic patterns, and the magnitude of these events (severity) poses a challenge to the financial management of catastrophic risk and a test of the effectiveness and reliability of existing prevention, protection, and compensation mechanisms in place. What is the scientific basis for assessing natural hazard risk? How well can the private sector and government predict natural disaster risks? How reliable and valid are current risk assessment models/methodologies and what are their implications for the pricing and availability of insurance and other risk spreading mechanisms?
2. **Reducing potential natural disaster losses.** A mega-catastrophic event striking a coastal region of the United States could impede interstate and foreign commerce and cause widespread economic hardship adversely affecting both the national and international economies. What is the current level of risk and its distribution between public and private sectors? What are the most cost effective ways to mitigate losses?
3. **Rethinking catastrophic risk management and financing strategies.** Is the present mix of private market and public policies the most efficient and equitable way of sharing risk? What is the potential for financial instruments to transfer risk, including insurance risk options/futures (e.g., weather derivatives), government-backed contracts, and state or regional insurance pools? Given the insurance risk transfer market's need for transparency and liquidity, what are the implications for regulation and federal intervention? Should Congress

allow insurers to establish pre-tax reserves by creating disaster protection funds for claims arising from future catastrophic events? Income allocated to the catastrophe reserves would be taxable as income only when withdrawn for the payment of losses.

THE U.S. EXPOSURE TO NATURAL CATASTROPHIC RISK

As stated earlier, the United States faces several types of natural catastrophic risk exposures that could result in lives lost and property and infrastructure damages. **Figure 1** shows private insured catastrophe property losses in the United States from 1989 to 2012.[12] Total losses are greater, sometimes more than two times greater, than insured losses.[13]

Table 1 shows the 10 costliest catastrophes—natural and technological—in the United States. Seven of the 10 most costly catastrophes were weather-related events affecting coastal states along the Gulf and Atlantic coast regions.

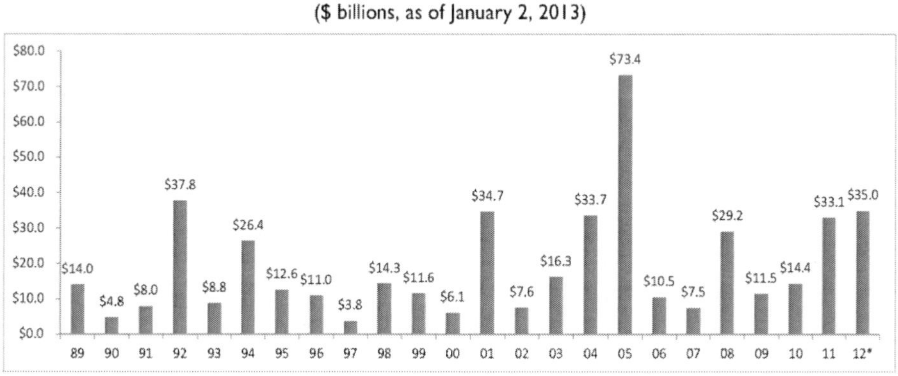

Source: Insurance Services Office's (ISO's) Property Claims Service and Insurance Information Institute

Note: 2001 figure includes $20.3 billion for 9/11 losses reported through December 31, 2001 ($25.9 billion in 2011 dollars). This figure includes only business and personal property claims, business interruption, and auto claims. Non-property/business insurance losses equal $12.2 billion ($15.6 billion in 2011 dollars). The $35.0 billion loss figure for 2012 includes $18.8 billion in gross loss estimate for Hurricane Sandy.

Figure 1. Total U.S. Catastrophe-Insured Property Losses, 1989-2012.

Table 1. Top 10 Most Costly Catastrophes in United States ($ in millions; as of January 18, 2013)

Rank	Date	Peril	Estimated Insured Property Losses	
			Dollars when Occurred	In 2012 Dollars
1	Aug. 2005	Hurricane Katrina	$41,100	$48,317
2	Sept. 2001	Fire, explosion: World Trade Center, Pentagon terrorist attacks	18,779	24,345
3	Oct. 2012	Hurricane Sandy	18,750	18,750
4	Aug. 1992	Hurricane Andrew	15,500	25,364
5	Jan. 1994	Northridge, CA, earthquake	12,500	19,365
6	Sept. 2008	Hurricane Ike	12,500	13,329
7	Oct. 2005	Hurricane Wilma	10,300	12,108
8	Aug. 2004	Hurricane Charley	7,475	9,085
9	Sept. 2004	Hurricane Ivan	7,110	8,641
10	Apr. 2011	Flooding, hail, and wind including the tornados that struck Tuscaloosa, AL, and other locations	7,300	7,451

Source: The Property Claim Services (PCS)—a unit of Insurance Services Office, a Verisk Analytics company.

Note: Does not include flood damage covered under the National Flood Insurance Program.

Recently, the series of weather-related events—Hurricanes Sandy and Isaac (2012), Irene (2011), Ike (2008), and Katrina and Rita (2005)—demonstrated the nation's vulnerability to coastal hazards. Sandy was the second-most costly natural disaster in U.S. history, behind Hurricane Katrina (2005) and close to Hurricane Andrew (1992). Sandy's torrential rainfall and flooding in 14 states in the Mid-Atlantic and Northeast, from North Carolina to Maine, caused significant property and infrastructure damages in the affected areas. Coastal areas of New York, New Jersey, and Connecticut were especially hard hit.

Types of Natural Disaster Losses

Table 2 and **Figure 2** show U.S. insured catastrophe property losses from 1992 through 2011 by type of natural hazard in table format and pie chart, respectively. According to the Insurance Services Office's Property Claims Service, an insurance industry group that collects data on catastrophes, the main types of natural catastrophes posing potential economic cost to the private insurance industry are hurricanes, tornadoes, earthquakes, and winter storms. Hurricanes and tornadoes resulted in 76% of all catastrophe losses. Wind and hail damage from hurricanes are also major contributors to insurance claim losses.

The rising cost of financing recovery and reconstruction following natural disasters is largely a result of increasing population growth and the rising concentration of property assets in vulnerable disaster-prone areas. For example, according to CoreLogic, a company that produces property information, analytics, and other services, more than 4.2 million homes along the U.S. Atlantic and Gulf coasts are located within storm-surge risk zones, totaling more than $1.1 trillion in property exposure.[14] CoreLogic indicated that, based on theoretical future rises in sea level, there has been a significant increase in both the total number of properties at risk of potential destruction associated with storm-surge flooding and the total value.[15]

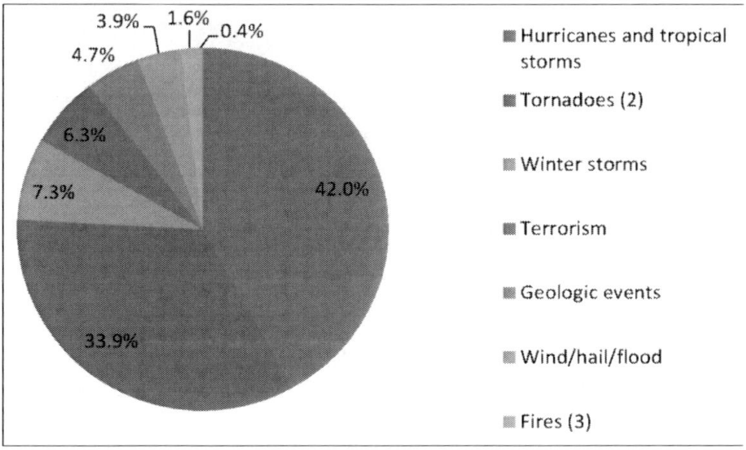

Source: ISO's Property Claim Services (PCS) and Insurance Information Institute.

Notes: Includes $18.8 billion gross loss estimate for Hurricane Sandy, as of January 2, 2013.

Figure 2. U.S. Catastrophe-Insured Losses by Cause of Loss, 1992-2011.

Table 2. Inflation-Adjusted U.S. Catastrophe-Insured Losses by Cause of Loss, 1992-2011

	Percentage	Losses ($ billions)
Hurricanes and tropical storms	42.0%	$161.3
Tornadoes	33.9	130.2
Winter storms	7.3	28.2
Terrorism	6.3	24.4
Geologic events	4.7	18.2
Wind/hail/flood	3.9	14.8
Fires	1.6	6.0
Other	0.4	1.4
Grand Total	100.0	384.5

Source: ISO's Property Claim Services (PCS) and Insurance Information Institute.

Notes: Adjusted for inflation through 2011 by ISO using the GDP implicit price deflator. Excludes catastrophes causing direct losses less than $25 million. Does not include flood damage covered by the federally administered National Flood Insurance Program. Includes losses from civil disorders, water damage, utility service disruptions, and any workers compensation catastrophes generating losses in excess of Property Claims Services threshold after adjusting for inflation.

Historically, floods were considered the most frequent and costly natural peril in the United States. In 1968, Congress established the National Flood Insurance Program (NFIP) to manage and finance the nation's flood risks at a time when the nation's flood hazards were largely associated with riverine (not coastal) flooding.[16] The NFIP is the second largest financial risk and liability of the federal government behind Social Security.[17]

Today, the costs associated with extreme weather and climatic events can overwhelm the NFIP. In short, from a cost perspective, the perils of coastal hazards now rival, and perhaps surpass, riverine flooding.[18]

Climate Change, Risk Management, and Adaptations

Most observers agree that climate change is a global phenomenon, with far-reaching economic, environmental, and fiscal implications for governments, risk management, and sustainability. A recent global-warming/climate-change study published by the United Nations World Meteorological Organization indicated that both land and ocean surface temperatures between 2001 and 2010 were the warmest since measurements began in 1850, and the global mean sea levels rose about twice as fast as the trend in the last century.[19] The analysis also suggested that greenhouse (carbon dioxide) gases are changing the climate such that the world is experiencing an extended period of accelerated global warming. Scientists report that global warming accelerated in the four decades of 1971 to 2010, and the decadal rate of increase from 1991 to 2000 and 2001 to 2010 was unprecedented.[20] Global warming, and its impact, has emerged as a pivotal, yet highly controversial issue in the disaster policy debate. Since the 1990s, and a series of increasingly costly natural disasters associated with extreme weather events, the potential impact of climate change on relevant natural hazards—hurricane-induced wind damage, coastal flooding, storm surge, thunderstorms/tornadoes, droughts, wildfires, and inland flooding due to both hurricanes and non-topical systems—has drawn increased attention from the public and U.S. policymakers. For instance, after Hurricane Sandy in 2012, there has been a growing awareness of the potential financial consequences of climate change and population growth in coastal shoreline counties (directly adjacent to the open ocean, major estuaries, and the Great Lakes) and U.S. coastal watershed counties (where the land area intersects coastal watersheds).

Unlike the effects of climate change on the erosion of beaches that are observable and easily measured, the broader impact of climate change on coastal hazards—that is, sea level rise, storm surge, and coastal flooding—and the U.S. economy is arguably less apparent and remains controversial. The issue is not whether climate change affects people and the environment. Instead, the policy challenge appears to be twofold. First, there is no consensus on an objective scientific basis for determining (and agreeing on) the magnitude and scope of the effects of global warming and climate variability/climate hazards on the U.S. economy. Second, there is no consensus concerning what to do about the adverse impact of global warming and climate adaptation (and resilience) in communities along vulnerable U.S. coastlines.

While the impact of global warming—especially the impact of climate-induced changes on natural disasters—remains controversial, a consensus seems be emerging around two major climate risk and disaster management strategies issues. *First*, there appears to be a growing consensus among policymakers in favor of enacting national climate adaptation and risk management strategies, such as retrofitting or raising existing structures and building dikes, levees, and pumping facilities, rather than requiring the abandonment of the present sites of climate hazards (coastal areas and waterfronts).[21] Opponents of the abandonment strategy argue that the coastal regions of the United States are economically vital to the nation's long-term economic growth.

Second, there is arguably a limited U.S. capacity for financing catastrophic risks. What has become clear in the post-Sandy rebuilding and recovery phase designed to produce a more sustainable coastline is that risk transfer and financing for public infrastructure, buildings, transportation systems, and communities against the impacts of climate change could involve significant costs to governments at all levels due to added storm protection needed from rising sea levels and protection from coastal erosion. Insuring increasingly vulnerable residential private property risks will likely require a substantial increase in risk transfer capacity that is currently beyond the existing property and casualty (P&C insurer) insurance industry's total claims paying capacity. Policymakers are currently examining the costs and benefits of comprehensive disaster risk management strategies that include possible private-public sector partnerships for producing new technologies, financial innovation in climate risk-assessment tools for determining damage potential, better planning in view of vulnerability (and recent storm histories), and catastrophe risk financing.

FINANCIAL MANAGEMENT OF CATASTROPHE LOSSES

The federal government has an established institutional framework for disaster preparedness, reduction, prevention, and response. Within this approach to disaster risk management, three programmatic elements stand out: disaster relief, insurance, and mitigation. Disaster relief assistance, for instance, meets the uninsured needs of disaster victims. The financial and technical resources provided through government relief are funded by annual and emergency supplemental congressional appropriations to the Disaster Relief Fund in the U.S. Treasury on behalf of (managed by) the Federal Emergency Management Agency (FEMA). Insurance is purchased by recipients in the private market or through state-sponsored, risk sharing programs. Mitigation consists of measures taken to prevent future losses, such as discouraging development in certain areas, or to reduce the losses that might otherwise occur.

Concerns about the financial burden of the rising response and recovery costs that may be anticipated from more severe future natural catastrophic events has led both Congress and the Obama Administration to explore alternative approaches to strengthen the nation's capacity to prepare for, respond to, and recover from natural catastrophic losses. Policymakers, for example, are rethinking existing U.S. preparedness policies and strategies for managing catastrophic disaster risks in the context of the *National Disaster Recovery Framework* designed to ensure a unified, collaborative, and effective recovery support to disaster-affected states, Tribes, Territorial and local jurisdictions. *The Presidential Policy Directive (PPD)-8* calls for FEMA to work with interagency partners to publish a recovery framework. This policy directive outlines specific steps to achieve the objective of "a shared understanding and a common, integrated perspective across all mission areas—Prevention, Protection, Mitigation, Response, and Recovery—in order to achieve unity of effort and make the most effective use of the nation's limited resources."[22]

Risk Mitigation and Risk Transfer

There are two main ways to reduce net economic losses from natural disasters: mitigating or reducing physical vulnerability to economic damage and managing the residual risk (financial vulnerability) with financial risk strategies, such as risk transfer instruments, securities, and federal disaster assistance.

Private insurance and federal disaster relief are complementary mechanisms to compensate disaster victims and provide for recovery after a natural disaster. Risk management theory, however, suggests at least three reasons why private insurance is more efficient than federal disaster relief for allocating the risk of large catastrophic losses:

- Federal tax and disaster relief assistance create negative incentives for risk mitigation (moral hazards) because the disaster victim's eligibility for compensation is not dependent on whether they have taken steps to reduce their exposure to loss. This inefficiency results in higher social and federal costs of disasters.
- From a welfare economics or resource allocation perspective, federal disaster relief is inequitable because taxpayers pay the costs of disasters regardless of their exposure to risk.
- Federal disaster relief is less efficient than private insurance and inclined to misjudgment because property owners oftentimes do not fully understand the risks they face, make risk management decisions

based on inaccurate information, and intentionally rely on disaster relief for compensation. Historically, insurance has been an efficient mechanism to deal with natural catastrophes; it establishes a price on the hazard, based on actuarial information, and creates economic incentives to mitigate losses.

The Limits of Insurability of Catastrophic Risks

The financial markets, which consist of the market for financial securities such as stocks, bonds, futures options, and insurance, allow the exchange of assets in the form of paper contracts and claims. They also allow the transfer and allocation of risk among different actors. Financial markets, however, are often "incomplete," which means they provide only a limited capacity to pool risk and shift or allocate that across individuals.

The unique characteristics of natural disasters represent a challenge to mitigating risk incident to economic activities (property damages), financing the remaining residual risk, and compensating disaster victims. The key policy question that emerges is whether catastrophe losses are insurable. Traditional insurance principles suggest that a risk is insurable if the insurance market is able to cover potential losses reliably—and profitably—at a premium rate that customers are willing to pay. The problem is that to cover catastrophic risk, insurers must (1) assemble a sufficient number of similarly insured objects to allow a reasonably close calculation of probable future losses; (2) estimate the probability of the risk events (timing, frequency, intensity); and (3) limit an exposure to simultaneous destruction (where many policyholders experience losses at the same time).

In the past, the solution to the catastrophic risk-financing problem has been for insurers to limit their overall catastrophic risk exposure to an acceptable level out of concerns about solvency and the cost of capital. Insurers accomplish this by means of (1) reinsurance, (2) pricing insurance rates using "catastrophe loads" to account for potential disaster-related losses,[23] and (3) alternative risk transfer instruments that allow insurers to transfer fully collateralized liabilities through insurance-linked securities (ILS) to the global capital markets. However, insurance securitization—ILS issuance and trading—lacks a clear, transparent, and tradable platform.

The Role of Traditional Reinsurance

Reinsurance is a form of insurance for insurance companies. Insurers usually hedge (or take offsetting risk positions) all or part of the risk assumed with the transfer ("cede") of that risk, along with the associated premiums, to a reinsurance company. Reinsurance companies, in turn, are free to purchase protection against catastrophe losses from other reinsurers ("retrocessionaire") and financial institutions.

Before discussing reinsurance transactions, four points are worthy of mentioning. First, reinsurance contracts are not standardized and the contractual terms and conditions can vary widely from line-to-line and from market-to-market. Second, primary insurers will transfer risk to a reinsurer for five basic reasons:

1. Stabilize underwriting results;
2. Provide protection against catastrophic losses;
3. Increase underwriting capacity or the limits of coverage an insurer can prudently assume based on its surplus and the nature of the business written;
4. Enable an insurer to write a greater number of policies by reducing the size of the company's liabilities; and
5. Provide a form of financing by increasing policyholder's surplus.

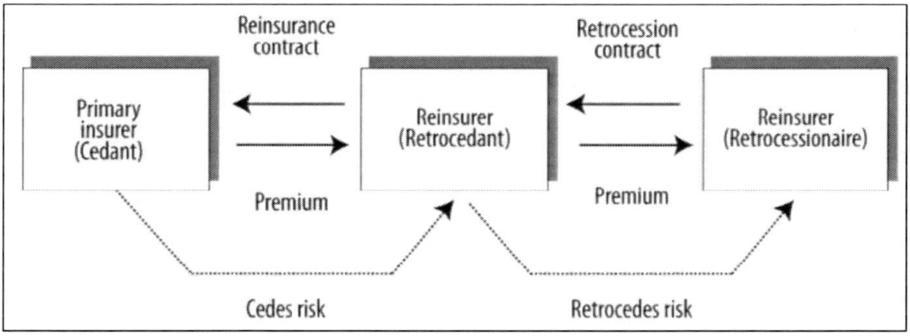

Source: CRS presentation.

Figure 3. Illustration of Reinsurance and Retrocessionaire Transaction.

Third, insurers typically purchase reinsurance from three sources: "professional" reinsurers, whose exclusive business is reinsurance; reinsurance departments of primary companies; and various organizations, such as reinsurance pools or syndicates, Lloyd's, and government-owned companies.

Fourth, the regulation of reinsurance transactions is limited. Regulation occurs in the state insurance regulator granting credit for reinsurance on the balance sheets of the primary or ceding insurer. However, professional reinsurers domiciled in the United States must meet statutory licensing requirements (e.g., solvency and annual statement filing) similar to those required of a primary insurer in the state in which it is applying for permission to do business.

Figure 3 illustrates the basic financial hedging strategy of insurers using a reinsurance contract. Under a typical reinsurance agreement, the primary or direct insurer (cedant) transfers to the reinsurer (retrocedant) a portion of the risk the primary insurer accepted in issuing insurance policies. The primary insurer agrees to pay the reinsurer a premium in exchange for the reinsurer's promise to indemnify the insurer, according to a specific formula. The expectation of indemnification (reinsurance "recoverables") from the reinsurer enables the primary insurer to plan for contingencies more effectively by limiting the liabilities they assume. This, in turn, allows the insurer to provide greater amounts of insurance coverage on a direct basis. The reinsurer, in turn, may transfer to another reinsurer (retrocessionaire) a portion of the risk they have taken on from the primary insurer.

Types of Reinsurance Agreements

There are two forms of reinsurance, which differ in the way primary insurers and reinsurers determine premiums and losses: proportional ("treaty") and non-proportional ("facultative"). Proportional reinsurance covers broad groups of policies. Proportional reinsurance arrangements cover all of a primary insurer's business or group of policies.

Proportional reinsurance agreements obligate the insurer and reinsurer to share losses and premiums in fixed proportions. The reinsurer retains the "faculty" or power to accept or reject all or part of any policy offered to it, and the insurer has the option to purchase reinsurance for a certain policy, and if so, when and from whom.

Non-proportional or "excess of loss" reinsurance agreements cover specific, individual risks. Under the arrangement, the ceding insurer is indemnified for the portion of a loss that exceeds a specific amount (the ceding insurer's net retention), subject generally to a fixed limit of reinsurance. The premium paid by the insurer for excess-of-loss reinsurance typically bears no proportional relationship to the original premium paid by the policyholder.

The rate is usually based on the potential for loss. Excess-of-loss agreements may cover policies on an individual basis or an occurrence, such as a tornado, an earthquake, or an aggregate of losses incurred over a period of time, usually a year.

The two types of proportional plans are "quota share" and "surplus share." Under a quota-share agreement, the insurer cedes a fixed percentage of each policy written in a certain line or class of business and receives a commission from the reinsurer for the business ceded. Under a surplus- share agreement, the primary insurer's retention is stated as a dollar amount. If the amount of insurance under a policy is less than the retention, no liability is ceded. If it is greater than the retention, the excess—the remainder of liability up to the liability limits—is reinsured. The premium is shared in the ratio of the retained liability to ceded liability.

The catastrophe insurance market includes risk transfer through insurance and reinsurance contracts as well as risk financing alternatives to reinsurance, namely, the securitization of insurable risk and insurance derivatives such as futures and options.

The next section analyzes the private insurance industry's risk transfer capacity; it excludes underwriting capacity from the reinsurance market and alternative risk transfer instruments.

Insurer Claims-Paying Capacity

The insurance industry's capacity to assume catastrophic natural disaster risk depends on how much capital and surplus exist on their balance sheets to absorb the annual variance in unexpected catastrophe losses. Within the context of a potential mega-catastrophic event, several scenarios could overwhelm the catastrophe insurance industry's claims-paying capacity. For example, according to Aon Benfield, a reinsurance intermediary, global reinsurance capital stood at $505 billion in 2012.[24] Although this level of capital might suggest the catastrophe insurance market industry is well capitalized, not all the global reinsurance capital is dedicated to financing U.S. catastrophic risks. Moreover, most disaster insurance experts agree that reinsurers appear no longer able to provide complete diversification of catastrophic risk both because catastrophic natural disasters appear to be correlated across risk and estimates of the probable maximum loss (PML) from catastrophes have risen dramatically.[25] Most experts argue that for the very highest layers of catastrophe risk, federal disaster relief (and consequently the taxpayer) is now, by default (due to limited private-sector capacity in the traditional reinsurance market), the insurer of last resort, particularly for uninsured property owners.

At the Congressional Research Service's (CRS's) request, AIR Worldwide Corporation, a catastrophe-modeling firm based in Boston, provided simulated estimates of potential insured catastrophe losses caused by U.S. hurricanes, earthquakes, and the fires that follow earthquakes. Loss estimates for the 1%, 0.4%, and 0.2% annual occurrence probabilities are illustrated in **Table 3**, which correspond to return periods of 100-, 250-, and 500-year losses, respectively.

As shown in **Table 3**, AIR Worldwide Corporation found that the national PMLs for hurricanes and earthquakes are $108.4 billion for the 1% return period, $164.5 billion for the 0.4% return period, and $217 billion for the 0.2% return period. The corresponding numbers for earthquakes and fire (combined) losses are $50 billion for 1% events, $90 billion for 0.4% events, and $119 billion for 0.2% events.

Table 3. Estimated Insured Hurricane and Earthquake Losses Nationally and for 10 States for 1-in-100-Year, 1-in-250-Year and 1-in-500-Year Catastrophes ($ in millions)

Rank	Area/State	100-Year Expected Loss (1%)	250-Year Expected Loss (0.4%)	500-Year Expected Loss (0.2%)
	United States	$108,387.18	$164,525.21	$217,031.79
1	Florida	87,764.37	144,249.92	200,125.61
2	California	38,955.37	66,317.74	94,020.46
3	Texas	21,314.38	32,808.29	44,156.20
4	Louisiana	12,121.11	18,552.82	24,530.98
5	New York	9,331.85	24,587.73	35,829.62
6	North Carolina	9,326.91	15,343.76	21,395.14
7	South Carolina	7,706.53	14,629.53	20,559.48
8	Alabama	6,022.22	11,402.77	16,255.20
9	Massachusetts	4,968.07	9,134.62	13,793.45
10	New Jersey	4,003.32	10,699.68	17,597.08

Source: AIR Worldwide, Inc.

Table 4 shows the operating financial budget for the U.S. property and casualty insurance industry—both commercial and residential—for 2008 through 2012. As shown in the table, the U.S. property and casualty industry had a $586.9 billion surplus in 2012. At first, it would appear that this surplus for unexpected losses would be sufficient for the property and casualty insurance industry, as a whole, to be able to underwrite the levels of catastrophe insurance needed to address the level of losses estimated in **Table 3**. However, only about 20% of the industry-wide policyholder surplus, a measure of capacity, is generally considered to be allocated to catastrophe property insurance lines of business. The remaining 80% is used (some would argue needed) to support non-catastrophic risks. This suggests that approximately $108 billion of policyholders' surplus is available for catastrophic property losses nationwide. When comparing this amount of insurer claim-paying capacity to the PML, arguably the insurance industry's financial resources could be insufficient to cover anything more than a 1-in-100 year loss.

Table 4. U.S. Property and Casualty Operating Results, 2008-2012 ($ billions)

	2008	2009	2010	2011	2012
Net Earned Premiums	$438.1	$419.0	$420.5	$433.9	$449.4
Incurred Losses & Loss Adjust Expenses	339.2	306.7	309.1	344.5	335.0
Expenses	118.1	113.4	119.5	124.0	129.0
Policyholder Dividends	2.0	2.0	2.3	1.9	2.1
Net Underwriting Gain (Loss)	(21.2)	(3.1)	(10.4)	(36.5)	(16.7)
Investment Income	51.2	47	47.2	49.0	47.7
Other items	(0.1)	0.8	1.0	1.2	2.3
Pre-Tax Operating Gain	29.9	44.7	37.8	14.8	3.3
Realized Capital Gain (Losses)	(19.8)	(8.0)	5.7	7.2	6.2
Pre-Tax Income	10.1	36.7	43.5	22.0	39.5
Taxes	7.7	8.4	8.9	2.9	6.0
Net After-Tax Income	**2.4**	**28.3**	**34.7**	**(19.2)**	**33.5**
Surplus (End of period)	455.6	511.5	556.9	550.3	586.9
Combined Ratio[a]	105.1	101.0	102.4	108.2	103.2

Source: Insurance Information Institute.

Notes: Figures may not add to totals due to rounding.

a. Insurers use the term "combined ratio" as a measure of underwriting profitability. It reflects the percentage of each premium dollar an insurer spends on claims and expenses. The combined ratio does not take investment income into account. A combined ratio above 100 indicates an underwriting loss.

To some, this line of reasoning arguably suggests federal intervention in catastrophe property insurance markets to address potential market failure in the range between the 0.4% to 0.2% return periods.[26] Some finance experts may also be concerned about projections that catastrophic losses will likely double every 10 years and the present government insurance approach might not be adequate.[27] John Seo, co-founder and managing principal at Fermat Capital Management, LLC, has asserted that a government insurance program might become challenged in its ability to cover losses for less than one generation's worth of exposure growth.[28] As an illustration, a $100 billion exposure is anticipated to become $200 billion after 10 years; $400 billion after 20 years; and $800 billion after 30 years. Ten years ago, a 1-in-100 event would have cost insurers $55 billion. Ten years from now a 100-year event could cost $220 billion.

In light of the concerns about the capacity of insurers to pay claims after mega-catastrophes, primary insurers have increasingly turned to private capital markets for risk-transfer capacity to complement traditional reinsurance markets. Professor Kenneth A. Froot of Harvard University has suggested that one reason for the search for alternatives to reinsurance has been the supply restrictions associated with capital market imperfections and market power exerted by traditional reinsurers.[29] This situation is a matter of basic economics of supply and demand: a limited number of reinsurers with specialized knowledge and unique access to global capital markets can exert substantial control over prices and supply. Given recent historical losses and concerns with future mega-catastrophes, there is some concern that catastrophe reinsurance capacity may be insufficient to meet societal demand.

State-Sponsored, Loss-Sharing Financing Mechanisms

The exclusion of wind, water (flood), and seismic perils in the standard homeowners' insurance policy led some states, beginning in the 1970s, to establish state pooling systems to finance natural hazard risks. These state-sponsored, so-called residual or involuntary property insurance pools include Fair Access to Insurance Requirements (FAIR) or Beach or Windstorm Plans and catastrophe funds that operate as insurers or reinsurers of last resort.

California, Florida, and Texas have created insurance companies—Florida Windstorm Underwriting Association, the Florida Citizens Property Insurance Company (CPIC), Texas Windstorm Insurance Association, and the California Earthquake Authority (CEA)—that provide wind and seismic insurance to high-risk property owners who may have difficulty obtaining such coverage from the voluntary property insurance market. Industry assessments support these entities.

FAIR Plans often provide property insurance in both urban and coastal areas, while state-run Beach and Windstorm Plans cover predominantly wind-only risks in designated coastal areas in states along the Gulf of Mexico and the Southeast Atlantic coast region. The CEA covers only primary residential buildings and provides limited coverage for building contents. Financing for the CEA comes from a combination of up-front and contingent insurer contributions, traditional reinsurance, and revenue bonds.

Florida has a unique program for financing catastrophe losses through implicit reinsurance contracts backed, in part, by the state's taxing authority. The Florida Hurricane Catastrophe Fund (Cat Fund) is a mandatory, state-sponsored catastrophe-reinsurance pool for property insurers writing business in Florida. Property insurers are required to maintain a retention—responsibility for a first dollar amount—against qualifying catastrophes in the state, but they may select to participate at one of three reinsurance coverage levels. The Cat Fund has the authority to spread the burden of unusual losses intertemporally through deficit financing—essentially imposing an intergenerational tax on future generations of state taxpayers.

In the wake of recent catastrophic losses, uncertainties surround the growing residual liabilities in state-run insurance pools and incentives to redistribute disaster losses to future generations (deficit financing). Some disaster insurance experts have proposed multistate pools on a regional or national level as a more effective mechanism for spreading and sharing disaster losses.[30]

Alternative Risk Transfer Techniques

After Hurricane Andrew in 1992 and the Northridge earthquake in 1994, there was recognition among insurers that existing capital within the insurance industry was inadequate to finance insurance risks. Some insurance industry participants were beginning to view the capital markets as a potential source of additional capacity. Deregulation of financial markets, the globalization of business, and innovation and technological advances in the 1980s and 1990s led to the evolution of derivatives as a risk management tool, and the application of securitization (the financial practice of pooling various types of assets into a security that can be purchased) to new insurance product lines, especially involving more esoteric or unique forms of insurance risk.

Consequently, capacity constraints in the insurance and reinsurance markets, corporate demand for more efficient risk financing (hedging) strategies, and the arrival of innovative capital market financial instruments created the market conditions whereby the insurance markets began to rethink the management of risk across traditional boundaries. This led to the development of alternative risk transfer (ART) techniques that could package insurance risk into discrete securities with finite risk, such that insurance risk could be traded and hedged in much the same way that interest rate risk is traded today.

In general, there are two categories of ART methods for financing catastrophic risk: (1) insurance- linked securities (catastrophe risk bonds) and exchange-traded insurance derivatives (catastrophe options and swaps); and (2) contingent risk financing. These ART techniques, driven by the need for risk management ("hedging"), balance sheet management, and capital management, have blurred the traditional distinction between insurance, securities, and banking.

The first catastrophe risk securitization was the introduction of insurance derivative contracts (index-linked catastrophe futures and catastrophe put and call options) traded on the Chicago Board of Trade (CBOT). By the late 1990s, several exchanges had introduced futures-and-options contracts on U.S. hurricane risk. Insurance securitization now represents a major risk-financing tool for transferring (hedging liabilities) windstorm and earthquake risk to investors in the capital markets.

Insurance-Linked Securities and Derivatives

Insurance-linked securities (ILS) permit the transfer of event risk assumed by insurers directly to investors through event-linked issuance of debt. For example, catastrophic risk (CAT) bonds are ILS that performs a risk transfer function similar to that of insurance and reinsurance. CAT bonds are purchased in the capital markets. With a Cat bond, investors place cash into a trust account from which they receive interest payments. The funds in the account are transferred to the insurer only on the occurrence of a defined catastrophic event. Also, exchange-traded insurance derivatives enable the trading of standardized, catastrophe event-linked futures and options contracts linked to some index to improve risk sharing.

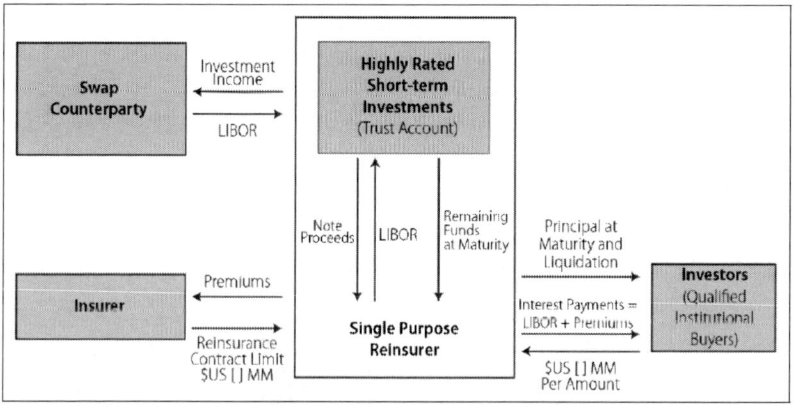

Source: Cummings, J.D. and Barrieu, P., "Innovations in Insurance Markets: Hybrid and Securitized Risk-Transfer Solutions," in Georges Dionne, ed., *Handbook of Insurance*, 2nd ed., Boston: Kluwer Academic Publishers, 2012.

Figure 4. Illustration of Catastrophe Bond.

Contingent Risk Financing

Contingent risk financing enables insurers and reinsurers to use contingent credit facilities to bridge financially the period between natural disaster events and the execution of post-event financing. Contingent financing instruments are designed to pre-finance insurance–related losses but without a transfer of the underlying insurance risks from insurer to capital market investors. The insurer only receives an inflow of capital to replenish its policyholders' surplus after it pays for the loss. The insurer pays a capital commitment fee to the party that agrees in advance to buy the equity or debt securities following a loss. Contingent capital can be available to insurers immediately after a catastrophe, when the insurer most needs that capital, through a wide range of alternative capital sources, such as contingent surplus notes, catastrophe equity put options, sidebars, or industry loss warrants.

The following discussion of ART instruments provides more in-depth information on the innovative uses of capital markets instruments, which are designed to achieve greater efficiency in catastrophic risk financing.

Catastrophic Risk Bonds

The most common form of insurance linked securities is a catastrophic risk (CAT) bond used to supplement the traditional reinsurance marketplace.

The securitized structure of a CAT bond is modeled on asset-backed securities transactions, such as mortgage loans, automobile loans, and student loans. The bonds are fully collateralized (eliminating concerns about credit risk), multi-year risk transfer financial (intertemporal diversification) instruments that allow for the direct transfer of catastrophic insurance risks from insurers, reinsurers, and corporations to investors in the capital market. The CAT bond typically covers the so-called high layers of reinsurance protection, for example, protection against events that have a probability of occurrence of 0.02% or less—that is, a return period of 50 years. CAT bonds provide an effective way for investors to target their investments and for insurers to access underwriting capacity from the larger capital markets.

Figure 4 shows a typical catastrophe bond issuance. The CAT bond transaction begins with the formation of a special-purpose reinsure (SPR)—a reinsurance company incorporated with the specific purpose of entering into a reinsurance agreement between the insurer ("cedent" or "bond sponsor") and the investor. The SPR issues bonds to investors and invests the proceeds in short- term securities, such as government bonds or AAA corporate securities held in a trust account. The insurer pays a premium to the investor, usually LIBOR (London Interbank Offered Rate) plus a risk premium in return for providing capital to the trust. To avoid interest-rate risk, the fixed returns on the securities held in the trust are swapped for floating returns based on LIBOR or some other widely accepted index. The bond pay-off is triggered (structured to pay off) by a defined catastrophic event. On the occurrence of the event, investors are subject to the loss of interest, principal, or both and the trustee for the trust account will release the principal in the SPR to help the insurer pay claims arising from the event. If no contingent event occurs, the trustee returns the principal to the investor upon the expiration of the bonds.

According to Guy Carpenter & Company, a provider of risk and reinsurance intermediation services, institutional asset managers—the custodians of trillions of dollars of investable assets— have largely accepted catastrophe risk as a component of mainstream investment strategy.[31]

Figure 5 and **Figure 6** show catastrophe bond issuance totaled $5.85 billion in 2012, up from $3.86 billion in 2011. Catastrophe bond risk capital outstanding rose from $12.14 billion to $14.83 billion during the same period. In 2013, financial experts expect the market to approach, or exceed, the record for annual issuance of $7.0 billion set in 2007. Total risk capital outstanding increased during the first quarter of 2013, reaching an all-time high of $15.0 billion. This marked the eighth consecutive quarter of growth in risk capital outstanding, up more than 17% since the end of the first quarter of 2012.

Although most disaster insurance risk experts see the expansion of the use of CAT bonds as an encouraging development in managing disaster risk, they also note that taxation, accounting, and regulatory barriers limit the likelihood of a rapid expansion of the insurance-linked securitization market.

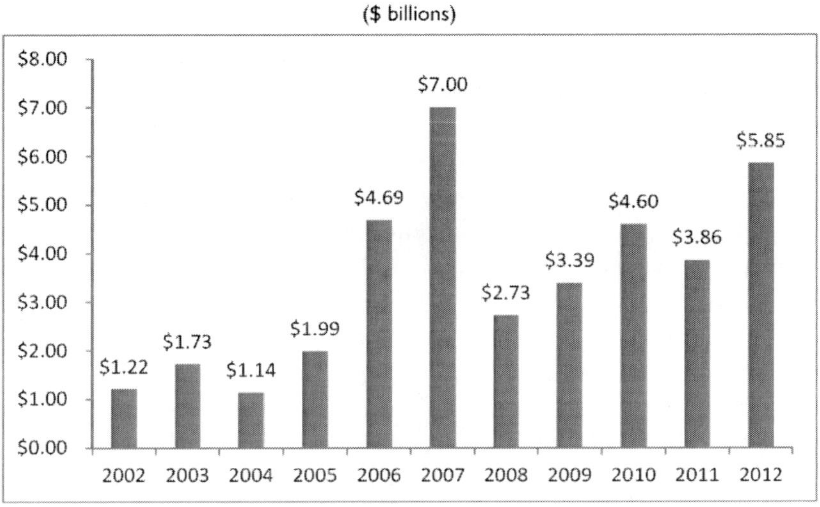

Source: Guy Carpenter & Company and Insurance Information Institute.

Figure 5. Catastrophe Bonds,Annual Risk Capital Issued, 2002-2012.

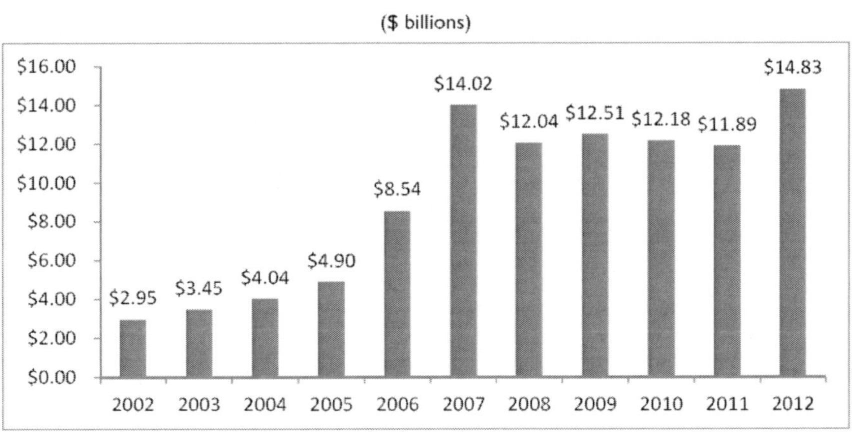

Source: Guy Carpenter & Company and Insurance Information Institute.

Figure 6. Catastrophe Bonds, Risk Capital Outstanding, 2002-2012.

Sidecars

Figure 7 shows a sidecar transition, which is an innovative financial vehicle established as a special-purpose vehicle (SPV) formed by an insurance or reinsurance company to provide additional capacity to write reinsurance. Reinsurers favor the sidecar because they provide additional capacity without diluting shareholders' equity. The SPV operates as a side vehicle— referred to as a "sidecar" company—to a larger established reinsurer's operation. The sidecar (1) diversifies or spreads an individual reinsurer's risk among the reinsurance community by issuing fully collateralized debt to its investors and (2) acts as a stop loss by partitioning reinsurers' risks to improve their financial strength ratings by reducing the volatility of their earnings.

Operationally, an insurer or reinsurer will establish a sidecar by transferring policies and premiums to an SPR that uses the funds as collateral for bonds, loans, and equity. Hedge funds and private equity investors have provided the bulk of the funds to capitalize these unusual insurance investment vehicles. Investors would agree, for example, to invest the funds for two to three years and typically earned 20% to 30% return or more on their investments. The reinsurer creating the sidecar receives a commission. Investors typically obtain a relatively high investment return through interest payments and dividends from the trust when the sidecar expires, assuming that all of the capital has not been used to meet claims payouts.

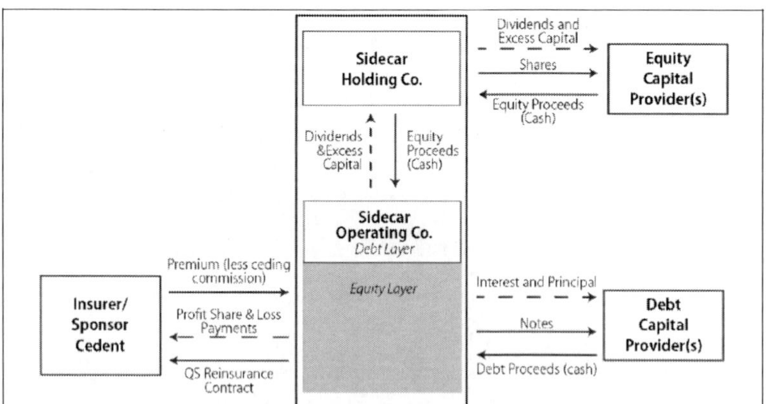

Source: Cummings, J.D. and Barrieu, P., "Innovations in Insurance Markets: Hybrid and Securitized Risk-Transfer Solutions," in Georges Dionne, ed., *Handbook of Insurance*, 2nd ed., Boston: Kluwer Academic Publishers, 2012.

Figure 7. Illustration of Sidecar Transaction.

Industry Loss Warrants

An industry loss warrant (ILW) is a contract between two insurers and is not pre-funded. Unlike traditional reinsurance, where the reinsurer pays a portion of the primary insurer's losses according to an agreed-upon formula, the ILW is triggered by a predetermined level of industry loss. However, the ILW has a second trigger based on indemnity losses. The contract "warrants" that the reinsurer will pay up to a specific amount toward the buyer's losses if the industry suffers a predetermined loss amount after the industry loss is triggered.

Industry loss trigger(s) are structured to provide prompt payment when, or if, aggregate industry losses for covered risks exceed a certain threshold for a single occurrence or sequential occurrences over the contract term. Importantly, since ILWs are priced and underwritten based on expectations of industry loss, underwriting information about the (re)insurance company is not needed, and the process and cost associated with these risk transfers is generally less significant than other options. The largest risk to the buyer of protection with these vehicles is basis risk. It is very possible that a (re)insurer could incur substantial losses, while the industry's losses do not exceed the payout trigger. Therefore, these contracts are typically very attractive to larger insurers that have exposures mimicking the broader industry.

Catastrophe Equity Puts

Catastrophe equity puts (Cat-E-Puts) are a form of contingent financing transaction in which the buyer has the option to issue preferred stock at a pre-agreed price on the occurrence of a contingent event. Insurers typically use Cat-E-Puts to raise equity capital at a favorable price after a catastrophe, when its stock price is likely to be depressed.

Cat-E-Puts are not asset-backed securities but options. A catastrophe equity put provides contingent capital on a post-loss basis, similar to a standby credit facility. A put option provides the option holder the right, but not the obligation to sell a security at a certain price at a future time. In this case, a reinsurer grants the option holder the right to sell its equity to the reinsurer at a set price in the event of a catastrophic loss.

The Cat-E-Put option buyer pays an option premium to the provider—option writer—of contingent capital. The option gives the buyer the right to obtain capital at pre-negotiated rates following the occurrence of a catastrophic event that exposes the company's capital beyond the insurance or reinsurance program in place at the time of the event. Catastrophe equity puts provide off-balance sheet risk capital at a lower cost than conventional reinsurance.

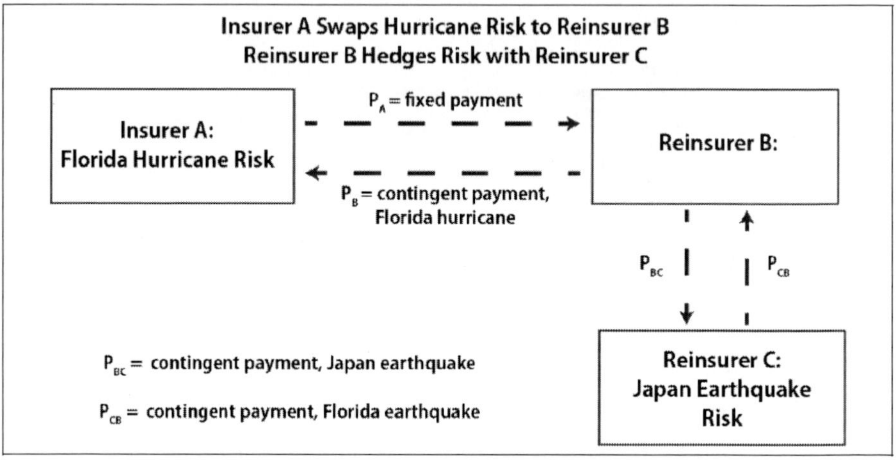

Source: Cummings, J.D. and Barrieu, P., "Innovations in Insurance Markets: Hybrid and Securitized Risk-Transfer Solutions," in Georges Dionne, ed., *Handbook of Insurance*, 2nd ed., Boston: Kluwer Academic Publishers, 2012.

Figure 8. Illustration of Catastrophe Swap.

Catastrophe Risk Swaps

Figure 8 provides an illustration of how catastrophe risk swaps are executed between two counterparties, which have agreed to exchange streams of cash flows, based on movements in the value of an asset, yield, or index, according to predetermined rules. The swaps are traded in the over-the-counter market. The swap is executed on a zero premium basis, provided the difference in riskiness can be agreed upon.

In a catastrophe insurance swap, insurers may exchange policies from one region of the country for policies in another region. Each swap is a reciprocal agreement between the two insuring entities. These transactions allow insurers to diversify their portfolios. For example, an insurer in Florida with a heavy concentration of hurricane-exposed risk can swap a portion of that business for a book of business in Illinois, where it is less exposed to the same risk.

A different kind of swap could involve an insurer exchanging a series of fixed predefined payments for a series of floating payments whose values depend on the occurrence of an insured catastrophic event. If the catastrophic event occurs, the insurer receives a higher cash flow from the floating payment stream, which can be used to offset claim payments. Catastrophe swaps make existing capital more efficient and provide an advantage to both parties because they result in reduced risk and improved diversification at no cost.

Key Challenges Facing Insurance Risk Securitization

Although catastrophe bonds trade with a somewhat higher spread over traditional debt, lack of standardized contracts, relatively limited trading volume due to a lack of liquidity, high cost, and uncertainty surrounding accounting, regulatory, and rating-agency treatment inhibit ILS market growth.

In general, the insurance-linked securitization market faces several challenges:

1. Uncertainty concerning the probability of catastrophic loss stemming from climate change, sea level rise, and storm surge;
2. Lack of uniform standards (e.g., language), institutional infrastructure, and methodology to evaluate the costs and benefits of risk transfer instruments that would facilitate comparison to conventional reinsurance;
3. Lack of standardized contracts for future delivery on organized exchanges (futures), and rights, but not guarantees for future delivery (options markets);
4. Unfavorable tax treatment of onshore securitization inhibits their utilization (regulatory recognition of offshore securitizations could encourage insurers to use this approach to manage their catastrophe risk);
5. Lack of tradable market indices (or granular data) for parametric transactions based on an index or a formula for payment; and
6. Limited secondary market makes insurance risk transfer instruments relatively illiquid.

Government Intervention in Risk-Transfer Markets

Since the mid-1990s, most policymakers and insurance industry participants have agreed that a catastrophic natural disaster could cause an unexpected and sudden large loss of insurers' capital reserves, leading to a rise in the price of insurance and a fall in supply. Given this risk scenario, some have called for an expanded role for the federal government in catastrophe insurance markets, arguing that such intervention is necessary to address market failure. Intervention could take any of several forms designed to expand the private sector's ability to provide catastrophe insurance, such as adding a high-end federal reinsurance backstop, providing short-term government liquidity loans, or offering federal multiple-peril homeowners insurance policies covering both wind and flood damages.

Arguments for Intervention

Proponents of federal intervention argue that the government is the *de facto* insurer of last resort for mega-catastrophes, largely because the government is presumed to be better positioned to bear catastrophe risk because of its broad resource base and borrowing capacity.[32] The federal government, however, currently lacks a comprehensive approach to manage the effects of catastrophic natural disasters, relying instead on ad-hoc disaster relief spending to facilitate recovery and rebuilding following a major disaster.

Federal financial intervention in the catastrophe reinsurance market, some contend, could reduce the burdens for future disaster relief expenditures, promote efficient risk management by property owners, and encourage individuals and states to take steps to reduce loss exposure, ultimately resulting, in theory, in overall lower social and federal costs. Some argue that an explicit *ex ante* federal government catastrophic risk financing approach would arguably be the best way to assess, budget, and plan for the future cost of catastrophe risks before such events occur.[33]

Arguments against Intervention

Opponents of federal intervention in catastrophe insurance markets insist that there is sufficient private insurance and reinsurance capacity to adequately cover catastrophic risks. They insist the federal government's role in disaster risk financing should be to ensure a framework that allows private market mechanisms to work without local regulatory interference (i.e., regulatory price constraints that seek to keep premium rates below actuarial rates).[34] In their view, federal intervention in catastrophe insurance markets is likely to have negative unexpected side effects, such as moral hazard, and reduces the economic disincentives for homeowners and businesses to locate in disaster-prone areas or neglect risk prevention. They argue that private insurers, state residual markets, and state catastrophe funds already protect coastal properties, and federal government intervention would only distort the insurance market by regulating the availability of coverage and level of premiums, displacing private capital deployed in insurance and reinsurance, and stifling innovative private sector solutions for managing and financing catastrophic risks.[35] Government insurance schemes, they say, would not reflect the risk level of the activity being insured, thereby eliminating a potentially powerful economic deterrent to risky behavior. Moreover, government intervention could force the public at large to cross-subsidize the risky behavior of residents in high-risk areas.

Potential Points of Agreement

Some consensus is that the federal government could use its regulatory authority to create incentives for private capital to flow into the property insurance market, such as establishing strong building codes, encouraging effective land planning techniques, and requiring a state insurance regulatory environment that fosters competition and risk-based pricing. In addition, there is some consensus that the federal government could help decrease barriers in the nascent markets for insurance-linked securities (ILS) and provide liquidity through temporary loans designed to stabilize the market after a mega-catastrophe. Other "common ground" topics include clarifying accounting rules for special-purpose reinsurers and changing the rules to require foreign and domestic reinsurers to meet the same collateral requirements.

LEGISLATIVE OPTIONS

Several catastrophic risk-financing legislative options are before the 113th Congress. For example, H.R. 737, the Homeowners' Defense Act of 2013, would establish a National Catastrophe Risk Consortium to facilitate both multistate pooling of catastrophic risks (covering a variety of event probabilities and types) and natural disaster-linked securitization, thereby strengthening the financial capacity of these programs.

H.R. 737 is designed to facilitate catastrophic risk transfer to capital markets and increase transparency (liquidity) in the market for catastrophic risk. The bill would establish the National Catastrophe Risk Consortium, a voluntary organization that states can choose to join that would be charged with facilitating financial innovation to allow participating states to transfer catastrophic risk to the capital market. The aim of the consortium would be to ensure the availability and affordability of homeowner's insurance coverage for catastrophic events. To facilitate catastrophe risk securitization, the consortium would use an integrated risk valuation method that identifies, tracks, and publicizes the risks embedded in financial transactions. The insurance risk securitization, serialization, bundling, and re-bundling of risk-adjusted assets within a single transaction process will be transferred to the capital market through a catastrophe risk interactive exchange platform.

In theory, the consortium would standardize natural catastrophe peril bond terms, tranches, and pay out formulae, which, in turn, would enhance the marketability/liquidity of risk-linked securities, such as catastrophe bonds structured to attract more capital. Credit rating agencies would rate the various tranches according to their expected loss. The consortium would issue catastrophe bonds, and other innovative financial instruments, using an electronic platform with a common legal structure and documentation. Securities would be issued by the consortium in an SEC 144A private placement to investors who are Qualified Institutional Buyers or similar classes of investors, and who sign an Investor Awareness Letter. Reinsurance credit would be granted by the insurance regulator based on the full collateralization of the reinsurance contract within a Regulation 112 trust, with suitable investment restrictions.

The consortium would transfer the catastrophe risk directly to international catastrophe reinsurance and capital markets on competitive terms. States would presumably grant reinsurance credit based on the full collateralization of the reinsurance contract within a Regulation 112 trust, with suitable investment restrictions. The consortium is structured to overcome regulatory and tax constraints to catastrophe risk transfer through securitization. Removal of regulatory and tax constraints associated with catastrophe bonds and other alternative financial instruments issued by the National Catastrophe Risk Consortium could, in theory, increase the capacity of the private capital market to assume more catastrophe risk.

H.R. 240, the Homeowners Insurance Protection Act of 2013, would create the National Commission on Catastrophe Preparation and Protection with the authority to establish a federal reinsurance program to make reinsurance coverage available to eligible state natural catastrophe insurance programs to improve the availability and affordability of coverage for homes, and the solvency and capacity of homeowners' insurance markets.

Congress could choose to provide tax incentives designed to expand the supply of capital reserves that stand behind private insurance. H.R. 549, the Homeowner Catastrophe Protection Act of 2013, would allow property and casualty insurance companies to make tax-deductible contributions to a tax-exempt policyholder disaster protection fund established for the payment of policyholders' claims arising from certain catastrophic events, such as windstorms, earthquakes, fires, or floods.[36] This tax law change would encourage the use of reinsurance by assessing the reserve amounts on net premiums.

Current tax provisions do not encourage insurers to reserve funds for unknown losses. Reserves for such contingencies can only be accumulated out of after-tax income. In contrast, reserves set aside for reported losses, or losses incurred but which have not been reported at the end of a given accounting period, are not taxed by the federal government. Allowing insurers to accumulate tax- deferred reserves for catastrophe perils would reduce federal tax revenue, and may involve tax benefits that favor one type of activity over another, raising issues of efficiency. Economists have raised the question of whether tax incentives for homeowners would be sufficient to get people to buy disaster insurance. Congress might decide to assess the cost-benefit of the provision for tax deductibility of catastrophe reserves against possible savings in ad hoc disaster relief outlays.

Congress might also choose to consider several other legislative options to address the financial consequences of catastrophic natural disaster losses. These include

- **Bipartisan Study Commissions.** Congress could choose to establish a bipartisan study commission to examine various proposals to improve capabilities of the insurance marketplace to provide sufficient capacity to facilitate the pooling and spreading of risk from catastrophic financial losses from natural disasters.
- **Implement a Federal Multiple Peril Insurance Program.** In the aftermath of the devastation caused by Hurricane Sandy, one policy option that Congress might consider would be to authorize the creation of multi-peril property insurance policies that cover wind perils under the National Flood Insurance Program (NFIP). Multiple peril insurance could eliminate the problem of uninsured property owners, but it could also create new uncertain liabilities for federal taxpayers.
- **Federal Catastrophe Liquidity Loan and Debt Guarantee Program.** Congress might decide to authorize the U.S. Treasury to guarantee municipal obligations of state sponsored and quasi-state sponsored municipal bonds and provide liquidity loans to state

"qualified reinsurance programs" for natural disasters. The loan program could dampen swings in insurance rates and address availability deficiencies caused by inefficient capital markets. The federal guarantees of debt issuance would complement existing state-sponsored measures that pre-fund insured property catastrophe exposures through insurance premiums and assessments on insurers.

CONCLUSION

In recent decades, the financial volatility of large-scale natural catastrophes and the cost of financing recovery have emerged as important policy issues for Congress. However, besides the Terrorism Risk Insurance Act of 2002,[37] Congress has not approved an explicit federal disaster insurance law, since the creation of the NFIP in 1968, because of a lack of consensus that a catastrophe risk-financing problem exists. Concerns expressed have included disagreements about what constitutes adequate provisions for mitigation, a desire to avoid unnecessary government intrusion into markets served by the private sector (crowding out), moral hazards associated with government guarantees or economic subsidies that distort market incentives and increase social costs, and the potential for expanded financial liabilities and burden on federal taxpayers.[38]

With this in mind, a key policy challenge for Congress is determining whether private insurers and their reinsurance partners have the financial capacity to absorb losses from a future mega-catastrophe and, if necessary, what reforms would improve insurers' access to capital to ensure adequate capacity. Is there a need to improve the nation's ability to finance catastrophe risk and, if so, how? Congress, for example, might choose to consider the appropriate roles and policies of the public and private sectors in addressing disaster risks.

Three key points of view usually emerge when debating catastrophe-funding issues. One view is that natural catastrophes are "uninsurable" in the private sector and the federal government should intervene to either directly underwrite catastrophe risks or provide a federal reinsurance backstop to private insurers, reinsurers, or state pools. This view has not been widely supported in the past because it was believed that the private sector had access to sufficient capital to enable it to finance the cost of providing catastrophic insurance.

A second point of view argues that catastrophe risk is insurable up to a point but federal involvement in the catastrophe insurance market would be required for a mega-catastrophic disaster. Many disaster insurance experts agree with this point of view; namely, for the very highest layers of catastrophe risk, the government (and consequently the taxpayer) is now, by default, the insurer of last resort. They support the idea of a public-private partnership in financing a mega-catastrophe. Such a public-private catastrophe insurance partnership would presumably leave the private sector responsible for underwriting property insurance and the federal government responsible for providing capital only when consumers and the private insurance and capital markets are unable to do so.

Under this arrangement, as envisioned by some disaster insurance experts, the government could facilitate a more effective risk spreading that achieves more effective pooling of losses over time and broader pooling of losses among risks through a borrowing mechanism (debt financing) and tax deferral of loss reserves for natural disasters. Broader pooling of losses among risks requires government-imposed mandatory purchase requirements. Economists note, however, that any scheme that imposes a mandatory insurance requirement for all property owners could create economic distortions, such as cross subsidization of risks, where low-risk individuals subsidize high-risk individuals.

A third point of view presupposes that financial resources in the private sector are sufficient to make federal intervention not necessary in catastrophe insurance markets. For risks to be insurable, however, they must be actuarially determined and risk-based, albeit potentially prohibitively high for the average household. However, if insurance rates are priced outside of the household budget of the average individual, the insurance product becomes essentially unmarketable—even with a government purchase mandate, as evidenced by the relatively low participation (purchase) rates in high-risk flood zones where a federal mandatory flood insurance purchase requirement exists.

In conclusion, several policy options for expanding the federal role in financing natural disaster losses are currently under consideration, but enactment into law will likely be based on whether it can be shown that potential catastrophe losses, in the absence of federal intervention, are beyond the capacity of private markets to diversify catastrophe risks.

End Notes

[1] Scientists define a natural environment hazard as a threat of a naturally occurring event that will have an adverse effect on people or the environment.

[2] This report does not address human-induced catastrophes. The Terrorism Risk Insurance Program provides a financial backstop for private insurers exposed to terrorism risks. For more information, see CRS Report R42716, *Terrorism Risk Insurance: Issue Analysis and Overview of Current Program*, by Baird Webel. In addition, the National Flood Insurance Program provides property insurance for flood risks facing property owners and small businesses in the United States.

[3] The U.S. insurance industry defines a catastrophe as an event that causes $25 million or more in insured property losses and affects a significant number of property/casualty policyholders and insurers.

[4] For information on estimates of total economic losses from Hurricane Katrina, see National Ocean Atmospheric Administration, National Weather Service, "Service Assessment, Hurricane Katrina, August 23-31, 2005," p. 1, located at http://www.nws.noaa.gov/om/assessments/pdfs/Katrina.pdf. For information on estimates of total economic losses from Hurricane Sandy, see National Ocean Atmospheric Administration, National Climate Data Center, "U.S. Billion- dollar Weather and Climate Disasters: Data Sources, Trends, Accuracy and Biases," located at http://www1.ncdc.noaa.gov/pub/data/papers/smith-and-katz-2013.pdf.

[5] In response to Hurricane Sandy, Congress passed the Sandy Recovery Improvement Act of 2013, which was included as Division B of P.L. 113-2, the Disaster Relief Appropriations Act, 2013. It provided $50.7 billion in disaster assistance. Congress also passed legislation (P.L. 113-1) to temporarily increase the National Flood Insurance Program's borrowing authority by $9.7 billion (from $20.725 billion to $30.425 billion). For more information on P.L. 113-2, the Sandy Recovery Improvement Act of 2013, see CRS Report R42991, *Analysis of the Sandy Recovery Improvement Act of 2013*, by Jared T. Brown, Francis X. McCarthy, and Edward C. Liu. For more information on Hurricane Sandy funding for disaster assistance see CRS Report R42869, *FY2013 Supplemental Funding for Disaster Relief*, coordinated by William L. Painter and Jared T. Brown.

[6] The *law of large numbers* is an important statistical theorem that, in essence, says the larger the number of exposure unites, the more closely will the actual results obtained approach the probable results expected from an infinite number of exposures. The theorem is important to the prediction of losses by insurance company actuaries and risk managers.

[7] Specifically, in economic theory, moral hazard refers to a tendency for an individual (or entity) to be more willing to take a risk, knowing that the potential costs or burdens of taking the risk will be incurred, in whole or in part, by others.

[8] Adverse selection, in economic theory, refers to the tendency for those exposed to a higher risk to seek more insurance coverage than those exposed at a lower risk.

[9] Guy Carpenter & Company LLC, "Influx of Convergence Capital Triggers Downward Pressure on Pricing at June 1 Renewals, June 3, 2013, located at http://www.gccapitalideas.com/2013/06/03/influx-of-convergence-capital-triggers- downward-pressure-on-pricing-at-june-1-renewals/.

[10] Guy Carpenter & Company, LLC, "Catastrophe Bond Update: First Quarter 2013," May 2013, located at http://www.guycarp.com/portal/extranet/insights/briefingsPDF/2013/ Catastrophe%20Bond%20Update%20First%20Quarter%202013.pdf;JSESSIONIDGCPORTALWCPORTALAPP=pjRQR2ZMLy5n2ppDpPxyl9lj5L5TdLYz4KTzdryXCkHpjs2bZg1p!-2116277995?vid=5.

[11] Having insurance capacity does not ensure private insurers will choose to sell insurance. Other factors like rates of return on investment (cost of capital) remains a key determinant in whether insurers will offer insurance coverage in a particular geographical area or state.

[12] Uninsured or underinsured public losses from natural catastrophes, including destruction of public buildings, infrastructure, and transportation systems are either retained or reimbursed by the public expenditure of funds or tax relief.

[13] For example, the National Hurricane Center typically doubles the estimated insured losses for an estimate of total damage losses in the United States.

[14] CoreLogic, "The 2013 CoreLogic Storm Surge Report," May 31, 2013, located at http://www.corelogic.com/ research/storm-surge/corelogic-2013-storm-surge-report.pdf.

[15] Ibid.

[16] For more information on the National Flood Insurance Program see CRS Report R42850, *The National Flood Insurance Program: Status and Remaining Issues for Congress*, by Rawle O. King.

[17] Timothy Beatle, David J. Brower, and Anna K. Schwab, *An Introduction to Coastal Zone Management* (Washington, DC: Island Press, 2002), pp. 94-95.

[18] National Ocean Atmospheric Administration, National Climate Data Center, "U.S. Billion-dollar Weather and Climate Disasters: Data Sources, Trends, Accuracy and Biases," located at http://www1.ncdc.noaa.gov/pub/data/ papers/smith-and-katz-2013.pdf.

[19] United Nations World Meteorological Organization, "The Global Climate 2001-2010: A Decade of Climate Extremes," located at http://www.unep.org/pdf/wmo_report.pdf.

[20] Ibid.

[21] For more information on New York's effort to rebuild and recover from Hurricane Sandy see New York City Mayor's Office, the "Special Initiative for Rebuilding and Resiliency," June 11, 2013, located at http://www.nyc.gov/ html/sirr/html/report/report.shtml.

[22] For more information, see CRS Report R42073, *Presidential Policy Directive 8 and the National Preparedness System: Background and Issues for Congress*, by Jared T. Brown.

[23] To price their products so that rates do not have to increase significantly whenever a catastrophe occurs, primary insurers estimate future expected losses from insured catastrophic events and calculates catastrophe loadings applicable to all property insurance rates. All homeowners' insurance rates include a component for this special catastrophe loading. Insurers offering insurance for catastrophic risk charge this load to build up reserves and purchase reinsurance. Catastrophe ratemaking procedures require the actuary to evaluate 30 years to 50 years of actuarial reported incurred loss data from many states subject to similar types of events, isolate the atypical catastrophic element, and then measure that catastrophic element against total losses. Data from the experience period losses rarely have direct impact on the catastrophe loading calculation for the current policy year, or in the state where the event occurred; instead, the recent catastrophe loss data are used to update the catastrophe loading calculation, which would be applicable to policies issued after the disaster. This process of spreading catastrophe losses on a state, regional, or national basis over a multiyear period has led in the past to the least disruption in insurance markets, in terms of price increases, insurer pullouts, and coverage restrictions.

[24] Aon Benfield, "Reinsurance Market Outlook: Reinsurance Capacity Growth Continues to Outpace Demand," January 2013, located at http://thoughtleadership.aonbenfield.com/ Documents/ 20130103_reinsurance_market_outlook_external.pdf.

[25] Hurricane Hugo was an unexpected but manageable $4 billion catastrophic loss event. After Hugo, the industry's probable maximum loss (PML) for a catastrophic hurricane event was $8 billion. Many disaster insurance risk experts say the market for catastrophic risk changed after Andrew and the Northridge earthquake in 1994. Insurers began to use computer simulation modeling in their pricing, requiring hurricane deductibles, and generally began to withdraw coverage from high-risk coastal areas if they could not price risk to cover significantly higher future expected catastrophic natural disaster losses.

[26] This analysis simplifies the complex worldwide market for catastrophe property insurance and is intended only to provide an indication of the industry's overall claims-paying capacity. This analysis, for example, does not determine the potential effect of natural catastrophes on the financial strength of insurers nor does it consider offsets from the broad spread and

syndication of risk through heavy use of reinsurance, much of it foreign. A significant share of the impact on surplus associated with a mega-catastrophic event would be transferred to the insurance industry balance sheet in foreign countries like Germany, Great Britain, Switzerland, and Bermuda. In addition, the analysis does not consider the total amount of catastrophe reinsurance provided by state residual markets or state catastrophe funds that would increase the overall ability to insure catastrophic risks. As stated above, some insurers and reinsurers are able to raise new capital after a major catastrophic event.

[27] Insurance Services Office, "Catastrophe Losses Will Double About Every 10 Years, Says Leading Catastrophe Modeling Expert at PCS Conference," located at http://www.iso.com/ index.php?id=2276&option=com_content&task= view.

[28] John Seo, "Telephone communication with the author," May 16, 2007.

[29] Kenneth A. Froot, "The Market for Catastrophe Risk: A Clinical Examination," *Journal of Financial Economics*, May 2, 2001, pp. 529-571.

[30] George L. Priest, "The Government, the Market, and the Problem of Catastrophe Loss," *Journal of Risk and Uncertainty*, 12: 219-237, 1996.

[31] Guy Carpenter & Company, LLC, "Catastrophe Bond Update: First Quarter 2013," May 2013, located at http://www.guycarp.com/portal/extranet/insights/briefingsPDF/2013/ Catastrophe %20Bond%20Update%20First%20Quarter%202013.pdf;JSESSIONIDGCPORTALWCPO RTALAPP=pjR QR2ZMLy5n2ppDpPxyl9lj5L5TdLYz4KTzdryXCkHpjs2bZg1p!-2116277995?vid=5.

[32] National Association of Insurance Commissioners, "Natural Catastrophe Risk: Creating a Comprehensive National Plan," June 15, 2009, located at http://www.naic.org/documents/ committees_c_natural_catastrophe_plan_final.pdf.

[33] Ibid.

[34] See Mark A. Hofmann, "Insurers, Reinsurers Oppose National Catastrophe Fund for Homeowners," March 24, 2013, located at http://www.businessinsurance.com/ article/ 20130324/NEWS04/303249981#; and Personal Letter from Chris Hackett, Director, Policy Development and Research, Property Casualty Insurers Association of America to Matthew A. McKenney, Federal Insurance Office, U.S. Department of the Treasury, June 24, 2013, located at http://www.pciaa.net/web

[35] Ibid.

[36] See CRS Report RL33060, *Tax Deductions for Catastrophic Risk Insurance Reserves: Explanation and Economic Analysis*, by Rawle O. King.

[37] P.L. 107-297; 116 Stat. 2322. For more information on the TRIA, see CRS Report R42716, *Terrorism Risk Insurance: Issue Analysis and Overview of Current Program*, by Baird Webel.

[38] U.S. Government Accountability Office, *Natural Disasters: Public Policy Option for Changing the Federal Role in Natural Catastrophe Insurance*, GAO-08-07 (Washington: November 26, 2007), located at http://www.gao.gov/ new.items/d087.pdf.

In: Natural Catastrophes
Editor: Oliver H. Rohde
ISBN: 978-1-62948-449-5

Chapter 2

FINANCING RECOVERY AFTER A CATASTROPHIC EARTHQUAKE OR NUCLEAR POWER INCIDENT*

Rawle O. King

SUMMARY

On August 23, 2011, a rare, powerful magnitude 5.8 earthquake and aftershocks hit Mineral, VA, shutting down two North Anna Power Plants located about 7 miles from the earthquake's epicenter. The earthquake was felt from Georgia to southeast Canada. Other earthquakes have also occurred in the area, as well as in surrounding areas. For example, on July 16, 2010, a 3.6 magnitude earthquake occurred in Gaithersburg, MD, about 110 miles from the epicenter. Seismologists report that although Virginia is classified as a "moderate" seismic risk zone, since 1977, the state has experienced 160 earthquakes, of which just 16% were felt. According to the U.S. Geological Survey (USGS), this earthquake was the strongest earthquake to hit the entire states since the 5.8 magnitude tremor in 1897.

Separately, on March 11, 2011, a massive 9.0 magnitude earthquake struck off the coast of Honshu, Japan. It was the most severe and likely the costliest earthquake to hit Japan in the 130 years of recorded history. The

---

* This is an edited, reformatted and augmented version of the Congressional Research Service publication, CRS Report for Congress R41968, dated August 25, 2011.

Japan earthquake and tsunami caused more than 10,000 casualties, widespread property and infrastructure damage, blackouts, fire, and nuclear meltdowns. The nuclear crisis has compounded the challenges faced by a nation struggling to clean up and recover from the earthquake and tsunami. Two weeks later, the disaster triggered a crisis at the nuclear power facility; Japan's government said there was a leaking reactor core at the Fukushima Dai- ichi nuclear reactor complex, releasing radioactive contamination into the atmosphere and groundwater.

In the aftermath of the recent East Coast earthquake (and shut down of the North Anna nuclear power plants) and Japan's technological and natural disaster, U.S. policymakers are asking if it could happen here and, if so, how associated costs would be financed. In the event of a major natural disaster, several catastrophe risk financing and insurance issues could arise, including (1) the need to revisit the nature, extent, and timing of potential earthquake and tsunami hazards in the United States; (2) the adequacy of nuclear third-party liability insurance capacity; and (3) the challenges of financing recovery from natural disasters and making earthquake insurance more affordable. The latter challenge is largely a function of the national financial markets' capacity to absorb the cost and economic burden of a devastating mega-earthquake.

Given the economic devastation in Japan, there is heightened congressional interest in finding ways to reduce disaster risk for homeowners, insurance companies, financial firms, and both federal and state governments. This report examines earthquake catastrophe risk and insurance in the United States in light of recent developments. It examines both traditional and non-traditional approaches for financing recovery from earthquake losses as well as challenges in financing catastrophe losses with insurance. The report also explores the feasibility of a federal residential earthquake insurance mechanism and assesses policy implications of such a program. Finally, the report examines legislation introduced in the 112th Congress that addresses issues related to earthquakes, including S. 637, the Earthquake Insurance Affordability Act. S. 637 would authorize the U.S. Treasury to guarantee up to $5 billion in bonds available to certified public entities, like the California Earthquake Authority (CEA), following a catastrophic seismic event. The entity would have to exhaust its claims-paying ability before the federal guarantee becomes available. The measure is designed to reduce earthquake insurance rates by reducing the need to purchase reinsurance. The bonds would be repaid with premiums.

This report examines catastrophic earthquake risk and insurance issues facing the United States in light of the recent devastating Japan earthquake and tsunami. It examines both traditional and non-traditional approaches for financing recovery from earthquake losses as well as challenges in financing catastrophe losses with insurance. Much of earthquake disaster and nuclear-accident liability is currently borne by taxpayers. This report explores the feasibility of a federal residential earthquake insurance mechanism and concludes with policy implications of such a program.

INTRODUCTION

Earthquakes and other seismic hazards (e.g., tsunamis and volcanic eruptions) are simultaneously a global phenomenon and a specific threat to the U.S. economy, its citizens, the built environment, and the insurance industry. Most Americans live in areas considered "seismically active," although the degree of vulnerability to earthquake risk varies greatly. Each year about 5,000 earthquakes occur in the United States, but only a relatively small percentage cause injuries or damage to property.[1] The U.S. Geological Survey (USGS) estimates that 40 states are subject to risk of earthquakes or volcanic eruptions. Several factors determine the extent of loss of property and life, including the amount of seismic energy released, duration of shaking, distance from epicenter, population and building density, and time of day.

On March 11, 2011, a massive 9.0 magnitude earthquake struck off the coast of Honshu, Japan. Although the earthquake was just the most recent seismic event to strike the planet, it represented both the most severe and costliest earthquake to strike in Japan in the 130 years of recorded history. The Japan earthquake and tsunami caused more than 20,000 deaths, widespread property and infrastructure damage estimated at about $235 billion by the World Bank, blackouts, fire, and nuclear meltdowns.[2] The release of radioactive contamination into the atmosphere and groundwater has compounded the challenges faced by a nation struggling to clean up and recover from the destructive earthquake and tsunami.

In the aftermath of the Japan earthquake, tsunamis, and nuclear incident, U.S. policymakers are asking whether a similar disaster could happen here and how the public and private sectors would finance the costs associated with such an event. In light of a magnitude 5.8 earthquake that struck the East Coast of the United States on August 23, 2011, there is heightened concern that a devastating earthquake could trigger a nuclear power plant accident, but the likelihood of such an event is generally considered minimal. Although the earthquake triggered the shutdown of North Anna Nuclear Power Plants, there was no apparent damage to the plants. Proponents assert that the nuclear facilities were designed for this kind of a seismic event.

Partly for this reason, with the exception of small business disaster loans, the federal government generally does not budget for future natural disasters. The United States has an economic structure in place to respond to emergencies after their occurrence and address issues of vulnerability to extreme events—but the nation has not established significant economic reserves for remediation and response. Federal law places most earthquake, tsunami, and nuclear-accident liability disaster recovery financing on the shoulders of taxpayers through ad-hoc supplemental appropriations for disaster relief assistance and tax credits—after accounting for private insurance and reinsurance that citizens finance through premiums.

This post-event catastrophe risk financing approach raises several broad questions:

- What are the appropriate roles of the private and public sectors in mitigating the possible consequences of a future earthquake, tsunami, or nuclear accident, and in providing the necessary funds for recovery?
- Is there a need for new institutional structures and (enforcement) mechanisms, as well as regulations and standards, for dealing with extreme events in an uncertain and increasingly interdependent world?
- What is the capacity of national financial markets to absorb the cost and economic burden of a devastating mega-earthquake or nuclear incident?

Given the economic devastation in Japan, there is heightened congressional interest in finding ways to reduce the direct and indirect impacts of extreme events and the social amplification of such risks (e.g., litigation and depressed economic activity) and ways to address these issues within a national risk management strategy. Whereas natural disaster losses have been financed on a post-event basis through taxpayer funded systems (e.g., the Robert T. Stafford Disaster Relief Act), the financing of recovery from a nuclear incident has been expected to be handled through nuclear recovery international liability (treaty) regimes and a federal government nuclear risk financing scheme. The earliest national liability laws were adopted in the United States in 1957 and in Europe in 1959.

The Price-Anderson Nuclear Industries Indemnity Act of 1957[3] supports commercial nuclear power in two ways. First, the act sought to encourage private investment in nuclear power generation despite the possibility of massive liability from an accident and the uncertain probability of such an accident occurring. The method chosen to encourage private investment in commercial nuclear power plants was to provide federal indemnification in the event of any liability and by capping total "public liability" per nuclear accident." Second, the act sought to make (insurance) funds available from reliable parties to pay up to the liability cap (rather than the power company declaring bankruptcy). It is argued, however, that by limiting the amount of primary insurance that nuclear operators must carry, the act reduces industry exposure to nuclear power's unique safety and security risks, but also leaves taxpayers responsible for the damages through ad hoc government disaster relief assistance, and arguably gives the industry a competitive advantage over other energy alternatives. (Although other energy alternatives do not seem to pose similar widespread threats.)

Congress could decide to explore how risk analysis could be used to better understand the challenges associated with extreme events so that more effective planning could be undertaken to reduce potential losses following a disaster. Members might also consider public-private partnerships and alternative policy strategies and financial instruments to help the private sector pre-fund and diversify disaster risk by financing catastrophic losses through insurance, reinsurance, and capital markets.

Recent Developments

East Coast Earthquake of 2011

On August 23, 2011, a rare, powerful magnitude 5.8 earthquake and aftershocks hit Mineral, VA, prompting the evacuation of buildings and the shutdown of two North Anna Power Plants located about 7 miles from the earthquake's epicenter.[4] The earthquake was felt from Georgia to southeast Canada.[5] Other earthquakes have occurred in the area, but not of this magnitude. According to the USGS, the recent earthquake was the strongest earthquake to hit the entire states since the 5.8 magnitude tremor in 1897. In addition, a 3.6 magnitude earthquake also occurred in Gaithersburg, MD (about 110 miles from the epicenter) on July 16, 2010. Seismologists report that although Virginia is classified as a "moderate" seismic risk zone, since 1977, the state has experienced 160 earthquakes, of which just 16% were felt.[6] The recent event was reportedly 160 times bigger than the 2010 event in Gaithersburg. Total estimates of injuries or physical damage caused by the East Coast earthquake, and its aftershocks, are not readily available. Engineers and disaster experts are assessing the damages.

Japan Earthquake and Tsunamis

Although Japan's losses will reach historic levels, various experts report that the country's relatively strict building codes and early warning system prevented even further destruction and loss of life. Japan is generally considered one of the best prepared nations in the world for earthquakes and tsunamis. Earthquake and tsunami warning systems are extensive there and disaster drills are part of everyday life. Following the 1995 Kobe earthquake, Japan engaged vast resources in developing new techniques to make structures sturdier, including retrofitting older and more vulnerable buildings.

Japan's total economic losses are likely to be much higher than insured losses because property owners without coverage will likely assume most of the burden of losses. Early estimates of the disaster's cost provided by the World Bank place the total losses of houses, factories, and public infrastructure in the range from $122 billion to $235 billion (2.5% to 4% of GDP).[7] The official Japanese government estimate of damage to housing, roads, utilities, and businesses across seven prefectures (states) is between $198 billion and $309 billion—a range that is in line with the World Bank's estimate.[8] In addition, the Japan earthquake and tsunami will be a costly event for the global insurance industry. On April 12, 2011, Risk Management Solutions (RMS), a private catastrophe modeling company, released a new report estimating that insurers will pay $21 billion to $34 billion in damages from the earthquake and tsunami in Japan, making the disaster the most costly for insurers since Hurricane Katrina in 2005.[9] RMS said that the powerful earthquake and the subsequent tsunami resulted in property losses of $18 billion to $26 billion, the most costly earthquake loss in history. RMS estimates that life and health insurance claims related to the disaster will total between $3 billion and $8 billion.[10] Japanese companies or cooperatives are expected to cover many of the home insurance claims while international insurers will cover many of the claims filed by businesses. RMS estimates that commercial and industrial payouts will represent 30% to 35% of property loss, or as much as $9 billion.[11] Financing for Japan's recovery will likely come from the issuance of Japanese government construction bonds, adding to the nation's already high fiscal debt.[12]

The Japanese government is likely to cover some of the damage to residential buildings and pay the liability costs related to the damaged Fukushima Daiichi Nuclear Power Plant. The national government serves as a backup to domestic home insurance and provides insurance covering nuclear plants for major natural disasters.

Nuclear power plant operators in Japan are required to register with the General Insurance Association of Japan and participate in a nuclear insurance plan operated by the Japan Ministry of Education, Culture, Sports, Science and Technology. Damages or claims related to earthquakes and tsunamis are not covered by the insurance association. Under Japan's 1961 Act on Compensation for Nuclear Damage, nuclear facilities operators are not liable for damage caused by their reactors due to "a grave natural disaster of an exceptional character or by an insurrection."[13] As a result, insurers of the nuclear power plant may not have to make payouts.

Japan's national earthquake program buys some external reinsurance coverage and local reinsurance programs are large and well-syndicated across most of the worldwide catastrophe markets. Historically, Japanese homeowners and businesses have been reluctant to buy earthquake insurance, which they perceive as too expensive. Consequently, the cost to insurers for residential property damage may be relatively limited.

U.S. Earthquake Risk Assessment and Exposure

Catastrophe risk management provides a policy framework for formal (e.g., decision analysis, cost-benefit analysis) and intuitive (e.g., rules of thumb) approaches to decision making. This promotes more effective planning to reduce potential losses and the direct and indirect impacts following a disaster. The first step in the risk management process is to define the event itself and the probabilities and consequences associated with it. Physical scientists and engineers provide data on the vulnerability of a region to different types of hazards and assess the risks to different structures and the surrounding environment. Although there are well-developed models specifying earthquake probabilities and consequences, many uncertainties remain regarding these risks, as well as nuclear damage risks.[14] Nevertheless, policymakers use available information to develop a set of risk management strategies for dealing with extreme events.

The remainder of this report provides information and analysis on risk assessment for extreme events and explores the U.S. exposure to seismic risk and the various methods of financing recovery from such losses. Challenges associated with financing earthquake losses with insurance and the feasibility of a federal earthquake insurance scheme are examined. The report concludes with some policy options and questions and summarizes legislative proposals under consideration in Congress.

Risk Assessment

Risk assessment combines information about a physical hazard (e.g., frequency, intensity, location) with information on vulnerability (e.g., exposed population, structures, critical facilities) to determine the likely impacts of a hazardous event.[15] This same risk assessment framework is used by scientists and engineers to develop uniform seismic hazard maps that provide a detailed description of the variations of shaking and damage, which is used to inform risk assessment and public policy on mitigation measures across the country.[16] The important factors to be considered in assessing the seismic hazard are past earthquake data and earthquake source characteristics in the region.

Seismic hazards may be analyzed deterministically by considering a particular earthquake scenario, or probabilistically, by considering the uncertainties involved in earthquake size, location, and time of occurrence.[17] The level of damage is directly proportional to the severity of ground acceleration. Calculating earthquake risk levels depends upon proximity to earthquake faults, the age and type of dwellings, and the soil types near those dwellings. Although progress has been made in the identification of earthquake risk, the delineation of local seismic hazards is still insufficient to accurately determine the risk in many areas. Earthquake maps are national-scale probabilistic estimates of maximum acceleration based on seismicity.

The U.S. Geological Survey National Seismic Hazard Maps display earthquake ground motions for various probability levels across the United States and are applied in seismic provisions of building codes, engineering design standards, estimating potential economic losses, preparing for emergency response, and insurance rates in areas of high risk. These probabilistic seismic hazard maps represent the best available science in earthquake hazards estimation for the United States; they are not intended for site-specific hazard analysis, but to provide a regional perspective on earthquake hazard.

Exposure

Figure 1 depicts a probabilistic earthquake risk map showing maximum horizontal ground acceleration (force per unit of mass) with a 2% probability of being exceeded in 50 years and the sites of operating nuclear power reactors in the United States.[18]

It suggests that potentially damaging earthquakes could occur in many parts of the United States, including the Pacific coast; the Mississippi valley around New Madrid in Missouri; Utah; Idaho; South Carolina; and the New England region around Boston.

Alaska, not shown on the map, is also subject to potentially damaging earthquakes. Scientists predict that there is a 90% chance of a major earthquake in California occurring in the next 30 years, with damage estimates ranging from $60 billion to $70 billion. Moreover, earthquakes can also strike in unexpected places. For example, in April 2002, a 5.1 magnitude earthquake struck the northeastern United States and parts of Canada. The event was centered on the town of Plattsburg, NY. In 1737 and again in 1884, New York City was hit by a 5.1 magnitude earthquake.[19]

Table 1 shows that, on average, more than 3,000 earthquakes strike the United States each year. According to the USGS, only a relatively few earthquakes cause large economic losses because most are small and occur in sparsely populated areas. Most Americans live in areas considered "seismically active," although the degree of vulnerability to earthquake risk varies greatly.[20]

Table 2 shows the 10 costliest world earthquakes and tsunamis ranked by insured losses. **Table 3** shows the deadliest world earthquakes and tsunamis ranked by the number of fatalities.

The world's deadliest seismic event occurred in Port-au-Prince, Haiti, on January 12, 2010, resulting in approximately $8 billion-$14 billion in economic losses but comparatively low insured losses. Because of Haiti's low income rates and limited insurance penetration, insured losses were a fraction of economic losses.[21]

(Peak Ground Acceleration for 2% Probability of Exceedance in 50 Years)

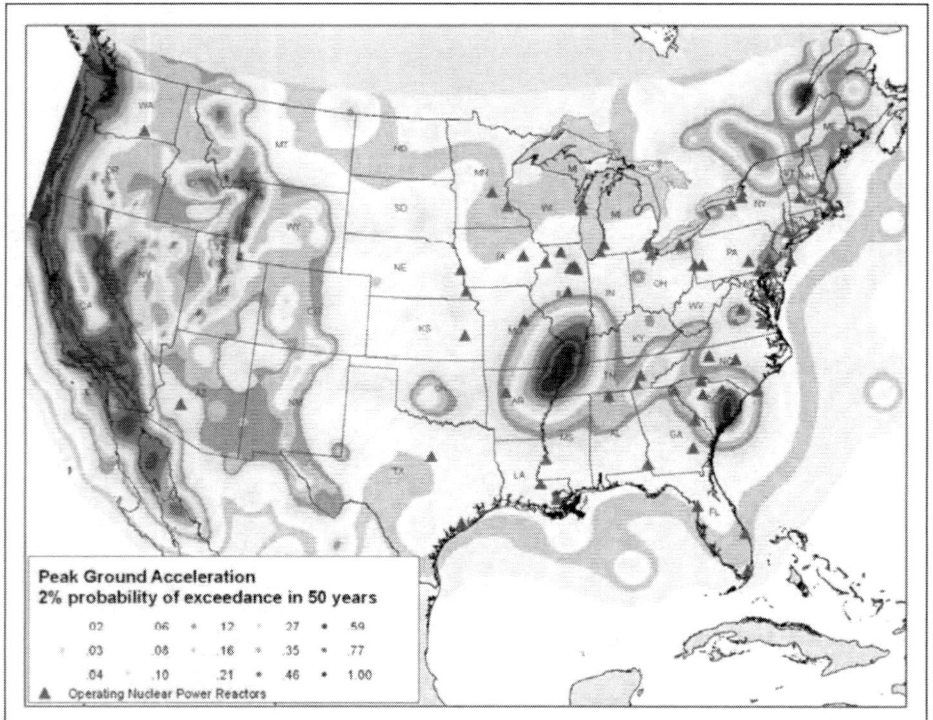

Source: Nuclear Regulatory Commission and United States Geological Survey, at http://pubs.usgs.gov/of/2008/ 1128/pdf/OF08-1128_v1.1.pdf.

Figure 1. Probabilistic Earthquake Hazard Map of the United States.

Table 1. Number of Earthquakes in the United States, 2000-2010

Magnitude	2000	2001	2002	2003	2004	2005	2006	2007	2008	2009	2010
8.0 to 9.9	0	0	0	0	0	0	0	0	0	0	0
7.0 to 7.9	0	1	1	2	0	1	0	1	0	0	0
6.0 to 6.9	6	5	4	7	2	4	7	9	9	3	1
5.0 to 5.9	63	41	63	54	25	47	51	72	85	53	1
4.0 to 4.9	281	290	536	541	284	345	346	366	432	290	16
3.0 to 3.9	917	842	1,535	1,303	1,362	1,475	1,213	1,137	1,486	1,449	40
2.0 to 2.9	660	646	1,228	704	1,336	1,738	1,145	1,173	1,573	2,335	39
1.0 to 1.9	0	2	2	2	1	2	7	11	13	25	1
0.1 to 0.9	90	0	0	0	0	0	1	0	0	1	0
Below 0.1	15	434	507	333	540	73	13	22	20	18	0
Total	**2,342**	**2,261**	**3,876**	**2,946**	**3,550**	**3,685**	**2,783**	**2,791**	**3,618**	**4,174**	**98**

Source: United States Geological Survey, *Earthquake Facts and Statistics*, available at http://earthquake.usgs.gov/earthquakes/eqarchives/year/eqstats.php.

Tsunami Exposure

Tsunamis occur infrequently in the United States. The communities at risk are along the U.S. West Coast, Alaska, and the Pacific region (Hawaii, American Samoa, Guam, Palau, the Federated States of Micronesia, and the Marshall Islands).[22] According to the National Oceanic and Atmospheric Administration (NOAA), during the past 204 years, 24 tsunamis have caused damage in the United States.[23] Although tsunamis pose a particular risk to coastal communities on the Pacific coast, historical records indicate that tsunamis occasionally hit the U.S. northeastern coastal states along the Atlantic Ocean. Tsunamis caused property damages in Puerto Rico in 1918 and Newfoundland, Canada, in 1922. Scientists are also reportedly concerned about the Cumbre Vieja volcano in Las Palmas (Canary Islands). Some geologists believe that a significant volcano eruption in this area could send a tsunami into the eastern seaboards of North and South America.[24]

Table 2. Ten Costliest World Earthquakes and Tsunamis Ranked by Insured Losses, 1980-2011 ($ in billions; before March 11, 2011)

Rank	Date/Year	Location	Losses When Occurred	
			Total	Insured
1	January 17, 1994	Northridge, CA	$44.0	$15.3
2	February 22, 2011	Christchurch, New Zealand	20.0	10.0
3	February 27, 2010	Maule, Chile	30.0	8.0
4	September 3, 2010	Christchurch, New Zealand	6.5	5.0
5	January 17, 1995	Kobe, Japan	100.0	3.0
6	December 26, 2004	Sri Lanka, Indonesia, India	10.0	1.0
7	October 17, 1989	Loma Prieta, CA	10.0	.96
8	October 23, 2004	Niigata, Japan	28.0	.7.
9	September 21, 1999	Nantou, Taiwan	14.0	.75
10	December 28, 1989	Newcastle, Australia	1.2	.67

Source: Munich Re. Geo Risks Research, NatCatService.

Unlike tsunamis that can sometimes be predicted—often (in sufficient time to give a public warning) using underwater sensors, floating data buoys, and radar data from orbiting environmental satellites, earthquakes currently cannot be predicted. However, scientists believe that one day earthquakes will be just as predictable as hurricanes, tornadoes, and other severe storms.[25]

Research to find ways to predict earthquakes is currently being conducted by the USGS and other federal and state agencies, as well as universities and private institutions. Some experts, particularly those at the National Earthquake Information Center, believe that scientists will ultimately be able to forecast earthquakes. In August 2005, a joint team of scientists from Stanford University and the USGS completed drilling a 2.4-mile-deep hole in the San Andreas fault in California to establish the first continuous monitoring probe from inside an active earthquake zone. The study is designed to determine if and how earthquakes can be predicted.

Table 3. Ten Deadliest World Earthquakes and Tsunamis Ranked by the Number of Fatalities, 1980-2011

Rank	Date/Year	Location	Losses When Occurred		
			Overall ($millions)	Insured	Fatalities
1	January 12, 2010	Port-au-Prince, Haiti	$8,000-$14,000	NA	222,500
2	December 26, 2004	Sri Lanka, Indonesia, India	10,000	1,000	220,000
3	October 8, 2005	Pakistan, India, Afghanistan	5,200	5	88,000
4	May 12, 2008	Sichuan, China	85,000	300	84,000
5	June 20-21, 1990	Manjil, Iran	7,100	100	40,000
6	December 26, 2003	Bam, Iran	500	19	26,200
7	December 7, 1988	Spitak, Armenia	14,000	NA	25,000
8	August 17, 1999	Izmit, Turkey	12,000	600	17,100
9	January 26, 2001	Gujarat, India	4,500	100	15,000
10	September 19, 1985	Mexico City, Mexico	4,000	275	9,500

Source: Munich Re. Geo Risks Research, NatCatService.

FINANCING RECOVERY FOLLOWING AN EARTHQUAKE

Financing economic recovery after a major earthquake in the United States is likely to be costly, complex, and involve both private markets and government. With respect to earthquake losses, the federal government is effectively an insurer of last resort for catastrophe risk. The emergence of a public-private earthquake insurance program that does not now exist would involve tradeoffs between moral hazard, adverse selection, loss potential, subsidy, and cost of insurance.

Standard residential homeowners' insurance and commercial casualty insurance coverage would be the most likely to be triggered as a consequence of a catastrophic event. However, because insurance policies protect the insured against a specified loss and insurance policies fall into the realm of private contracts, insurers generally have the authority to determine the scope of the coverage that they offer. As a result, most homeowners' and Commercial General Liability (CGL) policies offered by private insurers are an "all risk" policy, under which only those events that are specified are excluded from coverage. For example, floods and earthquakes typically get special exclusionary treatment.

In the absence of an explicit national earthquake insurance program or requirement, financing disaster recovery comes primarily from state and federal government disaster aid, private and public insurance (where in-force), private loans, contingent financing, and personal savings. Insurance is arguably the most efficient form of pre-disaster risk financing to mitigate potential losses and reduce the financial vulnerability of property owners and governments to earthquake risk exposure. The insurance, and ultimately the reinsurance, sector currently supports most of the costs of natural disasters. However, the capacity of national insurance markets, even backed by international reinsurance, is finite, and the insurance industry may, therefore, not always be in a position to provide sufficient protection in the event of a major natural disaster without endangering its financial viability.

Since the late 1990s, a combination of financial product innovation and deregulation ushered in a new wave of risk management mechanisms, including contingent capital instruments, securitizations, and notes and bonds based on insurance-related events. The idea behind so-called insurance-linked securities (ILS) was the issuance of securities that reference earthquake, hurricane, or windstorm risk to transfer exposures and create additional risk capacity. ILS transactions allowed domestic insurers to leverage retained capital to help increase insurance loss capacity and reduce their financial exposure to extreme events. Catastrophe bonds, for example, currently offer insurers and reinsurers an innovative approach to financing disaster losses by transferring some of the catastrophe risk to global financial markets.

The vast majority of businesses and individuals in seismic zones do not purchase earthquake insurance, preferring to take their chances rather than pay for protection at a cost that many consider too expensive for such a remote event. As a result, the government, through taxpayer- financed federal disaster assistance for disaster victim compensation, has become the de facto insurer of last resort and source of financial protection after a major disaster occurs.

Should a catastrophic earthquake hit the United States in 2011, there is a general consensus that a significant increase in capital is not likely to enter into the insurance market as it did after Hurricane Katrina in 2005. The reason is twofold: excess capital is not currently available in the world's financial markets and there is uncertainty about how and whether to socialize risk for natural disasters (earthquakes and tsunamis) and man-made disasters (nuclear power plant accidents). For example, concerns have been expressed about excessive taxpayer exposure to the risk of a nuclear catastrophe.

Residential Earthquake Insurance

Many people mistakenly assume that their residential insurance policies fully protect them against damage from earthquakes. This report's **Appendix** illustrates the earthquake hazard exclusion language in standard homeowners' insurance policies. Earthquake coverage is available either as an endorsement to an existing homeowner's or business owner's policy, or as a separate policy. It typically includes coverage for damage to the building's structure, contents or personal property, and loss of the structure's use. Commercial earthquake insurance typically also covers the loss of business income. Earthquake damage to vehicles is covered under the comprehensive automobile insurance policy.

According to the Insurance Information Institute, only about 12% of California residents currently have earthquake coverage, down from more than 33% in 1996. The relatively low coverage rate is due to a combination of factors:

- policy premiums are often viewed as too expensive;
- deductibles are perceived as relatively high, often 15% of the amount of the policy (not the loss);
- some homeowners lack knowledge that earthquake coverage is available or are misinformed concerning the terms of such insurance; and
- some homeowners lack incentives to take preventive action to reduce shaking losses, fire losses, and injuries.[26]

California is the only state that requires insurers that sell residential property insurance to offer earthquake coverage to their policyholders. After the 1994 earthquake in Northridge, CA, most insurers in California either stopped selling new homeowners' insurance policies or greatly restricted the sales of such policies. In 1995, as a result of insurers' reluctance to offer earthquake insurance because of the fear of insolvency, the California state legislature created a privately financed, publicly managed organization—the California Earthquake Authority (CEA)—to offer primary coverage for property losses arising from a seismic event. In offering earthquake coverage, insurance companies can become a member of the CEA and offer the CEA's residential earthquake policies, or they can manage the risk themselves. To date, companies that sell over two-thirds of the residential property insurance in the state have opted to become CEA participating companies. The CEA began providing residential earthquake insurance in December 1996 with a $10.5 billion funding package.

The Role of Reinsurance

The insurance industry could not function in its present form without access to traditional reinsurance. Reinsurance is purchased by insurers to hedge their own insurance portfolios. Almost all insurers purchase reinsurance. A reinsurer assumes part of the risk and part of the premiums originally taken by the insurer, known as the primary insurer. Reinsurance is sold in layers. Reinsurers have their own reinsurers, called retrocessionaries.

Under a typical reinsurance transaction, a primary insurer transfers a layer of the risks (and some of the premiums) to a reinsurer who, in turn, accepts a layer of risk and passes the remaining risk to a retrocessionary. As an illustration, under a 300/100 "excess-of-loss" facultative reinsurance agreement[27] between the primary insurer and a reinsurer, if losses from a specific earthquake exceed $300 million, the reinsurer will cover the next $100 million in losses. An earthquake that costs less than $300 million is paid entirely by the primary insurer. The reinsurer might choose to transfer to a retrocessionary a portion or layer of the $100 million. In return for assuming risk, the reinsurer (or retrocessionary) receives a reinsurance premium and agrees to indemnify the insurer (or reinsurer) for claims falling within the terms of the reinsurance agreement.

After the Northridge, CA, earthquake of 1994, large national insurers encountered difficulty in obtaining layers of reinsurance coverage at prices that they considered affordable. As a result, insurers were forced to find alternative sources of capital to underwrite catastrophe risk, which they found in the U.S. equity and debt markets that offered insurers liquidity to expand their capacity to sell catastrophe insurance. Investors, for their part, are attracted to securities that transfer catastrophe risk to the capital markets—the so-called ILS. They are drawn to ILS because the level of return depends solely on the occurrence of a catastrophe that triggers payment and is insensitive to economic factors like interest rates and credit default that give rise to systemic risk in other types of fixed income investments. Some of the existing barriers to the expanded use of ILS are that they tend to be more expensive than traditional reinsurance because the risk premium that investors demand for assuming unfamiliar types of risk is expensive to structure. Although the number of ILS transactions is still relatively small, the markets for these financial instruments are expected to grow.

Financing Recovery Following a Nuclear Incident

Nuclear energy plays an important role in the economy of the United States, but its generation involves certain risks. As the incident in Japan demonstrates, if a nuclear incident occurs, the damage to persons, property, and the environment can be substantial. Claims from a nuclear power incident could arise in several ways: (1) operating a reactor, (2) in the course of transporting nuclear fuel to a reactor site, (3) storage of nuclear fuel or waste at a site, and (4) the transportation of irradiated nuclear fuel and nuclear waste from the reactor. All property and liability insurance policies issued in the United States exclude nuclear accidents.

Three layers of defense exist to address potential nuclear damages: prevention, response, and the allocation of responsibility for repairing the damage and compensating victims. This is the function of nuclear liability law. The international liability regime relating to nuclear activities is quite unique. From the inception of the nuclear industry, countries realized that a special liability regime would be necessary, both nationally and internationally, due to the hazardous nature of nuclear activities and the complexities of the processes involved. The earliest national liability laws were adopted in the United States in 1957, and in Europe in 1959.

The centerpiece of nuclear legislation in the United States is the Atomic Energy Act of 1954, as amended. The federal government has assumed most of the responsibility for the regulation of nuclear energy. For example, federal legislation and administrative regulations govern facility licensing. States can regulate those nuclear activities that the federal government has chosen not to address so long as state regulation does not conflict with federal law.

Claims resulting from nuclear accidents are covered under the Price-Anderson Nuclear Industries Indemnity Act of 1957.[28] The 1957 act added Section 170 to the Atomic Energy Act of 1954 to address offsite nuclear accident liability and to encourage private industry to participate in the nuclear industry by assisting it with the costs of liability anticipated in the case of a nuclear incident occurring within the United States.

The act created a mixed system of compulsory commercial insurance coverage (to satisfy financial responsibility requirements) and emergency compensation funding to lessen the financial impact of post-accident litigation on holders of nuclear power plant licenses. It sought to ensure that adequate funds would be available to satisfy liability claims of members of the public for bodily injury, sickness, disease or death, or loss of or damage to property, or for loss of the use of property in the event of a nuclear accident involving a commercial nuclear power plant. The act helped encourage private investment in commercial nuclear power by placing a cap, or ceiling on the total amount of liability each holder of a nuclear power plant licensee faced in the event of an accident.

Recovery to accident victims is available through common law liability, coverage by private insurance, and government indemnification (reimbursement). Licensees must maintain financial security against offsite liability for a nuclear accident in an amount equal to that available through private insurance. This effectively represents a subsidy to the nuclear power industry. Without this protection, it is widely believed that commercial nuclear power development would not have developed as it has.

All nuclear reactor operators must participate in the program. The statute requires operators to obtain the maximum amount of private insurance coverage available. Under existing policy, owners of nuclear power plants pay a premium each year for $375 million in private insurance for offsite liability coverage for each reactor unit. This primary, or first tier, insurance is supplemented by a second tier. In the event a nuclear accident caused damages in excess of $375 million, each licensee would be assessed a prorated share of the excess up to $111.9 million. The "limit of liability" for a nuclear accident has increased the insurance pool to more than $12 billion. With 104 reactors currently licensed to operate, this secondary tier of funds contains about $11.6 billion. If 15% of these funds are expended, prioritization of the remaining amounts would be left to a federal district court. If the second tier is depleted, Congress is committed to determine whether additional disaster relief is required. Thus, the burden of exceeding the fund's limits could fall on the accident victims if the government chooses not to intervene.

Under the Price-Anderson Act, victims of nuclear accidents are free to pursue tort claims for property damage and personal injuries against the reactor operators or any other potentially responsible party in accordance with state tort law. The only limitation imposed by the act on recovery in such lawsuits is in the form of the total monetary cap on insurance funding. In the event of "extraordinary nuclear occurrence"[29] the act requires all claims to be consolidated in federal court. The act creates strict liability in tort for licensees involved in nuclear incidents and abrogates the defense of contributory negligence. Each individual claimant still bears the burden of establishing causation and particularized proof of economic loss and intangible harm.[30]

CHALLENGES IN FINANCING EXTREME EVENT LOSSES

The 112th Congress may choose to assess whether existing sources of funding of catastrophe losses will be adequate to finance recovery from a mega-catastrophe earthquake or other extreme events. In the aftermath of mounting natural disaster losses over the past two decades, property and casualty insurers have sought to limit their exposure to catastrophe risk while simultaneously exploring new and innovative sources of capital aimed at financing catastrophe losses.

Although private insurers are skilled at handling high-frequency, low-severity "non-catastrophic" events, like auto and home losses, that follow a relatively predictable claims frequency and magnitude, they face substantially greater difficulty when attempting to price and insure low- probability, high-consequence (LP-HC) risk. The problem is the finite amount of protection (capacity) that the insurance industry can offer against highly correlated risk that can produce catastrophic losses. The amount of private catastrophe insurance coverage is limited by the potential magnitude of possible insured losses, the sporadic and unpredictable nature of these events, and the ability to accurately estimate future losses and price coverage. Moreover, existing regulatory and accounting systems also result in catastrophe reserves being taxed as profits, discouraging insurers from accumulating loss reserves for catastrophes. Current tax laws discourage the establishment of financial reserve funds for a loss that has not yet occurred.

The private sector's coverage of catastrophe risk is limited by

- actuarial and rate-setting difficulties;
- industry capacity to meet the payout requirements resulting from a mega-catastrophic earthquake;
- difficulties in determining both the insurability of properties and the damages resulting from earthquakes;
- adverse selection and risk-spreading difficulties, including those associated with reinsurance;
- accounting and federal tax policy constraints on the accumulation of insurance company catastrophe loss reserves; and
- ineffectiveness of current loss-reducing activities (building-code enforcement and land-use zoning).

A general discussion of these interrelated challenges follows.

Actuarial and Rate-Setting Difficulties

One set of challenges facing private insurers involves actuarial and rate-setting difficulties that stem from the lack of sufficient data on past losses to accurately estimate probabilities of future losses and the potential for catastrophic losses that can jeopardize insurers' financial viability. Estimating future losses is difficult because earthquakes occur infrequently and the magnitude of losses is highly uncertain. Insurers must instead predict losses from technical studies and computer simulation models, which may arguably be no more reliable than actual prior historical loss data.

Insurers need to set a premium for each potential customer or class of customers to generate enough revenue to both cover the expected loss and earn a profit. Insurers must be able to estimate the frequency of specific events occurring and the magnitude of the loss should the event occur, a condition limited by the low-probability/high-consequence nature of earthquake risk and the difficulty in identifying what losses may occur. Insurance companies risk insolvency or being uncompetitive by underpricing or overpricing, respectively.

Adverse Selection and Risk Spreading

Insurers also face adverse selection and risk-spreading difficulties, including access to adequate reinsurance for earthquake peril. Their problem is that risk is not sufficiently spread over a larger geographical area, including areas which are relatively unlikely to suffer a catastrophic earthquake. Traditional insurance principles for insurability require that there is sufficient demand to yield appropriate levels of income revenue for insurers to supply the coverage. There is a tendency for mostly high-risk consumers to purchase policies. This results in a poor spread of risk and an inadequate premium base. Economists note that this "adverse selection" problem in insurance markets generally persists for two reasons: (1) the insured possess information on their particular risk, which is unknown to the insurer; and (2) consumers have short time horizons in determining the expected benefits relative to the up-front costs (rates and deductibles), or compare costs with potential benefits and conclude that loss-reduction measures are not good investments.

Tax, Accounting, and Regulatory Constraints

Another set of challenges to financing catastrophe risks involves tax policy and regulatory constraints on the accumulation of insurance company catastrophe loss reserves and the industry's ability to raise external capital during times of financial crisis. Under current federal income tax provisions, premiums collected by insurers and placed in a reserve fund for catastrophes are treated as excess profits and taxed at the corporate income tax rate. Insurers view this as a major impediment to the marketing of earthquake insurance, and they have supported a longer loss carry-forward period or tax-free reserves for potential earthquake losses.[31] Insurers might consider offering insurance coverage at a price level high enough to cover the high-end in the range of expected losses. The rate, however, would be so high that it may not be marketable to the average household and regulators may not approve extremely high catastrophe rates. At this point, insurers typically have opted to withdraw from lines of insurance in catastrophe-prone areas.[32]

A high percentage of property owners in areas prone to earthquakes do not have earthquake insurance, relying instead on good fortune or federal emergency disaster relief assistance to cover uninsured losses. Researchers have found that Americans are reluctant to purchase earthquake insurance because of the high cost of insurance and low likelihood of a disaster.[33]

Moreover, earthquake insurance is not required as a condition for federally secured mortgages, as it is currently in the case of flood insurance in federally designated flood zones. Fannie Mae and Freddie Mac require homeowners with federally backed mortgages to buy insurance for flood and windstorm damage, but not for earthquakes. Fannie and Freddie would arguably change the landscape for homeowners' property insurance if they required coverage for earthquakes. The penetration of earthquake insurance has been low, and the government, through disaster relief assistance, continues to serve as the predominant bearer of earthquake catastrophe risk.

In the event of a major disaster, lack of insurance or underinsurance against earthquakes could negatively affect bond and equity markets, the mortgage loan industry, and government budgets at all levels. With roughly 12% to 15% of exposed mortgage properties covered by earthquake insurance nationwide, a mega-catastrophe could leave a number of mortgages in default with lack of sufficient underlying market value. In the case of mortgages that are packaged and sold by federal mortgage agencies, uninsured losses are absorbed by the U.S. Treasury, a situation that could adversely affect the U.S. financial system and do little to help the owners of the distressed properties. In addition, federal, state, and local governments would likely be called upon to expend funds in emergency response and recovery at the same time as they lose tax revenues. Meanwhile, federal policymakers have focused on finding ways to enhance the private sector's ability to spread risk.

IS FEDERAL EARTHQUAKE INSURANCE FEASIBLE?

As stated earlier, a basic principle of insurance is the reduction of overall risk by pooling or spreading individual, independent risks. Insurance companies typically price risks where the frequency and severity of potential claims are limited, estimable, and stable. This principle and insurance practice tends not to hold when a single event affects many insureds simultaneously, as in the case of a major earthquake. In the event of uninsured losses, the federal government has become the de facto bearer of much of the burden for the uninsured cost of repairing or reconstructing buildings damaged by catastrophic earthquakes. Another option would be to create a national catastrophe fund (federal residential earthquake insurance program) to ensure adequate capacity and solvency of the insurance industry to meet consumer demand for protection against earthquake risks, which could, over the long term, minimize federal outlays for uninsured losses.

Advocates of an explicit government insurance program argue that it would offer several advantages: limited insurer insolvency risk, the ability of the government to spread risk over time, financing of short-run losses by borrowing, and lower requirements for federal disaster relief. The disadvantages would be the potential burden on taxpayers, weak underwriting incentives to keep the cost of claims low, preemption of existing and future private sector capacity, difficulty in implementing or sustaining risk-based pricing in a political environment, and potential impediments to capital market innovations, such as catastrophe bonds and options, that securitize catastrophe risk.

Since the late 1960s, the prevailing view among federal and state legislators and regulators has been that earthquake risks could be managed and financed in the private sector. Congress explicitly chose not to implement a federal earthquake insurance program because the justification that the earthquake hazards could not be insured by the private sector had not been convincingly made. Policy debate during and after the 88th Congress following the 1964 earthquake and accompanying tsunami at Alaska's Prince William Sound led to the creation in 1968 of the National Flood Insurance Program (NFIP).[34] Congress, however, waited until 1977 before addressing earthquake hazards with the creation of the National Earthquake Hazards Reduction Program (NEHRP).[35] NEHRP established for the first time a federal policy to encourage research on and implementation of methods to reduce earthquake losses.

Substantial progress has been made in the fields of earthquake science and engineering following the implementation of NEHRP, particularly with respect to seismic hazard identification and strategies to reduce seismic vulnerability of facilities and systems through land use practices and improvements in design and construction techniques. Disaster policy experts agree that despite the efforts of four federal agencies that collaborate under the NEHRP, one issue that has not been adequately addressed is the economic consequences of a catastrophic earthquake, and the efficiency and adequacy of present mechanisms for financing catastrophic earthquake recovery. NEHRP was not required to address this issue.

POLICY ISSUES AND QUESTIONS

The 112th Congress may choose to examine some of the following policy questions with respect to earthquake risk, insurance, and recovery:

- Is earthquake risk uninsurable in the private market?
- Is a federal residential earthquake insurance program feasible?
- What are the costs and benefits of government intervention in the catastrophe insurance market?
- Do benefits outweigh costs to taxpayers for providing a financial backstop for the insurance industry?
- Should federal earthquake insurance be compulsory, and, if so, what would be the enforcement mechanism?
- What role should land-use regulations and building codes have in mitigating disaster risk? Is current insurance regulation conducive to creating private sector incentives for mitigation?

Insurance market experts agree that the risk of a mega-catastrophic event could pose a significant capacity and liquidity problem for insurers who receive relatively stable premium flows but suddenly need large amounts of cash to cover disaster losses. A sudden loss of policyholder surplus, which is the statutory net worth or cushion available to insurers for handling the unexpected, could have an adverse effect on the financial strength of the property and casualty insurance industry. To better manage catastrophe risk, insurers have sought to raise premiums, impose a percentage deductible, and reduce the amount of concentration of their exposures. These changes have led to availability and affordability problems for many homeowners in disaster-prone areas.

The Japan earthquake and tsunami suggest several approaches to catastrophe risk and insurance issues, including (1) revisiting the nature and extent of earthquake and tsunami hazards in the United States and (2) addressing the challenges of financing recovery given limited capacity of national insurance markets to absorb the cost and economic burden of a devastating mega- earthquake. Given the economic devastation in Japan, there is heightened congressional interest in finding ways to reduce disaster risk for homeowners, insurance companies, financial firms, and federal and state governments. Members of Congress could decide to explore alternative policy designs and to consider ways to assist the private sector to pre-fund and diversify disaster risk by financing catastrophic losses through insurance, reinsurance, and capital from financial institutions and the investment community.

Finally, various government actions, such as those designed to increase access to federal disaster assistance or insurance, are likely to affect the behavior of individuals and firms in responding to catastrophe risk. For example, by reducing the financial risks of disaster-prone areas, new federal policies could create financial incentives for some people to move into harm's way, which would increase the potential for catastrophic property damages and economic losses. Hencc, Congress will find no shortage of issues to debate and resolve when considering proposals to establish a federal earthquake insurance program.

LEGISLATION

On March 17, 2011, Senators Barbara Boxer and Dianne Feinstein introduced S. 637, Earthquake Insurance Affordability Act. S. 637 would authorize the U.S. Treasury to guarantee up to $5 billion in bonds available to state certified public entities, like the California Earthquake Authority (CEA), following a catastrophic seismic event. The state entity would have to exhaust its claims-paying ability before the federal guarantee becomes available. The measure is designed to reduce earthquake insurance rates by reducing the need for insurers to purchase reinsurance. The bond would be repaid with premiums.

APPENDIX. STANDARD PROPERTY INSURANCE EARTHQUAKE AND FLOOD EXCLUSION LANGUAGE

We do not pay for loss resulting directly or indirectly from any of the following, even if other events or happenings contributed concurrently, or in sequence, to the loss:

(1) by earth movement, due to natural or man-made events, meaning earthquake including land shock waves, or tremors before, during or after a volcanic eruption, mine subsidence; landslide; mud-slide; mud flow; earth sinking; rising or shifting. Direct loss by Fire, Explosion, Sonic Boom, Theft, or Breaking of Glass resulting from earth movement, mine subsidence, landslide, mud-slide, mud flow, earth sinking, rising or shifting is covered.

(2) by water damage, meaning:

(a) flood, surface water, waves, tides, tidal waves or overflow of a body of water. We do not cover spray from any of these, whether or not driven by wind;

(b) water or sewage which backs up through sewers or drains; or

(c) water below the surface of the ground. This includes water which experts pressure on, or flows, seeps or leaks through any of a building or other structure, sidewalk, driveway, foundation, or swimming pool.

End Notes

[1] Geologists know very little about what causes earthquakes in some parts of the eastern United States; there is no clear association among seismicity, geological structure, and surface displacement. In contrast, seismic activity in the western United States, the mid-Atlantic, central Appalachian, and the Atlantic Coastal Plain regions are associated with movement along known earthquake faults.

[2] See *Japan Earthquake – Mourning the Death/Destruction and Returning to Normal*, located at http://earthquake- report.com/2011/03/28/japan-earthquake-mourning-the-deathdestruction-and-returning-to-normal-life-part-8/.

[3] P.L. 85-256; 71 Stat. 576.

[4] According to the Nuclear Regulatory Commission, the North Anna nuclear power plants lost power from the grid and switched to four diesel generators.

[5] The USGS received reports that the seismic waves were felt as far away as Montreal, Canada, and Jacksonville, Florida.

[6] Joel Achenbach, "5.8 Virginia Earthquake Shakes East Coast, Rattles Residents," *Washington Post*, August 23, 2011, at http://www.washingtonpost.com/earthquake-rattles-washington-area/2011/08/23/gIQATMOGZJ_print.html.

[7] Victoria Kim,"Japan Damage Could Reach $235 billion, World Bank Estimates," *Los Angeles Times*, at http://articles.latimes.com/2011/mar/21/world/la-fgw-japan-quake-world-bank-20110322.

[8] See, Jap*an Earthquake Damage*, at http://earthquake-report.com/2011/03/23/japan-earthquake-damage-catdat-did-come-up-with-a-reliable-estimate-only-90-minutes-after-the-earthquake/.

[9] *RMS Released Insured Loss Estimate for Tohoku Earthquake and Tsunami*, April 12, 2011, at http://www.rms.com/ news/NewsPress/PR_041211_TohokuEQ.asp.

[10] Ibid.

[11] Ibid.

[12] According to the *Central Intelligence Agency, The World Factbook*, Japan ranks first among nations in terms of public debt (i.e., cumulative total government borrowings) as a percentage of GDP, which stood at 225.8% in 2010. In contrast, the United States ranked 37th with 58.9%. Public debt is different from external debt, which reflects the foreign currency liabilities of both the private and public sector and must be financed out of foreign exchange earnings.

[13] Act No. 147 of 1961.

[14] For some hazards, like nuclear incidents and acts of terrorism, the estimation of the probability distributions is so uncertain that estimates of these risks are much less reliable. There is no universally accepted methodology for developing joint probabilities for multiple threats involving earthquakes, tsunamis, and nuclear incidents.

[15] Risk is usually defined in terms of a probability, consequence, potential threat or the possibility of deviation from the expected.

[16] Seismic hazard maps typically include the best available science, including information on fault slip rates, paleoseismologic data from fault trenching studies, earthquake catalogs, and strong-motion recordings from global earthquakes. Paleoseismology is used in the

calculation of seismic hazards by looking at geologic sediments and rocks for signs of ancient earthquakes.

[17] The seismic hazard maps do not include hazards from ground deformation such as liquefaction, landslides, or surface fault ruptures.

[18] The 2% probability of being surpassed in 50 years may be misleading because some parts of the country that have not experienced earthquakes for 200 years or more might be more susceptible to earthquakes than areas that have experienced recent earthquakes. The reason is that earthquake faults build up tension over long periods of time, which become earthquakes when that tension is released suddenly. It is theorized that relatively recent earthquake activity means that faults have released built-up tension—a lack of earthquake activity can mean that tension is still building and could be released at any time as an earthquake.

[19] "When the Earth Moves," *Reinsurance: Global Risk Analysis*, February 2005, p. 14.

[20] A.M. Best Company, Inc., *2006 Annual Earthquake Study*, October 16, 2006.

[21] London-based Axco Insurance Information Services Ltd. estimates that total non-life insurance premiums in Haiti amount to less than $20 million annually. See http://www.claimsmag.com/News/2010/1/Pages/Haiti-Lacks-Insurance-for-Earthquake-Losses.aspx.

[22] Tsunamis can also travel upstream in coastal estuaries and rivers, and cause damage further inland than the immediate coast.

[23] For more information on the U.S. exposure to tsunamis, see answers to questions posed to Admiral Conrad Lautenbaucher, Administrator of NOAA, available at http://whitehouse.gov/ask/print/20050114.html.

[24] Morgan O'Rourke, "Danger on the Coast: Coastal Catastrophe Risk," *Risk Management Magazine*, March 2005, p. 32.

[25] Center for Earthquake Research and Information, The University of Memphis, "100% Chance of an Earthquake Today," available at http://www.ceri.memphis.edu/ public/eqtoday.shtml.

[26] Howard Kunreuther and Paul R. Kleindorfer, "Managing Catastrophe Risk: Why Do Homeowners, Insurers, and Banks Not Use Simple Measures to Mitigate the Risk from Hurricanes and Earthquakes?" *Regulation*, vol. 23, iss. 4, March 8, 2001.

[27] The two most common types of reinsurance arrangements are treaty reinsurance and facultative reinsurance. Under treaty reinsurance, the reinsurer agrees to assume a certain percentage, up to preset limits, of all risks falling into the categories agreed in advance between the two parties. By contrast, a facultative reinsurer agreement is used for very large risks that treaties cannot absorb, and unique risks for which it is difficult to establish a reinsurance treaty. Under the facultative reinsurance agreement, the reinsurer is free to decline to cover a particular risk.

[28] P.L. 85-256; 71 Stat. 576, 42 U.S.C. §2012.

[29] "Extraordinary nuclear occurrence" is defined as "any event causing a discharge or dispersal of source, special nuclear, or byproduct material…in amounts offsite, or causing radiation levels offsite," 42 U.S.C §2014(j).

[30] 10 C.F.R §140.81.

[31] For more information, see CRS Report RL33060, *Tax Deductions for Catastrophic Risk Insurance Reserves: Explanation and Economic Analysis*, by Rawle O. King.

[32] In 1996, the California Legislature created the California Earthquake Authority (CEA) to sell residential property insurance in California. Insurers in the state can choose to offer their own privately funded earthquake insurance product or they can become a participating insurance company of the CEA. Only participating insurance companies can offer CEA earthquake insurance policies.

[33] Howard Kunreuther and Paul R. Kleindorfer, "Managing Catastrophe Risk: Why Do Homeowners, Insurers, and Banks Not Use Simple Measures to Mitigate the Risk from Hurricanes and Earthquakes?" *Regulation*, vol. 23, iss. 4, March 8, 2001.

[34] The National Flood Insurance Program was established under the National Flood Insurance Act of 1968 (P.L. 90- 448, title XIII, §1360, August 1, 1968, 82 Stat. 476, codified at 42 U.S.C. §§4001-4128).

[35] The NEHRP was established by the Earthquake Hazard Reduction Act of 1977 (P.L. 95-124; 91 Stat. 1098; Oct. 7, 1977). The NEHRP involves four agencies: Federal Emergency Management Agency (FEMA); National Institute of Standards and Technology (NIST); National Science Foundation (NSF); and United States Geological Survey (USGS). The goals of NEHRP are to (1) reduce earthquake losses, (2) improve techniques to reduce seismic vulnerability of facilities and systems, (3) improve seismic hazards identification and risk-assessment methods and their use, and (4) improve the understanding of earthquakes and their effects.

In: Natural Catastrophes
Editor: Oliver H. Rohde

ISBN: 978-1-62948-449-5

Chapter 3

THE NATIONAL FLOOD INSURANCE PROGRAM: STATUS AND REMAINING ISSUES FOR CONGRESS*

Rawle O. King

SUMMARY

In late October 2012, Hurricane Sandy caused widespread flood-related property damage in coastal areas of states throughout the Northeast and the mid-Atlantic region. The storm exposed vulnerabilities in the region's public transportation and infrastructure and underscored the nation's growing exposure to extreme weather events, sea-level rise, and coastal flooding. Although the full economic cost of Sandy will not be known for years, the storm has resulted in substantial federal disaster recovery assistance, including tens of billions for flood and hurricane protection and coastal restoration, and the rebuilding of mass transit systems and housing.

Government payouts under the National Flood Insurance Program (NFIP) are estimated to be between $12 billion and $15 billion in flood insurance claims. In the immediate aftermath of Sandy, this amount quickly exceeded the $4 billion in cash and remaining borrowing authority from the Treasury Department. By January 2013, the NFIP had processed more than 140,000

---

* This is an edited, reformatted and augmented version of the Congressional Research Service Publication, CRS Report for Congress R42850, dated February 6, 2013.

claims for Sandy-related damages totaling about $1.7 billion. To protect the financial integrity of the NFIP and ensure that the NFIP has the financial resources to cover its existing commitments following the devastation caused by Sandy, the Obama Administration requested that Congress pass legislation to increase the NFIP's borrowing authority. On January 4, 2013, Congress passed, and the President two days later signed into law, H.R. 41 to provide a $9.7 billion increase in the NFIP's borrowing authority, from $20.725 billion to $30.425 billion, to pay flood claims related to Hurricane Sandy.

Policymakers have expressed views on several flood management challenges facing the NFIP. These challenges include finding ways to (1) improve the accuracy of flood risk assessment and mapping of hurricane and coastal storm hazard areas; (2) strengthen the financial sustainability of the NFIP in the face of expected future extreme weather events (climate change), sea-level rise, and coastal flooding; (3) address potential affordability challenges associated with mandatory purchase requirements and implementation of full actuarial premium rates, beginning in 2014; (4) reduce the likelihood of future emergency supplemental spending to finance recurring recovery expenditures by making communities stronger and more resilient; (5) address uncertainty surrounding human settlement patterns and the NFIP's ability to contain the nation's growing exposure to floods; and (6) explore the creation of effective hazard-reduction strategies—linked to land use planning techniques (and construction standards)—to direct development and people out of, and away from, flood-prone areas.

Early in 2012, Congress passed and President Barack Obama signed into law the Biggert-Waters Flood Insurance Reform Act of 2012, P.L. 112-141. The law reauthorized the NFIP through September 30, 2017, and made a number of reforms to strengthen the future financial solvency and administrative efficiency of the NFIP. In the wake of Sandy, Congress might choose to consider policy options to achieve greater sustainability and cost savings by addressing long-term flood management challenges. Options include the use of flood policies (10-20 years, rather than 1 year), privatization of flood risk, issuance of community based flood insurance contracts, and regulatory and tax changes to encourage financial innovation in financing recovery from large- scale natural disasters.

This report provides an analysis of flood risk management, summarizes major challenges facing the NFIP, and outlines key reforms enacted in the Flood Insurance Reform Act of 2012. The report identifies and presents some key remaining flood management issues for congressional consideration, and concludes with a discussion of policy options for the future financial management of flood hazards in the United States.

On October 29, 2012, Hurricane Sandy hit the East Coast, flooding some coastal areas and causing massive economic disruptions in states throughout the Northeast and the mid-Atlantic region. Communities in New York, New Jersey, and Connecticut were particularly hard hit. In the wake of disaster recovery from Hurricane Sandy, policymaker attention has refocused on the effectiveness of the existing unified national program for floodplain management in reducing the loss of life and property from weather-related coastal hazards (hurricanes, storm surges, and tornadoes), aging coastal protection infrastructure and increasing vulnerability to storm impacts, persistently low insurance participation in the National Flood Insurance Program (NFIP), and the escalating cost of flooding to taxpayers.

Despite billions spent on preparedness and structural[1] and non-structural[2] mitigation measures to reduce disaster-related losses, the nation faces growing exposure to flood-related losses. Some argue that storms of Sandy's strength and intensity will occur more frequently, resulting in increasing incidents of major flooding and damage. This situation raises at least five policy concerns and questions. First, is federal flood insurance that complements land use management still a workable method of managing flood risk, reducing the costs and human suffering from floods, and distributing burdens equitably among those protected by flood insurance and the general public? Second, is flood risk possible for private insurers to underwrite? Third, could flood risk be effectively transferred to the private sector through reinsurance or to capital markets through catastrophe bonds? Fourth, should the NFIP debt to the Treasury be forgiven? Fifth, are the consequences of flood risks and the level of protection offered by hurricane protection systems communicated effectively to the public? These are some of the issues of contention that remain after recently passed NFIP-reform legislation in Congress.

This report provides an analysis of U.S. flood risk management policy, summarizes major challenges facing the NFIP, and outlines key insurance reform provisions in the Biggert-Waters Flood Insurance Reform Act of 2012 (Flood Insurance Reform Act of 2012).[3] The report also identifies and presents some key remaining flood management issues of contention for congressional consideration, and it concludes with a discussion of policy options for the future financial management of flood hazard costs.

Background

The United States is a geographically diverse nation exposed to hydro-meteorological (weather, climate, and water-related) perils that each year cause widespread physical and economic damage and threaten human life and fragile ecosystems. Already the most costly and prevalent natural disaster risk in the United States, incidents of flooding appear to be increasing.[4] The traditional method of flood hazard mitigation has been to build levees and other flood control structures to keep water away from population centers and agricultural areas. Beginning in the 1950s and 1960s, with the nation facing higher-than-expected flood losses from weather-related disasters and breached levees, policymakers shifted focus from purely structural flood controls toward a system that included both structural and non-structural risk mitigation strategies.

The Regulatory Flood Management "Fix"

In 1968, Congress established the NFIP as a unified floodplain management strategy to reduce property losses from flood peril and public spending to compensate disaster victims. Today, the Department of Homeland Security's (DHS's) Federal Emergency Management Agency (FEMA) administers the program by developing flood hazard maps that are used to set flood insurance rates, regulate floodplain development, and inform those who live in the "100-year" floodplain of potential flood hazards.[5]

FEMA reports that the existing "unified floodplain management strategy" saves the nation an estimated $1.6 billion annually in avoided flood losses.[6] These savings are achieved, for example, when buildings are constructed in compliance with NFIP building standards.[7] However, new social and economic challenges, such as the growth in population and property values in coastal areas, have arisen that complicates the existing challenges facing U.S. flood management policy. These challenges could require congressional oversight and possible regulatory reforms.

Issues of Contention

From a policymaker's perspective, the fundamental flood management challenge facing the NFIP is finding the best mix of strategies to reduce the nation's long-term exposure to flood losses while ensuring the program's solvency and statutory mandate to provide affordable flood insurance to the general public. These two policy objectives raise several broad post-reform policy questions:

- How can FEMA balance the program's fiscal soundness and actuarial rates with the affordability of flood insurance?
- How can the nation reduce the escalating cost of flooding and need for taxpayer- financed disaster assistance or weather-induced catastrophic floods?
- How to incentivize potentially at-risk property and business owners in coastal watershed counties or floodplain areas to purchase flood insurance protection while encouraging state and local governments to make appropriate land use adjustment to constrict the development of land in high risk flood zones?
- How can the private-sector's role be expanded in assuming NFIP flood risk?

Hurricanes Katrina and Rita (2005) and Sandy (2012) illustrate the potential cost and consequence of the nation's growing exposure to hurricane-induced coastal flooding and the tens of billions of tax dollars that would likely be spent on compensating flood victims and coastal reconstruction in the aftermath of storms. In this context, five issues are worthy of mention.

First, under the current flood risk management regulatory framework, residents who have a federally backed mortgage and live in a floodplain are required to have insurance against flood. However, these individuals often do not purchase the mandatory insurance coverage. Estimates are that only 15% to 25% of at-risk properties in Special Flood Hazard Areas (SFHA) in the Northeast were insured for flood losses.[8] Only 38,785 residential and business policies were in force in New York City, out of an estimated 7.2 million households (2010 census), as of August 31, 2012; and only 8,129 households (out of about 39,000 households) and businesses in Atlantic City, NJ, had federal flood insurance coverage.[9] Nationally, recent reports suggested that only 18% of Americans in flood zone areas have flood insurance, which raised the possibility of high uninsured flood-related losses.[10] The transition toward full-actuarial rates could create an increasing financial burden on federal taxpayers who often fund emergency supplemental appropriations for disaster relief assistance.

Second, individuals tend to misunderstand flood risk, thinking that after a 100-year flood occurs, they are safe for another 100 years. Behavioral scientists have noted that many individuals in flood-prone areas often dismiss low-probability catastrophic events, misunderstand the risk- spreading function of insurance, and tend to be optimistic regarding the prospects of damage to their property.[11] The reality is that a 100-year flood only refers to a probability and that multiple "100-year" floods could occur in a row.[12] Some disaster experts believe a better way of portraying flood risk would be to refer to the 100-year flood in probabilistic terms as the "1% annual chance flood."

Third, NFIP insurance rates might not adequately reflect the actual flood risk. There is some anecdotal evidence which suggests that if property owners had to incur more of the cost of locating in flood-prone areas, they would make more efficient location decisions. One recent study suggested that NFIP's current rates are about a third of the true market-risk cost of flood insurance.[13] Congress established the NFIP with the statutory mandate that coverage be widely available and affordable. Rates are affordable because, unlike private insurers who are subject to state insurance regulatory requirements, the federal flood insurance program does not buy reinsurance or have to set rates to cover the cost of capital, taxes, and contingent reserves. The federal government serves as a direct primary insurer of last resort, diversifying (spreading) flood risk geographically through the mandatory purchase requirement and over time with the program's authorization to borrow from the Treasury.

Separately, FEMA's new digital flood maps might not meet certain flood hazard data quality standards.[14] For example, the maps do not adequately delineate areas of storm water and groundwater flooding or capture increases in localized storm water runoff flooding resulting from development, deforestation, and other land use changes.

FEMA has indicated it recognizes this challenge and has undertaken many changes in its flood map assessment and mapping standards to accurately reflect risk on flood maps, but more changes might be needed.[15] A potential reform could be to adopt a different regulatory standard of protection, such as the 1-in-250-year or 1-in-500-year flood events, and to replace FEMA flood maps with those that contain high-accuracy and high-resolution land surface elevation data.

Adopting accurate flood maps that require new or sharply higher insurance premiums associated with greater risk exposure could cause unintended consequences that would require congressional oversight to ensure households and businesses are able to comply with the regulatory changes.

Policymakers will likely be called upon to balance the presumed tradeoffs between keeping insurance affordable and widely available, as it has been since the NFIP's inception, and the regulatory changes needed to ensure the long-term financial viability of the NFIP. Driving debate surrounding this tradeoff is the reality of the large and growing segment of the U.S. population subject to the 1% annual chance coastal flood hazard[16] and the increasing frequency and severity of hurricane-induced floods.

Fourth, the increasing public cost of post-disaster recovery financing is another issue of contention that may merit future congressional oversight. Rebuilding of infrastructure like roads, bridges, and utilities in disaster-prone areas in the aftermath of Hurricane Sandy is expected to cost taxpayers tens of billions of dollars, but an exact figure is still not known. Some experts have expressed concerns about taxpayer-financed rebuilding that duplicates the vulnerability that existed before Hurricane Sandy. The policy challenge may be to identify those disaster-prone areas that it no longer makes sense to rebuild (in light of future coastal hazards) and to develop a culture of building construction that reduces the nation's increasing flood risk vulnerability.

A related issue of contention is the notion that many at-risk property owners do not think flood insurance is a good investment or opt to finance post-disaster reconstruction with federal-disaster assistance, albeit insurance is generally considered the most effective way to finance post-disaster recovery. The Flood Insurance Reform Act of 2012, P.L. 112-141, includes a provision to raise historically low premiums and reduce homeowners' incentives for rebuilding in flood risk zones.

Some critics point out that the costs—financial risk and ecological damage—are widely distributed to taxpayers across the country and the benefits, by contrast, are disproportionately enjoyed by wealthy counties and by owners of vacation homes.[17] However, not all beneficiaries of the NFIP are wealthy, and primary homes are also affected by the NFIP.

Fifth, hazard mitigation is considered an important element in reducing flood losses, but it is not always incorporated in risk management decision making at all levels of the government and in the private sector. For example, while local community officials might understand that for every hazard mitigation dollar spent five dollars are saved, the reality is that restrictive land-use zoning regulations and building requirements are not always enforced when such actions conflict with local plans for economic development. Moreover, the cost-sharing mitigation funding requirements on property buy-outs and relocation of at-risk properties and restoration of floodplains that provide benefits beyond flood control could be a financial burden for many local communities across the country already facing difficult budgetary choices. Many of these communities might also lack adequate financing to repair locally owned flood levee systems and, therefore, might not have them certified by the government as providing adequate protection against the 1% annual chance flood.[18] Without FEMA levee (or USACE) accreditation, the area behind the levee is mapped into a mandatory flood insurance purchase area.

RECENT DEVELOPMENTS

The Effect of Hurricane Sandy on the NFIP

On October 29, 2012, Hurricane Sandy struck the East Coast, causing massive floodwater inundation and economic disruptions in states throughout the Northeast and the mid-Atlantic region.[19] Given the geographic scope of heavily flooded areas and residential take-up rates (number of flood policies divided by an estimate of total households) in affected coastal communities that participate in the NFIP, government payouts under the NFIP are estimated to be from $12 billion to $15 billion in flood claims. At that time, the projected amount exceeded the $4 billion in cash and remaining borrowing authority from the Treasury Department for the program. By January 2013, the NFIP had processed more than 140,000 flood claims totaling about $1.7 billion.

Table 1 provides a list of the top 20 flood events in the United States in terms of NFIP payouts. With expected insured flood losses of $12 billion to $15 billion, Sandy could become the second-largest flood disaster for the NFIP behind Hurricane Katrina, which was a pivotal event in the history of federal flood-control policy. Beginning with Hurricanes Katrina and Rita in 2005, and continuing through Hurricane Irene and Tropical Storm Lee in 2011 and Hurricane Sandy in 2012, public awareness has been focused on the destructive impacts of hurricane-induced coastal flooding.

On December 7, 2012, the Office of Management and Budget (OMB) submitted to Congress a request for a FY2013 supplemental budget appropriation for an additional $60.4 billion to respond to the impacts of Hurricane Sandy in all affected states. The OMB supplemental budget appropriation request included an additional $9.7 billion in NFIP borrowing authority. On January 4, 2013, Congress passed, and President signed into law, H.R. 41 to provide a $9.7 billion increase in the NFIP's borrowing authority (from $20.725 billion to $30.425 billion) to pay flood claims related to

Hurricane Sandy. The law was considered the first step toward providing supplemental disaster relief to flood victims affected by Sandy.

On January 15, 2013, the House approved the Disaster Relief Appropriations Act of 2013, H.R. 152, to provide $17 billion to fund FEMA's Disaster Relief Fund, the Transportation Department's Federal Transit Authority Emergency Relief Program, and the Community Development Block Grant program. The House also agreed to an amendment to H.R. 152 that provided an additional $33.4 billion in disaster funding for various long-term recovery and rebuilding efforts. On January 29, 2013, President Barack Obama signed into law H.R. 152. Passage of the emergency disaster relief supplemental legislation (H.R. 152, as amended) combined with the enacted flood insurance bill (H.R. 41) totaled the $60.4 billion in Sandy relief requested by the Administration.

COST AND CONSEQUENCE OF RECENT CATASTROPHIC FLOODS

Hurricanes Katrina and Rita in 2005 caused approximately $200 billion in economic losses, of which $21.9 billion related to insurance claims under the NFIP. Katrina financially overwhelmed the program. Then, in 2008, the Atlantic hurricane season was among the costliest on record for flood losses. Hurricane Ike alone caused about $2.7 billion in NFIP claims in coastal areas of Texas and Louisiana and further inland, including many areas not typically subject to tropical rain events. Extensive 500-year floods affected more than 11 million people in nine Midwestern states as major rivers in Illinois, Indiana, Iowa, Kansas, Michigan, Minnesota, Missouri, Nebraska, and Wisconsin overflowed their banks and levees. Especially hard hit states were Iowa, Indiana, and Illinois, where the river levels surpassed levels reached in the Great Flood of 1993.

FEMA has the responsibility to identify areas of special flood, mudslide, or flood-related erosion hazards within communities; complete a Flood Insurance Study (FIS); and issue a Flood Insurance Risk Map (FIRM) showing the applicable risk premium rate zones. In the aftermath of Hurricane Katrina, FEMA focused on properly identifying properties facing residual risk behind levees and providing residents with adequate risk-based coverage. To ensure that FIRMs accurately reflected current flood hazards, particularly weather-related coastal hazards, FEMA began a nationwide FIS designed to remap the nation's floodplain. The FIS required FEMA to certify all levees appearing on FIRMs as meeting the 100-year protection regulatory standard. FEMA was able to produce digital flood hazard data for more than 88% of the nation's population and produce accurate flood hazard maps that reflected current flood hazards.

Table 1. Top 20 Significant Flood Events Covered by the National Flood Insurance Program (1978-November 30, 2012; $ nominal)

Rank	Event	Date	Number of Paid Losses	Amount Paid	Average Paid Loss
1	Hurricane Katrina	Aug. 2005	167,671	$16,264,188,476	$97,001
2	Hurricane Ike	Sept. 2008	46,412	2,664,167,040	57,391
3	Hurricane Ivan	Sept. 2004	27,658	1,590,436,206	57,504
4	Hurricane Irene	Aug. 2011	43,848	1,302,111,631	29,696
5	Tropical Storm Allison	June 2001	30,663	1,103,877,235	36,000
6	Louisiana Flood	May 1995	31,343	585,071,593	18,667
7	Hurricane Isabel	Sept. 2003	19,869	493,452,308	24,835
8	Hurricane Rita	Sept. 2005	9,517	472,774,099	49,677
9	Hurricane Floyd	Sept. 1999	20,437	462,252,753	22,618
10	Tropical Storm Lee	Sept. 2011	9,748	442,259,918	45,369
11	Hurricane Opal	Oct. 1995	10,343	405,527,543	39,208
12	Tropical Storm Isaac	Aug. 2012	10,126	407,251,178	40,218
13	Hurricane Hugo	Sept. 1989	12,840	376,433,739	29,317
14	Hurricane Wilma	Oct. 2005	9,614	365,030,822	37,975
15	Nor'Easter	Dec. 1992	25,142	346,150,356	13,768
16	Midwest Flood	June 1993	10,472	272,819,515	26,052
17	PA, NJ, NY Floods	June 2006	6,423	228,743,070	35,613
18	Torrential Rain – TN	Apr. 2010	4,108	228,248,545	55,562
19	Nor'Easter	Apr. 2007	8,636	225,657,504	26,130
20	Hurricane Fran	Sept. 1996	10,315	217,843,972	21,119

Source: U.S. Department of Homeland Security, Federal Emergency Management Agency, *Significant Flood Events as of November 30, 2012*, located at http://www.fema.gov/policy-claim-statistics-flood-insurance/policy-claim-statistics-flood-insurance/policy-claim-13-9.

But the issuance of new or revised FIRMs posed a challenge for many families and communities remapped into Special Flood Hazard Areas (SFHA). This situation prompted widespread criticism about the accuracy of the underlying flood hazard engineering data and scientific methodology used in developing the FIRMs. During congressional debate that led to the passage of the Flood Insurance Reform Act of 2012, individual property and business owners, local officials, and some Members of Congress representing areas remapped into a SFHA raised concerns about the accuracy of the maps and affordability of coverage, and they sought to delay or avoid the implementation of the new or revised flood maps, in many cases making it easier to ignore flood risk.

Efforts made to stall implementation of new or revised flood maps and mandatory purchase requirements reflected the political and regulatory environment in 2011. Hurricane Irene and Tropical Storm Lee struck the Northeast and the nation experienced higher-than-normal rainfall and flooding in states along the lower Mississippi River Valley and the upper Midwest adjacent to the Missouri River not seen since the 1930s.[20] According to the National Oceanic and Atmospheric Administration's National Weather Service (NWS), there were 12 weather events that each caused at least $1 billion in damage.[21] Direct flood damages in 2011 totaled $8.41 billion.[22] To put this amount in context, flood damages in 2011 were 108% of the 30-year average (1980-2010) of $7.82 billion (adjusted for inflation).[23]

The devastating flood damage following Hurricane Katrina in 2005, Midwest floods in 2008 and 2011, and Hurricane Ike in 2008 prompted legislative efforts in Congress to reform and reauthorize the NFIP and transition the program toward a more resilient, sustainable, and comprehensive approach to flood management.

The Biggert-Waters Flood Insurance Reform Act of 2012

After almost four years of debate, Congress passed and President Barrack Obama signed into law, on July 6, 2012, the Biggert-Waters Flood Insurance Reform Act of 2012, P.L. 112-141, which reauthorized the NFIP through September 30, 2017. The law made a number of reforms to strengthen the future financial solvency and administrative efficiency of the program by raising historically low premiums and reducing homeowners' incentives for rebuilding in flood risk zones. See **Appendix B** for a summary of the major provisions of this law.

In brief, several post-reform issues of contention remain for possible congressional consideration.

- **Revised Analysis and Mapping of Non-Accredited Levees**. FEMA has agreed to assess and map residual risk (levee protection) below the 100-year standard that would give communities "credit" for levees that provide a level of protection less than the 100-year regulatory protection standard. There are inherent complexities and technical challenges in determining levee-specific risk (probabilities of flooding at a particular point in a levee) and establishing a corresponding risk premium.
- **Actuarial Soundness, Program Solvency, and Affordability**. Insurance premium adjustments designed to strengthen the financial solvency of the NFIP could have an unintended consequence of property owners having to drop their policies because the premiums are not affordable. Public debate on the affordability issue will likely focus on the cost effectiveness and feasibility of implementing means-tested insurance premium increases that preserve some level of subsidization for low-income households.
- **Debt Forgiveness**. FEMA is currently obligated to repay about $17.5 billion owed to the Treasury Department from having to issue notes and other debt obligations to pay claims from Hurricane Katrina in 2005. Many insurance analysts believe FEMA will not be able to repay the current debt in the next 10 years.
- **Development of an Integrated Disaster Risk Management Approach.** Given the similarity in coastal and riverine hazard risks and water resources management challenges facing the nation, Congress may wish to consider options for a comprehensive integrated watershed management framework of risk perception, risk management, and disaster strategy that go beyond floodplain development management.
- **Private-Sector Role in Financing Flood Risk**. Is it feasible to expand the role of the private sector in assuming a portion of the NFIP's flood risk? Will private reinsurance companies be willing to assume primary insurer's flood risk and transfer it to the capital markets through alternative risk financing instruments?

A Nation Exposed to Flood Risk

Historically, flooding along river banks has been a major national public policy issue for which the government has played a substantial role as an insurer of last resort and a provider of disaster assistance to flood victims and communities. FEMA spends an average of $4.3 billion each year responding to a wide range of disasters.[24] These funds, which are intended to address immediate and longer-term impacts of disasters on individuals and communities, are in addition to the funds spent each year on compensation for flood victims for uninsured losses and mitigating future flood losses under the NFIP.

Statistical data from FEMA, the National Oceanic and Atmosphere Administration (NOAA), and private organizations suggest an increasing frequency of catastrophic flood events linked to extreme weather and climatic events like hurricanes, storm surge, or tornadoes. The nation arguably continues to face increasing exposure to flood risks as evidenced by the fact that floods that would historically occur once every 20 years are now projected to happen every 4 to 6 years.[25] Urban populations and property assets and public infrastructure appear to be more vulnerable to coastal flood hazards and levee flood hazards. Concerns have been raised that more than half of the U.S. population now lives in coastal watershed counties or floodplain areas and approximately 50% of the nation's gross domestic product is generated in Gulf and Atlantic coastal areas.[26] One estimate from Lloyds of London and Risk Management Solutions (RMS) predicts that flood losses along the Gulf and Atlantic coastlines would increase 80% by 2030 with a one-foot rise in the sea level.[27]

Economic Regulation and Recovery from Flood Disasters

Congress has a responsibility through the "general welfare" and "interstate commerce" clauses of the U.S. Constitution to promote national economic growth. One factor affecting the nation's economic well-being is the proper functioning of markets for natural disaster risk. In deciding whether to intervene in private insurance markets, policymakers typically ask several questions: Do economic markets provide a sufficient amount of insurance against flood hazards? To the extent that flood insurance exists, are the insuring firms sufficiently capitalized so that widespread insolvency would not occur? Would federal disaster insurance crowd out private insurers and reinsurers and create unintended federal liabilities for taxpayers? Would insurers engage in "cherry-picking" the most appealing risks and leave the "less appealing" risk to the federal government?

The U.S. government has at times regulated private economic activity for the purpose of promoting economic recovery and protecting or supporting particular economic groups. For example, economic uncertainty stemming from widespread flooding in the mid-1960s, the need for economic relief and recovery for flood victims, and calls for a reduction in the financial burden on taxpayers led to economic regulation of the nation's floodplains and insurance markets.

On September 9, 1965, Hurricane Betsy, a Category 3 hurricane, hit the Louisiana coast, causing Lake Pontchartrain to overflow its banks and resulting in widespread flooding. Betsy was the first natural disaster to generate more than $1 billion in damages. At the time, there was little flood insurance because private insurers were unwilling to offer protection to offset flood losses. In response, Congress created the NFIP in 1968 as a quid pro quo program that would regulate the nation's floodplains with land-use controls and building requirements that communities located in SFHA must adopt and enforce for property owners to be eligible for insurance under the program.

Under the NFIP, the government became a de facto regulator of certain economic activity in flood-prone areas. In the absence of a sufficient supply of insurance to meet societal demand, the government took action to safeguard the economic interests of consumers, private businesses, communities, and taxpayers. Economic regulation was accomplished in two ways. First, the government acted to address the cost and consequences of risky economic activity in flood-prone areas. Depending on whether a building is located in a government-designated SFHA, flood insurance may be required as a condition of obtaining a federally secured mortgage loan. Homeowners typically discover they need flood insurance during the home-buying process, which normally includes a disclosure of where the property is located relative to the SFHA that is mapped on a FIRM.[28]

Second, economic regulation was accomplished through "managerial regulation," with the government providing subsidized flood insurance for individuals and private businesses in communities that undertook specific steps to regulate the floodplain through land-use zoning ordinances and building standards.[29] The government later made the purchase of flood insurance mandatory for federally insured mortgages.

In general, there were four broad underlying causes for economic regulation—government intervention—in the market for flood insurance in the

1960s. *First*, people insisted that social and ethical values as well as economic values should be reflected in the operation of the economy. Persons suffering economic distress or dislocation from flood hazards sought and received governmental aid in dealing with their problem. The aid was in the form of disaster relief assistance, subsidized flood insurance, and government spending on flood risk identification and mapping.

Second, government action was viewed as being necessary to more efficiently coordinate and use resources. Economic regulatory programs were thought to be needed to prescribe certain land-use zoning ordinances and building-code standards to govern economic or business behavior to reduce the physical and economic risks associated with coastal hazards.

Third, as the nation experienced widespread flooding in the 1960s, people became interested in shifting some of the risk from themselves to government. In response, policymakers changed the way economic risk of flooding was defined and the means of achieving security for the individual. Disasters, whether man-made or natural, were initially considered inevitable or "acts of God" but came to be viewed as public problems that required government action to protect individuals, businesses, communities, and taxpayers. Government assistance in the form of subsidized insurance premiums was viewed as a solution to reduce the future costs and risks of investing in flood-prone areas.

Premium subsidies were initially considered necessary because residents in flood-prone areas often did not understand the flood risk when they built in floodplains (flood maps were not available), there were no public safeguards restricting construction on the floodplain, and premium subsidies on pre-FIRM structures could provide an incentive for local communities to participate in the program and discourage unwise future floodplains construction. Premium subsidies were intended to be phased out over time as the number of pre-FIRM properties gradually diminished when they were damaged and rebuilt or relocated under stronger floodplain management and building codes.

Fourth, sole reliance on insurance markets for flood risks was not an option. This situation provided a rationale for possible government intervention in the economy to ensure that the costs of living in flood-prone areas were not ignored. Individuals and insurers at risk of flooding, however, have in the past lacked the information necessary for the market system to operate effectively. Insurers did not always have flood hazard maps, as they do now, and thus had no reliable, consistent, and cost-effective way to identify and assess flood risk. Homeowners did not (and sometimes still do not) have the information needed to make rational economic decisions about real estate investments. All of this resulted in a misallocation of resources that required and still arguably requires government intervention to protect the public interest.

Financial Management of Flood Risk

Flood hazards are deemed commercially uninsurable in the private-insurance market given that only those most exposed to loss tend to purchase coverage, the possibility of catastrophic losses, and concerns about the insurer's ability to correctly price the contracts of insurance because of limitations in hazard assessment. Traditional insurance principles indicate that financial intermediation through insurance contracts tends to work best when the insurer is able to gather a large enough pool of independent risks to allow the actuarial technique of "law of large numbers" to diversify the risk. Because the nature of flood risk is that many property owners simultaneously face the same flood hazard when the event occurs, their risks tend to be highly correlated—not independent. Correlated risk means the insurer must charge higher premiums to reflect a larger risk load or administrative costs that account for the uncertainty faced by the insurer in predicting future losses of the pool. The premium level that private insurers needed to adequately underwrite flood hazards would be so high that few would be willing to purchase coverage.

The NFIP was a public-policy response to the flood peril and escalating costs of taxpayer-funded disaster relief for flood victims. Government mapping of areas prone to flooding, subsidized flood insurance, and floodplain management regulations were key to the program's structure and function.[30] Federally backed flood insurance was made available to homeowners and businesses in communities that voluntarily agreed to adopt and enforce floodplain management ordinances designed to reduce flood-related property losses. The creation of the NFIP marked a significant shift in U.S. flood control policy. The shift was away from a "levee-only" flood reduction approach toward a risk identification, risk financing, and floodplain management approach that was intended to foster individual responsibility and build local self-sufficiency in terms of land-use zoning ordinances and construction standards.

Federal flood insurance was considered to be an economically efficient way to indemnify flood victims and to have them internalize some of the risk of locating property in the floodplains.[31] The federal government would use its capacity to spread losses over time with the NFIP's ability to borrow money from the U.S. Treasury to offset program deficits. A federal government insurance program, it was thought, could also link the availability of flood insurance to land-use regulation and building codes that would, in theory, reduce long-term flood risk.

The NFIP has undergone major changes largely in response to significant flood events over the years. As an illustration, the program was created after Hurricane Betsy devastated the Gulf Coast in 1965. After Hurricane Agnes in 1972, recognizing the low market penetration of flood insurance, Congress passed the Flood Disaster Protection Act of 1973[32] to establish a mandatory flood insurance purchase requirement for structures located in identified SFHAs. After the 1973 act, federally regulated lenders were obligated to require flood insurance on any loan secured by improved real estate in a FEMA-designated SFHA in a participating community. After the Midwest floods of 1993, it became increasingly apparent to Congress that homeowners were still not adequately complying with the mandatory insurance purchase requirement. The flood provided the impetus for strengthening lender compliance through the mandatory purchase provisions in the 1994 National Flood Insurance Reform Act.[33] Recognition of the impact of properties prone to repetitive flooding on the financial condition of the program led to the passage of the Flood Insurance Reform Act of 2004,[34] which established a pilot program for the mitigation of severe-repetitive-loss properties (SRLPs) and the funding of mitigation activities for individual SRLPs.

After the 2008 and 2011 catastrophic floods, Congress focused attention on long-term reforms and reauthorization of the NFIP to ensure the financial viability of the program, ensure continued comprehensive coverage for all property in floodplains, and explore a private-sector role in financing flood risks. These efforts led to the passage of the Flood Insurance Reform Act of 2012.

Identifying and Mapping Areas of Special Flood Risk

Accurate flood maps with the latest engineering and flood modeling digital mapping technologies help to reduce future flood losses and ensure that rates reflect actual risk, which, in turn, promotes the fiscal soundness of the NFIP.

Accuracy of Maps

Flood maps could become outdated and inaccurate when they fail to reflect floodplain and wetland altered by watershed development that destroys the natural system that contains flooding.[35] The altering of rivers and streams by construction of dams, levees, and other flood- control structures arguably increased the risk of inland floods and development throughout the affected floodplains. Similarly, the construction of roads and buildings creates impermeable surfaces that reduce the natural environment's ability to absorb or delay water flows and changes in drainage patterns—a situation that could increase flood risk in the affected area. Flood maps might not adequately consider coastal-flood hazards, such as cumulative shoreline erosion or the loss of wetland, which serves as a natural buffer to storm surge and reduces downstream flooding in inland areas.[36]

Basic Mechanics of Flood Mapping

A typical Flood Insurance Study (FIS) begins with modeling of rainfall and storm tide records for the local areas. The data are then simulated to determine the likely discharge that could result from storms of various probabilities. These discharge data are applied to a cross section of the floodplain to estimate flood depths at various locations. Once FEMA determines water surface elevation data in various areas in the community, the next steps are to calculate the depth of flooding for buildings in the area and calculate the dollar damages using a vulnerability function (state-damage curve) derived from past flood events.[37] The Base Flood Elevation (BFE) of the first floor of the structure relative to the flood depth on the floodplain determines property- specific flood risk data to guide construction and insurance decisions. FEMA used these flood hazard data to create FIRMs that delineate areas determined to have a 1% chance of flood in any given year (the "100-year floodplain"). The 1%-annual-chance flood is a flood insurance standard, not a public safety standard.

Flood Risk with Respect to Levees

The Flood Insurance Reform Act of 2012 requires FEMA to develop risk models, flood zones, and insurance rates that account for several typical non-accredited levee scenarios. This regulatory reform stems in part from the consequences of the breaching of the levee system protecting the city of New

Orleans in 2005 and the massive flood inundation it caused, which led to the most costly flood event in the history of the NFIP. Residents in the SFHA had to purchase flood insurance if they had a federally insured mortgage. FEMA assumed the levee system would prevent the flow of water on the landward side of the levee during the 1%-annual-chance flood event and, therefore, did not adequately price the risk of levee failure or overtopping. FEMA assumes non-accredited levees do not meet the federal standard for reducing the risk associated with a major flood and, therefore, prices this risk.

Funding Flood Hazard Mapping Activities

Table 2 shows recent funding levels for FEMA's flood mapping program. In 2003, FEMA began the Flood Map Modernization (Map Mod) program to update the nation's inventory of FIRMs to digital FIRMs (DFIRMs) for areas of the United States with the greatest flood risk. Map Mod provided updated DFIRMs for more than 92% of the U.S. population.

FEMA's Risk Maps, Assessment, and Planning (Risk MAP) Program

The Map Mod program successfully developed and delivered a new digital platform that has enabled FEMA to make flood hazard data more widely available while providing opportunities to focus on enhancing data accuracy and resolution issues. Other technologies were also developed to provide opportunities to focus efforts on raising risk awareness and building a risk management framework to achieve sustainable actions to reduce and better manage flood risks going forward.

In 2009, FEMA's Map Mod program became the Risk Mapping, Assessment, and Planning (Risk MAP) program that builds on flood hazard data and maps produced during the Map Mod program.[38] Risk MAP is an integrated flood risk management approach that weaves NFIP flood hazard data into watershed-based risk assessments that serve as the basis for local hazard mitigation plans and support community actions to reduce risk.

Under the Risk MAP program, FEMA initiated projects for 37% of the U.S. population through FY2011 and anticipated increasing that number to 43% by the end of FY2012. In addition, FEMA had also anticipated providing to communities New, Validated or Updated Engineering (NVUE) data for 54% of the miles mapped under the NFIP. By the end of FY2012, FEMA had initiated studies to cover approximately 61% of the miles mapped. FEMA continues to update the nation's coastal-flood hazard studies.

Table 2. FEMA Flood Mapping Program Funding Levels: FY2011- FY2013 ($ in thousands)

Program	FY2011 (Enacted)	FY2012 (Enacted)	FY2013 Pres.Budget
Flood Hazard Mapping & Risk Analysis, Risk Map	$204,131	$97,712	$89,329
National Flood Insurance Fund, FIF, Flood Studies & Surveys	$113,509	$117,706	$116,000
Total	**$317,640**	**$215,418**	**$205,329**

Source: U.S. Department of Homeland Security, FEMA's Office of Legislative Affairs.

FINANCIAL STATUS OF NFIP

This section examines the current financial status of NFIP, including borrowing from the U.S. Treasury and remaining financial issues for Congress.

Table 3 shows that the NFIP currently has about 5.6 million policies in force nationwide covering approximately $1.3 trillion in property. The NFIP has almost 20,000 participating communities, and policyholders paid $3.48 billion in premiums in 2011. The NFIP experienced 6 catastrophic loss years—defined as payouts of $1 billion or more—in its 44-year history that severely tested the financial resiliency of the program. These years include 1995, 2001, 2004, 2005, 2008, and 2011.

Table 3. NFIP Program Statistics (as of December 31, 2011; $ nominal)

Calendar Year	Number of Policies in Force	Total Written Premium	Total Face Value of Coverage	Total Number of Claims Paid	Total Payments Made to Policyholders
1972-1977	NA	NA	NA	4,441	$18,035,658
1978	1,446,354	$111,250,585	$50,500,956,000	29,122	$147,719,253
1979	1,843,441	$141,535,832	$74,375,240,000	70,613	$483,281,219
1980	2,103,851	$159,009,583	$99,259,942,000	41,918	$230,414,295
1981	1,915,065	$256,798,488	$102,059,859,000	23,261	$127,118,031
1982	1,900,544	$354,842,356	$107,296,802,000	32,831	$198,295,820

Calendar Year	Number of Policies in Force	Total Written Premium	Total Face Value of Coverage	Total Number of Claims Paid	Total Payments Made to Policyholders
1983	1,981,122	$384,225,425	$117,834,255,000	51,584	$439,454,937
1984	1,926,388	$420,530,032	$124,421,281,000	27,688	$254,642,874
1985	2,016,785	$452,466,332	$139,948,260,000	38,676	$368,238,794
1986	2,119,039	$518,226,957	$155,717,168,000	13,789	$126,384,695
1987	2,115,183	$566,391,536	$165,053,402,000	13,400	$105,432,378
1988	2,149,153	$589,453,163	$175,764,175,000	7,758	$51,022,523
1989	2,292,947	$632,204,396	$265,218,590,000	36,245	$661,658,285
1990	2,477,861	$672,791,834	$213,588,265,000	14,766	$167,896,816
1991	2,532,713	$737,078,033	$223,098,548,000	28,549	$353,681,702
1992	2,623,406	$800,973,357	$236,844,980,000	44,650	$710,225,154
1993	2,828,558	$890,425,274	$267,870,761,000	36,044	$659,059,461
1994	3,040,198	$1,003,850,875	$295,935,328,000	21,583	$411,075,128
1995	3,476,829	$1,140,808,119	$349,137,768,000	62,441	$1,295,578,117
1996	3,693,076	$1,275,176,752	$400,681,650,000	52,677	$828,036,508
1997	4,102,416	$1,509,787,517	$462,606,433,000	30,338	$519,537,378
1998	4,235,138	$1,668,246,681	$497,621,083,000	57,348	$886,327,133
1999	4,329,985	$1,719,652,696	$534,117,781,000	47,247	$754,970,800
2000	4,369,087	$1,723,824,570	$567,568,653,000	16,362	$251,720,536
2001	4,458,470	$1,740,331,079	$611,918,920,000	43,589	$1,277,002,489
2002	4,519,799	$1,802,277,937	$653,776,126,000	25,312	$433,644,094
2003	4,565,491	$1,897,687,479	$691,786,140,000	36,838	$780,492,440
2004	4,667,446	$2,040,828,486	$765,205,681,000	55,825	$2,232,042,331
2005	4,962,011	$2,241,264,140	$876,679,658,000	212,778	$17,713,105,660
2006	5,514,895	$2,604,844,133	$1,054,087,148,000	24,592	$640,623,771
2007	5,655,919	$2,843,422,049	$1,141,242,230,000	23,129	$612,351,594
2008	5,684,275	$3,066,729,200	$1,197,659,846,000	74,266	$3,450,249,017
2009	5,704,198	$3,202,267,224	$1,233,005,263,000	30,821	$772,390,723
2010	5,559,313	$3,348,222,091	$1,227,932,424,400	27,165	$708,992,043
2011	5,585,797	$3,477,338,993	$1,264,043,634,800	65,315	$1,847,881,892

Source: U.S. Department of Homeland Security, FEMA's Office of Legislative Affairs.

Figure 1 shows that over the period from 1978 to 2011, the NFIP experienced nine loss years in which flood loss payments exceeded premiums written.[39] In 2005, Hurricanes Katrina- and Rita- related losses easily dwarf all other loss years. The flood-related losses from the 2005 and 2008 hurricane seasons resulted in substantial NFIP borrowing from the U.S. Treasury that led to the current $17.75 billion in cumulative debt. (See Table 4.)

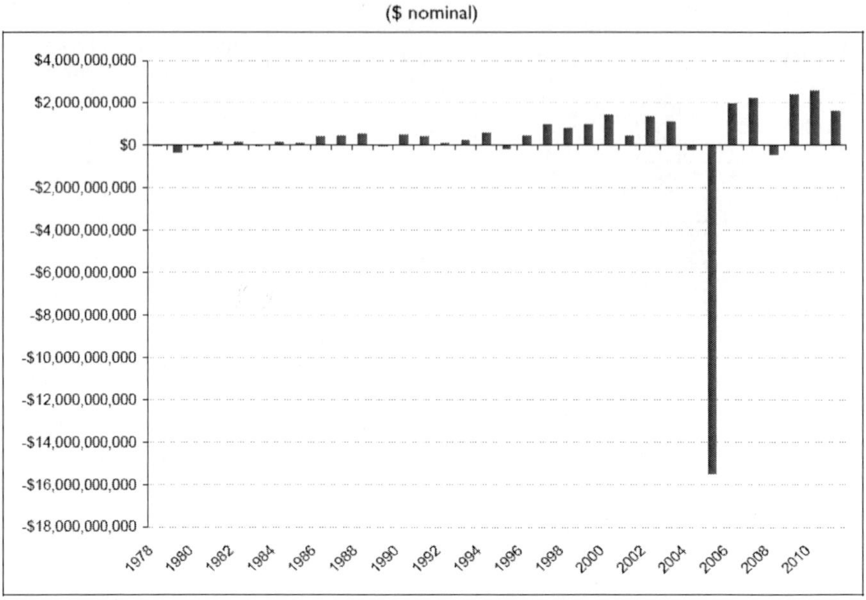

Source: CRS presentation based on data from the Federal Emergency Management Agency.

Figure 1. Difference Between Total Premiums Written and Total Payments Made to Policyholders Under the National Flood Insurance Programs: 1978-2011.

Table 4. History of U.S.Treasury Borrowing Under the National Flood Insurance Program (as of June 30, 2012; $ nominal)

Fiscal Year	Amount Borrowed	Amount Repaid	Cumulative Debt
Prior to 1981[a]	$917,406,008	$0	$917,406,008
1981	$164,614,526	$624,970,099	$457,050,435
1982	$13,915,000	$470,965,435	$0
1983	$50,000,000	$0	$50,000,000
1984[b]	$200,000,000	$36,879,123	$213,120,877
1985	$0	$213,120,877	$0
1986-1993	$0	$0	$0
1994[c]	$100,000,000	$100,000,000	$0
1995	$265,000,000	$0	$265,000,000
1996	$423,600,000	$62,000,000	$626,600,000
1997	$530,000,000	$239,600,000	$917,000,000
1998	$0	$395,000,000	$522,000,000
1999	$400,000,000	$381,000,000	$541,000,000
2000	$345,000,000	$541,000,000	$345,000,000

Fiscal Year	Amount Borrowed	Amount Repaid	Cumulative Debt
2001	$600,000,000	$345,000,000	$600,000,000
2002	$50,000,000	$640,000,000	$10,000,000
October 2002	$0	$10,000,000	$0
2003 (Nov.-Sept.)	$0	$0	$0
2004	$0	$0	$0
2005[d]	$300,000,000	$75,000,000	$225,000,000
2006	$16,660,000,000	$0	$16,885,000,000
2007	$650,000,000	$0	$17,535,000,000
2008	$50,000,000	$225,000,000	$17,360,000,000
2009	$1,987,988,421	$347,988,421	$19,000,000,000
2010	$0	$500,000,000	$18,500,000,000
2011	$0	$750,000,000	$17,750,000,000
Total	**$23,707,523,955**	**$5,957,523,955**	**$17,750,000,000**

Source: CRS presentation based on data from the U.S. Department of Homeland Security, Federal Emergency Management Agency's Office of Legislative Affairs.

Notes: Borrowings through 1985 were repaid from congressional appropriations. The NFIP did not borrow from 1986 through 1993. Since 1994, borrowings are repaid from premium and other income. The existing debt outstanding is expected to be repaid with premium income or with congressional appropriations.

a. Balance forward from U.S. Department of Housing and Urban Development.

b. Figure for the $213.1 million in cumulative debt in 1984 provided by FEMA reflects additional cost outside of the insurance program.

c. Of the $100 million borrowed, only $11 million was needed to cover obligations.

d. NFIP borrowed $300 million in 2005 to pay claims from the 2004 hurricane season, but Hurricanes Katrina, Rita, and Wilma struck after late August 2005, and claims were submitted after the 2006 fiscal year began.

Treasury Borrowing

Table 4 shows the history of U.S. Treasury borrowing and repayments under the NFIP from 1981 through 2011. The NFIP was self-supporting from 1986 until 2005, covering all administrative expenses and claim payments out of premium income and fees. Since Hurricane Katrina struck in August 2005, FEMA has had to borrow $19.64 billion, which includes $2.6 billion over the 2007- 2009 period, to pay claims from Hurricane Ike and the Midwest floods of 2008.[40] The NFIP's borrowing authority was increased to $20.725 billion on March 23, 2006, and to $30.425 billion on January 6, 2013.

The Flood Insurance Reform Act of 2012 requires FEMA to establish a reserve fund, beginning in FY2013, to offset claims during catastrophic loss years to reduce the likelihood of the NFIP having to borrow from the

Treasury.[41] Although the 2012 Reform Act does not forgive any portion of the NFIP debt, it requires FEMA to create a repayment schedule for funds borrowed from the Treasury and directs FEMA to include catastrophic loss years when assessing flood risk in order to set annual premium rates.[42] The latter requirement allows the program to collect risk- based premiums that, in theory, would reduce the likelihood of the program encountering financial deficits that result in program borrowing from the Treasury. Some experts believe that even if FEMA increased flood insurance rates up to the maximum amount allowed under the new law (20% per year), the program would still not have sufficient funds to cover future obligations for policyholder claims, operating expenses, and interest on debt.

Factors Affecting Financial Soundness of the NFIP

In considering the NFIP's financial solvency, it may be useful to recognize two things: (1) the NFIP was not capitalized at inception by Congress and (2) the program does not operate under the traditional insurance definition of fiscal solvency that requires the insurer to have statutory reserves as a condition of receiving authorization to sell insurance in a given state.

Premium Subsidies

Before the passage of the Flood Insurance Reform Act of 2012, the NFIP faced a long-term solvency challenge because the program did not have a financing mechanism for handling catastrophic losses and it charged less-than-actuarial rates for pre-FIRM structures.[43] Annual premiums were not likely to cover the program's long-term expenses, claim costs, and interest and principal debt repayment to the U.S. Treasury. Therefore, taxpayers faced financial exposure from recurring catastrophic flood events.[44] FEMA's old rate-setting structure was designed to generate premiums at least sufficient to cover losses and loss adjustment expenses relative to the "historical average loss year."[45] There was no contingent amount added to premiums to build a surplus. When losses and expenses exceeded premiums, the program was authorized to borrow from the U.S. Treasury but had to repay the funds with interest.

Many experts insisted that the NFIP would not be financially sound until actuarial risk-based rates were charged. FEMA reports that 78% of policyholders already pay actuarial premiums, albeit there is some debate about whether rates reflect the true flood risk to people and property.[46]

Charging rates that fully reflect flood risk arguably would discourage development in the most risky areas.

The new law eliminated subsidized premium rates and allowed rates to be adjusted to reflect true risk, taking into consideration historical loss data, including catastrophic loss years and other factors, such as coastal storm surge and climate change.[47] To address the affordability issue, the new law authorized a study of the feasibility of an insurance voucher system or similar means tested assistance.[48] As indicated earlier, the Flood Insurance Reform Act of 2012 established a catastrophe fund to stabilize catastrophe losses from year to year.[49]

Repetitive Flood Loss Properties

Properties that experience repetitive flood losses, known as a "repetitive loss properties" (RLP) and "severe repetitive loss properties" (SRLP), account for a disproportionately large share of all the flood insurance claims filed and paid under the NFIP.[50] Historically, it is estimated that approximately 1% of the properties insured under the NFIP have accounted for over a third of claims paid. About 1 in 10 homes that suffer repetitive flood damages have cumulative flood insurance claims that have exceeded the value of the house.[51] FEMA estimates that 90% of all RLPs were built prior to December 31, 1974, or before the adoption of a FIRM—and, hence, have been subject to premium discounts. Importantly, the annual increase in new RLPs is outpacing FEMA mitigation efforts by a factor of 10 to 1. After the 1993 Midwest flood, FEMA and other federal government agencies spent hundreds of millions of dollars to remove frequently flooded structures from the floodplain.

Table 5. Total Repetitive Flood Loss Properties in the NFIP: 1978-2011 (as of December 31, 2011: $ nominal)

Building Payments	$9,332,087,006
Contents Payments	$2,768,293,788
Total payments	$12,100,980,774
Average payment	$24,388
Number of Losses	496,178
Number of Properties	166,368

Source: U.S. Department of Homeland Security, Federal Emergency Management Agency.

Table 5 shows that since 1978, a total of 166,368 RLPs have had 496,178 claims paid, which has cost the National Flood Insurance Fund a total of $12.1 billion in nominal dollars. **Appendix A** shows RLPs by state. The average claim for these properties was $24,388.

FEMA has undertaken several actions over the years to address the RLP problem. The initial strategy, announced in 1999, was to identify the nation's inventory of RLPs and focus on structures that were substantially damaged (i.e., damaged 50% or more of market value), at which time they would be reconstructed, elevated, or flood-proofed to prevent future damage. One reported difficulty has been reluctance and inconsistency at the local community level in declaring structures substantially damaged, which triggers the requirement to rebuild to a higher flood construction standard.

FEMA also pursued a strategy of phasing out premium subsidies on RLPs through voluntary buyouts or the imposition of full actuarially based rates on RLP owners who refuse to accept FEMA's offer to mitigate the effect of flood damage. In addition, the agency incorporated special incentives into the Community Rating System and provided data to states and communities to help them address the RLPs.

The Flood Insurance Reform Act of 2004[52] required FEMA to establish the Repetitive Flood Claims (RFC) and the Severe Repetitive Loss (SRL) Grant programs to provide funding to reduce or eliminate the long-term risk of flood damage under the NFIP. The RFC program offers grants to states and local governments to mitigate future flood losses. Mitigation projects typically include demolishing, relocating, elevating, or flood-proofing structures. However, the SRL program has proven to be cumbersome for communities and states to administer. Currently, there are more than 12,300 SRL policies being serviced in the NFIP-Special Direct Facility (NFIP- SDF).

The Flood Insurance Reform Act of 2012 streamlined and reauthorized the Flood Mitigation Assistance Program (FMA), the RFC, and the SRL to allow federal funds to be used for mitigation of repetitive- or severe-repetitive-loss structures to improve their effectiveness and efficiency.[53]

Low NFIP Program Participation

The intent and success of the NFIP rests on making affordable flood insurance widely available to the general public and protecting communities from potential damage through floodplain management. Since 1973, federal regulations have required flood insurance on structures located in identified Special Flood Hazard Areas (SFHAs) that have a federally backed mortgage.

Also, since 1994, recipients of certain flood disaster assistance have been required to purchase and hold flood insurance to protect against future flood losses, under penalty of receiving no federal disaster aid in subsequent floods.[54] Despite the existence of this mandatory flood insurance purchase requirement, take-up rates for flood insurance have historically been low and the federal government's exposure to uninsured property losses from flooding remains substantial. Many homeowners do not completely recognize or internalize their flood risk and are overly optimistic about the magnitude of the flood risk to which they are exposed. Consequently, the NFIP has not achieved the level of individual participation originally envisioned by Congress.

Researchers indicate that there are at least five possible explanations for the low market penetration for flood insurance: (1) flood insurance is not seen as being worth the cost (i.e., a poor investment); (2) individuals have misperceptions about low-probability risks and lack information about the NFIP;[55] (3) private insurance agents do not market NFIP policies; (4) lack of compliance with the mandatory purchase requirement or failure to ensure that property owners maintain coverage for the life of the loan; and (5) many homeowners in risky areas either do not have a mortgage or have a mortgage from a lender that does not enforce the mandatory purchase requirement.

FEMA lacks nationwide data on the number of properties in floodplains, which makes it difficult to accurately determine insurance market penetration. Available evidence suggests that penetration rates in the 100-year floodplain are consistently low. A 2006 study of the NFIP's mandatory purchase requirement nationwide conducted by the Rand Corporation indicated that only about 49% of single-family homes in SFHAs are covered by flood insurance.[56] In the absence of flood insurance, the cost of repairing flood-damaged property is usually borne by either the property owner from their own financial resources or with assistance through federal relief programs, instead of by flood insurance payments. This situation has resulted in billions of dollars of uninsured property losses and arguably results in higher social costs.

The Flood Insurance Reform Act of 2012 addressed the lack of enforcement of the mandatory insurance purchase requirement by increasing the amount of civil penalties that can be imposed against regulated lending institutions that fail to require flood insurance from $350 to $2,000 per violation.[57]

Inaccurate Flood Hazard Maps

FEMA is responsible for identifying and mapping the nation's floodplain areas and identifying flood-risk zones in such areas. Flood Insurance Rate Maps (FIRMs) are used for setting flood insurance rates, regulating floodplain development, and communicating information about the 1%-annual-chance flood hazard to those who live in floodplains. FIRMs also are used to determine whether property owners are required by law to obtain flood insurance as a condition of obtaining mortgage loans or other federally related financial assistance. Without accurate and updated flood hazard maps, property owners and small businesses could underestimate their exposure to flood risks and make poor financial decisions about protecting their properties (i.e., where to build and whether to purchase flood insurance or take other measures to protect their properties).

The Flood Insurance Reform Act of 2012 authorized several regulatory changes to improve the accuracy of flood maps and established a process to allow communities to request a remapping based on the standards recommended by a newly established Technical Mapping Advisory Council and adopted by FEMA.[58] The new law also authorized the creation of an independent Scientific Resolution Panel consisting of experts on flood hazard maps and flood insurance to address mapping-related concerns from communities that are dissatisfied with the outcome of their appeal to FEMA.[59]

Lack of Enforcement of Floodplain Management Regulations

The Flood Insurance Reform Act of 2012 requires FEMA to conduct a study of the impact, effectiveness, and feasibility of including widely used and nationally recognized building codes as part of the floodplain management criteria. The new law would also allow the use of funds under the Community Development Block Grant Program (CDBG) to include community building code administration grants.[60]

Under the NFIP, FEMA is prohibited from providing flood insurance to property owners residing in communities not participating in the NFIP.[61] Local communities must adopt and enforce certain minimum floodplain management ordinances as a condition for participation in the NFIP. However, efforts to guide construction and development away from high-risk areas through community-based land-use and zoning ordinances have reportedly been subordinated to building and elevation requirements that lead to further development of the floodplains.[62] Even in hazard- prone floodways and coastal areas, building and rebuilding are allowed under NFIP standards, with the cost of insurance varying with property elevation.

Coastal Flood Hazard Risk Assessment and Mapping

One issue of contention that emerged from the controversy and litigation surrounding Katrina- related wind versus water insurance claims disputes was whether the NFIP should be expanded to allow policyholders to purchase optional wind coverage. Following the storm, individuals and businesses in Louisiana, Mississippi, and Alabama protested against what they claimed were inappropriate obstacles to the payment of their property damage insurance claims. When insurance adjustors and damage experts assessed the properties damaged by Hurricane Katrina, they were faced with the issue of allocating damages between wind (a covered loss) and flood (an excluded loss). Post-Katrina insurance claims litigation and the delays and economic uncertainty generated for consumers and insurers raised concerns about post-event judicial interpretations of the scope of insurance coverage.

Proponents of optional wind coverage under the NFIP argued that this policy change was necessary because of the difficulties property owners faced in obtaining affordable private wind coverage in states along the Gulf and Atlantic Coasts. Private insurers had increased premiums and deductibles and reduced coverage or withdrawn altogether from these areas out of concern about catastrophic risk exposure.

Opponents of adding wind coverage to the NFIP believed there was adequate wind coverage capacity in every state through either the traditional private market or through the state residual market program (e.g., wind pools). Critics maintained that expanding the NFIP to add wind coverage would dramatically increase the financial exposure of the NFIP and, hence, federal taxpayers. Concerns were also expressed about the NFIP's ability to determine actuarially sound rates for the windstorm portion of this coverage and avoid wide-scale financial deficits in the program following a catastrophic flood event.

Moreover, there were concerns that even actuarial rates may not produce sufficient premium income to cover the program's administration costs and losses in the event of a catastrophic event. The Government Accountability Office (GAO) issued a report in 2008 that outlined some difficulties that FEMA could face in implementing an optional wind coverage provision. Some of the obstacles included (1) the concern about "adverse selection" or the likelihood that only those property owners at highest risk would purchase coverage; (2) wind hazard prevention standards that communities would have to adopt to receive coverage; (3) uncertainty about the adoption of programs to accommodate wind coverage; (4) difficulties in establishing a new rate-setting process; (5) enforcement of new building codes; and (6) administration and oversight of the program.[63]

The Flood Insurance Reform Act of 2012 established the Consumer Option for an Alternative System to Allocate Losses (COASTAL) program to authorize the use of scientific coastal hazard data collected by NOAA in conjunction with engineering formulas to be developed by FEMA to accurately assess flood insurance claims for total-loss, "slab" properties.[64] The aim of the COASTAL program is to better estimate wind versus water risks and allocate insured losses following a major hurricane, storm surge, or tornado.

Moral Hazard and Federal Disaster Assistance

According to the written testimony of Administrator Craig Fugate of FEMA, most owners of flood-prone property in NFIP-participating communities opted to not purchase flood insurance prior to a purchase mandate, choosing instead to rely on federal disaster assistance to finance their recovery.[65] As discussed above, the low-penetration rate of NFIP continues and suggests that many people may still rely on federal disaster assistance instead of flood insurance. In economic theory, the assurance of federal assistance in the event of repeated disaster-related losses may create a "moral hazard" by lowering the incentives to take appropriate steps to mitigate loss. This situation counteracts one of the original objectives of the NFIP, which is to develop mitigation plans and implement measures (insurance linked to land management) to reduce future flood damages and the cost of taxpayer-funded disaster assistance.

In 1977, President Jimmy Carter signed into law Executive Order 11988 to require federal agencies to avoid direct and indirect support of floodplain development in coastal velocity zones—the so-called V zones on FIRMs—by taking action "to reduce the risk of flood loss, to minimize the impact of floods on human safety, health and welfare, and to restore and preserve the natural and beneficial values served by floodplains in carrying out its responsibilities."[66] Under E.O. 11988, FEMA staff must (1) determine eligibility and the required elevation of all new construction in coastal high-hazard areas on the Gulf Coast and (2) decide whether new structures, the costs of repair, or the replacement of facilities in V zones are eligible for FEMA funding.

Although regulatory guidelines for E.O. 11988 are outlined in 44 CFR Part 9, there has arguably been a lack of clarity in interpreting those guidelines to determine whether officials are to support recovery and community development in V zones. Access to federal assistance for recovery and hazard mitigation projects undertaken in V zones could emerge as an important issue in the aftermath of Hurricane Sandy. The decision to approve and obligate FEMA recovery funds for public assistance projects located in V zones could be an essential consideration in the reconstruction or redevelopment of some coastal areas devastated by Hurricane Sandy.

Remaining Issues for Possible Congressional Oversight

Since 2008, when the NFIP lost its authorization, Congress has passed 17 short-term extensions and the program has lapsed 4 times (see **Appendix C**). The Flood Insurance Reform Act of 2012 did not resolve all flood management issues pertaining to the NFIP. The law reflects a consensus as of that moment in time with respect to the financial stability and administrative efficiency of the NFIP, the need to have those who reside in flood-prone areas to pay for that risk, and the need for strengthening the mapping program. However, several policy issues and questions remain for future congressional consideration. These remaining issues and questions include the following:

The nation's increasing flood risk vulnerability in an era of frequent extreme weather and climatic events and population growth in flood-prone areas

- What are the true costs borne by the federal government under the NFIP with consideration of both the direct effects and indirect social and economic costs?
- What additional steps, if any, should the federal government undertake to effectively manage and mitigate flood disasters and discourage overdevelopment in flood vulnerable areas?
- How best to strengthen coordination among the nation's water resources and floodplain management agencies at the federal, state, and local levels of government?
- Is there a need to plan for the sustainability of the NFIP in an environment of increasingly frequent catastrophic flooding across the country?

Affordability of insurance coverage in era of actuarial (full-risk) premium pricing

- Will the changes in premium structure made under the Flood Insurance Reform Act of 2012 be adequate to address solvency concern?
- What is the feasibility of vouchers for low-income NFIP policyholders who are not able to pay actuarial flood insurance rates?
- What is the best approach to balance the government's need to increase the NFIP's future income versus making the insurance coverage affordable and widely available?
- Would the privatization of flood risk make insurance more affordable or less so? Is the private sector up to the task? Is there capacity to underwrite this risk?

Debt forgiveness

- Should Congress eliminate the NFIP's debt to the Treasury?
- What are the distributional consequences across different stakeholders of debt forgiveness?
- Will the NFIP reserve fund be sufficient to offset future catastrophic loss years?

Accuracy of flood hazard maps and risk assessment methods

- In the aftermath of recent catastrophic flood events, what should be the scope of coastal hazard mapping and risk assessment and property damage mitigation in U.S. Atlantic and Gulf of Mexico coastal communities that are inherently at risk from hurricanes, sea-level rise, erosion, and coastal flooding?
- Is there a need for consistency between U.S. Army Corps of Engineers and FEMA levee certification, that is, a definition of flood protection? What is the best way to improve risk communication with respect to flood control structures?
- What is the feasibility of NOAA and FEMA developing accurate and consistent coastal hazard risk assessment and mapping tools and methodologies?

- What would it take to produce both flood risk and coastal hazard vulnerability maps?
- What will be the effectiveness of FEMA's efforts to have the level of risk reflected in flood insurance rates?

Movement toward a comprehensive integrated watershed management framework of risk perception, risk management, and disaster response strategy

- Is it time for a more encompassing water resources and mitigation planning process that encourages flood and water resources planning and flood mitigation on a watershed basis? How best to promote a comprehensive approach to resource management on a watershed basis?
- What is the best approach to strengthening local floodplain management and planning and guide development and building practices in regulated floodplains to save lives and reduce property damage?

Feasibility of catastrophic disaster insurance

- What is the best approach to address misperceptions about the nature of the NFIP and barriers to public understanding of flooding and flood risk?
- Should the NFIP cover all claims associated with catastrophic losses or just claims in the average annual loss year?

Federal disaster assistance and moral hazard

- Does the presence of federal disaster assistance introduce moral hazard in flood management in a way that inappropriately shifts risk to taxpayers?[67] Property owners may choose not to purchase the coverage, relying instead on federal disaster assistance to finance recovery. Is there a need to better coordinate the need for insurance coverage rather than access to government relief for post- flood recovery? Separately, some experts have suggested that access to federal disaster assistance under the Stafford Act could have the unintended consequence of shielding communities from the full implications of their decisions on land use and families from the financial consequences of rebuilding in disaster-prone areas.

Options for Managing and Financing Flood Risk

Despite billions invested in flood management, the United States has not been able to curb the rising costs of flood damage and public and private development in flood risk areas. This was the conclusion of the Gilbert F. White National Flood Policy Forum held in November 2007 at George Washington University.[68] The forum brought together 92 diverse experts to consider the future of floodplain management under a "business-as-usual scenario" and under an alternative scenario of aggressive action to address increasing flood risk in the nation. The experts at the forum concluded that an unprecedented set of conditions (e.g., population growth and migration, changes in climate, and degradation of water-based resources) now faces the United States that could increase flood losses more rapidly in the future. Several policy options emerged, and are listed below.

Long-Term Flood Insurance Contracts

Long-term flood insurance contracts (LTFIC) coupled with mitigation loans arguably would encourage investment in risk-reduction measures.[69] The idea is for private insurers to offer 5-, 10- or 20-year flood insurance contracts combined with long-term mitigation loans (e.g., for retrofitting, elevation, and flood-proofing of structures) tied to the mortgage. Mitigation loans would be offered to help finance the high upfront costs associated with investing in mitigation measures. The long-term flood insurance policies would have a maturity that corresponds to the length of the mortgage on the property and the policy would not terminate when the property owner sells the property.

The economic rationale for using LTFI to pre-fund disaster costs is that insurers, generally, need guaranteed premiums for a long time period if rates are to be based on expected losses. By lengthening the term of the property insurance contract, and spreading the risk through a mandatory purchase requirement, LTFI contracts could implicitly permit insurers to compensate for their present inability to prepare adequately for rare and unpredictable flood events.

Privatization of Flood Risk

FEMA has a responsibility to examine the NFIP's contingent liabilities and recommend ways to provide financial stability to the federal flood insurance program. This activity is performed in conjunction with the program's annual rate-setting process. In 2000, FEMA undertook a study with the assistance of accounting firm Deloitte & Touche to explore alternative financing arrangements to reduce the need for U.S. Treasury borrowing.[70] FEMA was concerned about the NFIP's erratic cash flow and the potential for catastrophic losses within a short period of time.

Since Hurricane Katrina in 2005, recognizing the shortcomings of the current financing arrangement under the NFIP, two basic alternatives have emerged: a multi-peril insurance approach and a reinsurance pool approach (i.e., standing facility provided for in the original 1968 act) that would expand the private-sector involvement in the NFIP. With the development of computer simulation catastrophe risk models and remote sensing technologies, some private- sector firms have argued that reinsurance and catastrophe bonds are good ideas that should be explored.

In this context, FEMA could require private insurers to "make available" private flood insurance policies at actuarially determined prices in flood-prone areas with the federal government providing federal reinsurance (see discussion on "Multi-peril Insurance" below). The Flood Insurance Reform Act of 2012 requires FEMA and GAO to study the option of privatizing the program and to report to Congress within one year of enactment.[71] The new law also mandated the director of the Federal Insurance Office to study the current state of the market for natural disaster insurance in the United States.[72]

Multi-Peril Homeowners Policies Covering the Flood Peril

Along the lines of privatization, Congress might choose to encourage private insurers to offer multiple-peril insurance policies covering the flood peril, and to have this risk segmented for the insurers' other book of business and transferred through reinsurance transactions to the federal government. Under this arrangement, the federal government would operate as a reinsurer, rather than a direct writer as it does currently under the Write Your Own Program. The underwriting of flood risk by private insurers would be exempt from state insurance law. Rates, flood maps, and the criteria (regulation) for land management and use would continue to be the responsibility of the federal government. States and local communities would continue to enforce floodplain management regulations developed by the federal government. Lending institutions would continue to enforce the NFIP mandatory flood purchase requirement.

In theory, the main benefits of the "multi-peril policy" option would be enhanced efficiency in risk financing through greater pooling and diversification of flood risk. The flood coverage would be distributed more broadly through the larger homeowners' insurance market, resulting presumably in more contracts issued, and losses spread more broadly among all insurers.

On the other hand, this option could give rise to questions of fairness, the potential for new liabilities for federal taxpayers, and institutional and practical issues surrounding the way private and social risks are managed and financed (e.g., rate setting processes, data quality, coverage for catastrophic losses, oversight, and "who benefits and who pays for development at risk").

Community-Based Flood Insurance Policy Contracts

Congress might choose to explore the feasibility of group flood insurance either for entire communities, identified-floodplain areas, or residual-risk areas behind levees. The group policy would be purchased by the community on behalf of all residents. Premiums would be collected either through property taxes or as a utility-type payment. In the 112th Congress, the House of Representatives passed H.R. 6186 to require FEMA to undertake a study of the feasibility of voluntary community-based flood insurance options and how such options could be incorporated into the NFIP. The bill required the GAO to review and provide an analysis of the FEMA study and to report its findings and recommendations to Congress within one year. To address the affordability of insurance for low-income property owners, Congress might also explore the feasibility of providing means-tested flood insurance vouchers.

Integrated Watershed-Based Risk Management Strategy

In recent years, FEMA has undertaken a long-term flood risk management strategic planning effort. This effort included studying the feasibility of a more integrated watershed-based risk management strategy designed to weave flood hazard data developed in support of the NFIP into watershed-based risk assessment. The goal has been to increase the public's awareness and understanding of risk management and to address the nation's increasing vulnerability to flood risk and water resources management challenges. This integrated (some call it "holistic") approach to flood risk management draws on floodplain management with natural resources (i.e., water resources and waste water) management; it requires coordination among federal, state, and local authorities, businesses, and individuals homeowners.

Many disaster experts believe effective flood risk management policy will require intergovernmental coordination of natural resources management with floodplain management activities that reduce the vulnerability of people and economic assets to catastrophic flooding. Policymakers have been moving in this direction for several years.

Technological Innovation in Financing Large-Scale Natural Disasters

The series of extreme weather events since 2005 underscores some social and economic challenges to U.S. disaster risk management policy. The costs of reconstruction and compensation for flood victims are financed through tax revenue, dedicated disaster funds, and, to a lesser extent, private insurance payments. Private disaster insurance, however, has become less available and affordable because of insurability problems posed by uncertainties surrounding extreme risks, such as catastrophic flood events.

The Biggert-Waters Flood Insurance Reform Act of 2012 authorized FEMA to study the capacity of private insurers, reinsurers, and financial markets to assist communities in managing financial risk associated with flooding.[73] One possible public-private initiative for financing catastrophic flood risk is for the government to encourage private-sector technological innovation—through tax and regulatory policy changes—in financing recovery from large-scale natural disasters. Given the nation's increasing flood exposure, and the desire to alleviate taxpayers' responsibility for flood losses (i.e., post-disaster relief), some disaster experts have expressed an interest in finding alternative ways to finance residual flood risk through the standardization of insurance- linked securities that transfer flood risk on an electronic platform to the capital markets. This approach would reduce the government's current role under the NFIP.

In November 2012, at an annual meeting of the National Association of Insurance Commissioners, Center for Insurance Policy Research (NAIC/CIRP), regulators and stakeholder groups with an interest in catastrophe risk financing explored new standards for transparency, compliance, and accountability with respect to two kinds of large scale disasters: environmental (i.e., catastrophe risk) and financial (i.e., residential mortgage back securitization).

One speaker at the meeting, David M. Rowe, concluded that in order to efficiently transfer risk to capital markets via the issuance of financial instruments, two obstacles must be overcome: (1) a computer system challenge that involves data storage, communication issues, and computer processing analytics and (2) finding ways to make risk exchanges and transaction platforms more efficient.[74]

Eric Nordman, director of Research for the NAIC, and coordinator of the study released at the 2012 NAIC/CIRP meeting, suggested that the two risk management challenges identified by David M. Rowe could be addressed through regulatory changes in the way insurance companies invest in certain financial instruments, including residential mortgage-backed securities.[75]

During the NAIC/CIRP panel discussion, Michael Erlanger, managing principal of Marketcore, a company that developed an electronic system architecture for aggregating risk elements in a way that facilitates valuations for complex risk transfers, stated that legislation introduced in previous Congresses, the Homeowners Defense Act,[76] had, among other things, called for a change in regulatory structures that deliver consistent micro-to-macro risk-detailing views in near real time, assuring transparency in the market for catastrophe risk, including flood risk.

He pointed out that the act called for the creation of a *National Catastrophe Risk Consortium* to (1) encourage data capture that leads to catastrophe risk differentiation and (2) expand the ability of private-sector financial and capital market firms and state residual property insurance pools to underwrite and bear the risk of an extreme event, such as a catastrophic flood event.

The Consortium, Erlanger stated, could, in theory, establish a holistic risk assessment framework that results in ever more granular market information induced by financial and strategic incentives for risk disclosure by all market participants.

The standardized "granular risk data" at the contract level could be aggregated and the risk transferred via the Consortium's electronic platform to investors in the capital markets. This structure arguably would induce transparency, provide market liquidity for catastrophe risk financing, and track all changes in the underlying contracts (e.g., flood policies) in real time.

In theory, driving transaction volume and associated liquidity to a new exchange by leveraging the most valuable thing the new exchange provides, namely, the reliable, timely, and detailed information it creates, could enable financial markets to supply the necessary pressure for sellers (private insurers, reinsurers, and capital markets participants) to make their offerings increasingly more transparent.

Opposition to the Homeowners' Defense Act of 2010 in the 111th Congress had come from representatives of insurance and reinsurance groups, and several organizations including the National Fire Protection Association, National Flood Determination Association, National Wildlife Federation, Heartland Institute, Taxpayers for Common Sense, and Competitive Enterprise Institute.

These groups argued the legislation would encourage coastal development in environmentally sensitive areas by lowering costs, bail out wealthy owners of beachside vacation homes, and crowd out the private insurance market.

CONCLUSION

The current system of managing and financing flood risk (NFIP) is more than $20 billion in debt. The Flood Insurance Reform Act of 2012 made significant changes in the financial, operational, and management structures of the NFIP.

Specifically, this law would work to achieve several outcomes: (1) implement a phase out of premium rate subsidies that have undermined the financial viability of the program; (2) ensure that flood risk maps are updated and accurate and take into account anticipated sea-level rise and residual risk behind levees so that people understand and can better prepare for their risks; (3) encourage broad participation in the NFIP; and (4) streamline and strengthen federal mitigation programs to protect flood-exposed homes, businesses, and communities better, which helps to decrease future flood losses.

Some experts question whether the NFIP still provides appropriate protection against the peril of flood losses and helps build resilient communities. The success of the NFIP will be judged in part by how it handles five major challenges:

- **Extreme weather events and coastal flooding.** Most experts expect coastal storm surge and storm impacts will intensify as sea levels continue to rise. According to FEMA, flood and flood damage associated with extreme rainfall events have risen from $6 billion to $10 billion each year, despite billions spent on flood control.
- **Accurate Flood Risk Maps.** The accuracy and reliability of FEMA's flood mapping process. FEMA's Risk Mapping, Assessment, and Planning (Risk MAP) provides flood hazard data and tools to increase public awareness and help people make better decisions to protect themselves and communities to enforce floodplain management regulations that support the building of sustainable and resilient communities.[77]
- **Financial Sustainability of the NFIP.** The financial soundness of the NFIP requires flood insurance premiums to fully reflect a building's actuarial risk. Some experts have argued that subsidized insurance rates facilitate development in flood-prone areas that put people and property at risk. Compensating flood victims with federal disaster relief is costly and a potential burden on federal taxpayers. But requiring property owners to pay full actuarial rates that reflect actual risk could make flood policies less affordable.
- **Residual Flood Risk from Levees.** The existing regulatory framework for residual flood risk behind certified 100-year levees has created a perceived safety zone that spurs development behind the levee systems.[78] Individuals might think a flood occurring once in a 100-year period could not harm them and, therefore, choose not to seek financial protection against this risk. Most disaster experts would agree that resolution of the nation's flood management challenge must involve hazard-mitigation measures that get people and communities to retreat or avoid living in flood-prone areas while supporting the building of hazard-resilient coastal communities.
- **Distributional Effects of the NFIP.** There is a perception of the inequitable distribution of the NFIP's costs and benefits across income groups and geographic regions.

Appendix A. National Flood Insurance Program's Repetitive Flood Loss Properties

Table A-1. Repetitive Flood Loss Properties in the National Flood Insurance Program (as of December 31, 2011; $ nominal)

State Name	Building Payments	Contents Payments	Total Payments	Average Payment	Losses	Properties
Alabama	$402,612,962.16	$81,730,441.39	$484,343,403.55	$35,084.64	13,805	4,833
Alaska	$972,686.23	$137,448.10	$1,110,134.33	$13,375.11	83	31
Arizona	$7,732,063.08	$1,372,949.13	$9,105,012.21	$15,251.28	597	258
Arkansas	$37,637,695.99	$9,726,561.34	$47,364,257.33	$21,249.11	2,229	808
California	$155,312,672.34	$37,638,334.53	$192,951,006.87	$21,175.48	9,112	3,299
Colorado	$1,010,193.40	$354,498.51	$1,364,691.91	$10,338.58	132	57
Connecticut	$72,987,538.72	$21,270,677.91	$94,258,216.63	$18,053.67	5,221	1,667
Delaware	$24,442,431.44	$13,222,588.18	$37,665,019.62	$34,778.41	1,083	395
District Columbia	$613,444.22	$16,919.85	$630,364.07	$19,101.94	33	14
Florida	$1,074,522,754.69	$283,995,996.57	$1,358,518,751.26	$32,274.99	42,092	16,546
Georgia	$103,724,414.09	$26,811,644.87	$130,536,058.96	$29,768.77	4,385	1,604
Guam	$363,009.86	$52,467.45	$415,477.31	$13,849.24	30	14
Hawaii	$10,801,779.20	$2,274,003.49	$13,075,782.69	$24,953.78	524	187
Idaho	$591,608.96	$100,132.05	$691,741.01	$10,980.02	63	24
Illinois	$124,766,766.99	$27,723,077.14	$152,489,844.13	$12,761.72	11,949	3,954
Indiana	$54,697,450.19	$10,569,246.21	$65,266,696.40	$16,143.14	4,043	1,467

Table A-1. (Continued)

State Name	Building Payments	Contents Payments	Total Payments	Average Payment	Losses	Properties
Iowa	$52,098,900.80	$12,491,664.61	$64,590,565.41	$23,694.26	2,726	1,033
Kansas	$21,231,625.75	$9,189,450.32	$30,421,076.07	$24,278.59	1,253	445
Kentucky	$89,312,937.78	$28,477,331.70	$117,790,269.48	$19,459.82	6,053	1,817
Louisiana	$2,029,521,249.82	$646,722,728.26	$2,676,243,978.08	$27,472.04	97,417	29,472
Maine	$10,313,173.36	$2,844,104.99	$13,157,278.35	$20,917.77	629	235
Maryland	$43,185,640.35	$15,594,237.25	$58,779,877.60	$25,259.94	2,327	959
Massachusetts	$131,940,529.86	$28,353,371.58	$160,293,901.44	$17,776.86	9,017	3,045
Michigan	$13,402,503.32	$5,179,082.14	$18,581,585.46	$10,975.54	1,693	655
Minnesota	$22,679,730.39	$3,707,955.03	$26,387,685.42	$16,298.76	1,619	644
Mississippi	$456,372,579.11	$132,138,941.21	$588,511,520.32	$33,232.34	17,709	6,139
Missouri	$224,032,976.31	$98,902,428.05	$322,935,404.36	$18,040.08	17,901	5,124
Montana	$1,899,435.24	$225,584.67	$2,125,019.91	$13,889.02	153	68
Nebraska	$9,232,709.39	$3,031,207.41	$12,263,916.80	$12,909.39	950	380
Nevada	$6,955,148.57	$3,435,927.12	$10,391,075.69	$59,377.58	175	76
New Hampshire	$17,452,959.68	$2,677,136.28	$20,130,095.96	$23,111.48	871	338
New Jersey	$715,423,006.56	$209,398,401.52	$924,821,408.08	$21,836.03	42,353	12,432
New Mexico	$1,187,339.29	$60,885.43	$1,248,224.72	$13,716.76	91	39
New York	$385,475,945.74	$104,436,883.54	$489,912,829.28	$16,433.96	29,811	10,712
North Carolina	$404,534,147.25	$69,935,397.40	$474,469,544.65	$19,658.17	24,136	8,664
North Dakota	$23,279,423.10	$2,517,270.79	$25,796,693.89	$29,448.28	876	379
Ohio	$91,459,636.06	$29,487,550.73	$120,947,186.79	$19,237.66	6,287	2,268

State Name	Building Payments	Contents Payments	Total Payments	Average Payment	Losses	Properties
Oklahoma	$45,972,663.99	$14,183,242.06	$60,155,906.05	$19,405.13	3,100	958
Oregon	$17,795,025.67	$5,818,442.24	$23,613,467.91	$26,237.19	900	339
Pennsylvania	$446,636,272.49	$127,959,807.52	$574,596,080.01	$25,615.02	22,432	7,878
Puerto Rico	$17,228,403.79	$39,202,639.67	$56,431,043.46	$9,027.52	6,251	2,040
Rhode Island	$26,195,718.48	$13,469,137.25	$39,664,855.73	$35,798.61	1,108	396
South Carolina	$70,906,728.62	$15,600,759.95	$86,507,488.57	$22,958.46	3,768	1,486
South Dakota	$5,712,923.39	$686,932.13	$6,399,855.52	$16,161.25	396	175
Tennessee	$50,621,555.88	$13,993,951.06	$64,615,506.94	$20,512.86	3,150	1,077
Texas	$1,325,875,765.26	$468,960,530.48	$1,794,836,295.74	$27,567.06	65,108	20,395
Utah	$942,899.43	$202,236.88	$1,145,136.31	$17,350.55	66	27
Vermont	$5,712,953.83	$1,323,304.01	$7,036,257.84	$21,257.58	331	133
Virgin Islands	$13,714,143.86	$24,171,345.01	$37,885,488.87	$46,887.98	808	294
Virginia	$281,880,147.26	$54,258,059.06	$336,138,206.32	$20,827.70	16,139	6,101
Washington	$86,791,060.88	$17,829,587.55	$104,620,648.43	$26,777.74	3,907	1,360
West Virginia	$92,557,791.85	$40,038,260.89	$132,596,052.74	$17,001.67	7,799	2,991
Wisconsin	$20,125,657.08	$4,758,741.43	$24,884,398.51	$17,055.79	1,459	624
Wyoming	$236,225.06	$32,264.07	$268,489.13	$9,588.90	28	12
Total	$9,332,687,006.11	$2,768,293,768.01	$12,100,980,774.12	$24,388.39	496,178	166,368

Source: U.S. Department of Homeland Security, Federal Emergency Management Agency.

APPENDIX B. KEY PROVISIONS IN THE BIGGERT-WATERS FLOOD INSURANCE REFORM ACT OF 2012

On July 6, 2012, President Barack Obama signed into law the Flood Insurance Reform Act of 2012[79] to extend funding for the NFIP to September 30, 2017. This legislation includes several key provisions:

Actuarial Soundness, Program Solvency, and Affordability

Premium Rate Structure Reform and Affordability

- Immediately eliminate pre-FIRM insurance premium subsidies on second properties, severe repetitive loss properties and properties that have incurred flood-related damage that exceed the fair market value of the property, and commercial properties that have undermined the financial stability of the program.[80]
- Gradually phase in actuarial rates for structures newly mapped into special flood hazard areas.[81]
- Increase in the annual cap on premium rate increases from 10% to 20%.[82]
- Authorize a new way of defining "average loss year" when setting annual flood insurance rates that include catastrophic loss years and raise the cap on premium increases.[83]
- Study the economic costs and benefits to taxpayers of providing flood insurance vouchers to lower-income property owners.[84]

Privatization

- Study of the capacity of the private reinsurance market to assume a portion of the NFIP insurance risk,[85] and clarify FEMA's authority to secure reinsurance from the private market to minimize the probability that the program would need to borrow Treasury funds.[86]
- Require FEMA to obtain reinsurance proposals to lay off a portion of the risk.[87]
- Require the director of the Federal Insurance Office (FIO) to study and report to Congress on the claims-paying capacity of the private insurance market for natural catastrophic insurance in the United States.[88]

Program Solvency and Debt Forgiveness

- Create a $12 billion catastrophe reserve fund to more effectively spread overtime losses from catastrophe loss years over time while reducing the likely need for borrowing from the Treasury.[89]
- Authorize FEMA to create a repayment schedule for funds borrowed from the Treasury.[90]

Flood Map Accuracy

- Establish a Technical Mapping Advisory Council (TMAC) to advise the administrator of FEMA on risk-based approaches to assessing future flood risk vulnerability[91] and an independent appeals board, Scientific Review Panels, for homeowners and communities to challenge revisions to their FIRMs with conflicting technical and scientific data.[92]
- Establish a process for communities to request a remapping based on standards developed by the TMAC and adopted by FEMA.[93]
- Establish a Federal Protection Structure Accreditation Task Force to better align the data that the U.S. Army Corps of Engineers collect during levee inspection with the data required under FEMA's accreditation program.[94]
- Establish a process and formula (COASTAL—Consumer Option for an Alternative System to Allocate Losses) for settling wind-related versus water- related property damage claims disputes by using scientific data currently collected by the National Oceanic and Atmospheric Administration (NOAA), academic institutions, and private entities, in conjunction with engineering formulas to be developed by FEMA, to help allocate total losses between the two perils or causes of loss after a major storm.[95]

Mitigation Funding Program Reform

- Combine and streamline FEMA's flood hazard mitigation programs and move toward risk-based mitigation planning and activities that result in sustainable action that reduces risk to life and property from floods.[96]

NFIP Management and Operational Efficiencies

- Impose civil penalties or enforcement actions for non-compliance with mandatory flood insurance requirements.
- Set procedures for monitoring contracts and claims records.
- Require federal agencies to work together and share data to improve flood mapping.[97]
- Authorize a study of ways to improve interagency and intergovernmental coordination of flood mapping.[98]

APPENDIX C. CHRONOLOGY OF PUBLIC LAWS THAT REAUTHORIZED THE NATIONAL FLOOD INSURANCE PROGRAM: 2008-2012

Presidential Signing Date	Public Law	Last Day of Effective Program Authority	Lapse in NFIP Authority
September 30, 2008	P.L. 110-329; 122 Stat. 3575 H.R. 2638 (Price)—Consolidated Security, Disaster Assistance, and Continuing Appropriations Act, 2009 (Sec. 145)	March 6, 2009	
March 6, 2009	P.L. 111-6; 123 Stat. 522 H.J.Res. 38 (Obey)—Continuing Appropriations Resolution, 2009	March 11, 2009	
March 11, 2009	P.L. 111-8; 123 Stat 988 H.Res. 184 (Obey) —Omnibus Appropriations Act, 2009	September 30, 2009	
October 1, 2009	P.L. 111-68; 123 Stat 2047 H.R. 2918 (Wasserman Schultz)—Legislative Branch Appropriations Act, 2010 (Sec. 129)	October 31, 2009	
October 28, 2009	P.L. 111-83; 123 Stat. 2142 H.R. 2892 (Price)—Department of Homeland Security Appropriations Act, 2010	October 31, 2009	
October 30, 2009	P.L. 111-88; 123 Stat. 2904 H.R. 2996 (Dicks)—Department of the Interior, Environment, and Related Agencies Appropriations Act,2010 (Sec. 102)	December 18, 2009	
December 19, 2010	P.L. 111-118; 123Stat. 3409 H.R. 3326 (Murtha)—Department of Defense Appropriations Act, 2010 (Sec. 1005)	February 28, 2010	March 1, 2010
March 2, 2010	P.L. 111-144; 124 Stat 45 H.R. 4691 (Rangel)—Temporary Extension Act of 2010 (Sec. 8)	March 28, 2010	March 29, 2010

Presidential Signing Date	Public Law	Last Day of Effective Program Authority	Lapse in NFIP Authority
April 15, 2010	P.L. 111-157; 124 Stat 1116 H.R. 4851 (Levin)—Continuing Extension Act, 2010 (Sec. 7)	May 31, 2010	June 1, 2010
July 2, 2010	P.L. 111-196, §2(a); 124 Stat 1352 H.R. 5569 (Waters)—National Flood Insurance Program Extension Act	September 30, 2010	
September 30, 2010	P.L. 111-250, §2(a); 124 Stat 2630 S. 3814 (Vitter)—National Flood Insurance Program Extension Act of 2010	September 30, 2011	October 1, 2011
October 5, 2011	P.L. 112-36 §130; 125 Stat. 390 H.R. 2608 (Graves)—Continuing Appropriations Act, 2012	November 18, 2012	
November 18, 2011	P.L. 112-55; 125 Stat 710 H.R. 2112 (Kingston)—Consolidated and Further Continuing Appropriations Act, 2012, Div. D (Sec. 101)	December 16, 2011	
December 16, 2011	P.L. 112-67; 125 Stat. 769 H.J.Res. 94 (Rogers)—Making Further Continuing Appropriations for Fiscal Year 2012, and for Other Purposes	December 17, 2011	
December 17, 2011	P.L. 112-68; 125 Stat. 770 H.J.Res. 95 (Rogers)—Making Further Continuing Appropriations for Fiscal Year 2012, and for Other Purposes	December 23, 2011	
December 23, 2011	P.L. 112-74, Div. D, Title V, §573; 125 Stat. 985 H.R. 2055 (Culberson)—Consolidated Appropriations Act, 2012	May 31, 2012	
May 31, 2012	P.L. 112-123; H.R. 5740 (Biggert)—National Flood Insurance Program Extension Act	July 31, 2012	
July 6, 2012	P.L. 112-141; 112 Stat. 916; Div. F, Title II, H.R. 4348 – Biggert-Waters Flood Insurance Reform Act of 2012	September 30, 2017	

Source: Congressional Research Service.

End Notes

[1] Structural measures (levees, dams, floodwalls, channels modification) are those that change or control flood water flow to reduce the probability of flooding.

[2] Non-structural measures (flood-proofing, acquisition/relocation, and retrofitting structures) focus on floodplain management and flood warning to reduce risks associated with flooding and moving above and away from flood water.

[3] P.L. 112-141; 126 Stat 916.

[4] Testimony of Craig Fugate, Administrator of Federal Emergency Management Agency before the Senate Committee on Banking, Housing, and Urban Affairs, *National Flood Insurance Program Reform*, June 9, 2011, p. 3.

[5] The financial management of flood hazards also involves (1) funding mitigation activities and (2) providing direct federal disaster assistance to individuals, private businesses, and communities to help rebuild destroyed property, provide temporary housing to displaced victims, and compensate uninsured victims. These costs are usually financed through emergency supplemental appropriations or dedicated disaster funds under the Robert T. Stafford Act.

[6] Testimony of Craig Fugate, Administrator of Federal Emergency Management Agency before the Senate Committee on Banking, Housing, and Urban Affairs, *National Flood Insurance Program Reform*, June 9, 2011, p. 2.

[7] Department of Homeland Security, Federal Emergency Management Agency, "National Flood Insurance Fund: Fiscal Year 2013, Congressional Justification," at http://www.fema.gov/pdf/about/budget/ 11h_fema_nfi_fund_dhs_fy13_cj.pdf.

[8] Anita Lee, "Sandy Catches Northeasterners without Flood Coverage," *The Sun Herald*, November, 2, 2012, at http://www.weather.com/news/sandy-northeasterners-no-insurance-201211.

[9] Ibid.

[10] Susan Stellin, "Reconsidering Flood Insurance," *The New York Times*, November 8, 2012, at http://www.nytimes.com/2012/11/11/realestate/reconsidering-flood-insurance-after-hurrican-sandy.html?pagewanted=all&_r=0.

[11] See Howard Kunreuther and Paul Slovic, "Economics, Psychology, and Protective Behavior," *The American Economic Review*, vol. 68(2); 1978, p. 64-69.

[12] R.A. Pielke, "Nine Fallacies of Floods," *Climatic Change*, vol. 42(2), 1999, p. 413-438.

[13] Property Casualty Insurers Association of America, "True Market-Risk Rates for Flood Insurance," June 2011, at http://www.pciaa.net/web/sitehome.nsf/lcpublic/304/$file/NFIP_White_Paper_June2011.pdf.

[14] *The National Academy of Science*, "Mapping the Zone: Improving Flood Map Accuracy," 2009, at http://www.nap.edu/openbook.php?record_id=12573&page=13.

[15] FEMA, for example, shifted focus to coastal hazard mapping with its *Risk MAP 2010-2014 Multi-Year Plan*, March 2009, built on the Flood Map Modernization program. Risk MAP is an integrated flood risk management approach that weaves NFIP flood hazard data into watershed-based risk assessments that serve as the basis for local hazard mitigation plans and support community actions to reduce risk. As part of Risk MAP, FEMA has provided to communities New, Validated or Updated Engineering (NVUE) data for 54% of the miles mapped in the NFIP flood hazard inventory.

[16] FEMA estimated that about 8.7 million people or 3% of the U.S. population (based on the 2000 U.S. Census) live in Coastal AE Zones and VE Zones (i.e., areas subject to the 1% annual chance coastal flood hazard). See *An Estimate of the U.S. Population Subject to the One-Percent Annual Chance (100-year) Coastal Flood Hazard* by Mark Crowell and Kevin Coulton, Proceedings of Coastal Zone 09, Boston, Mass., July 19, 2009, at http://www.csc.noaa.gov/cz/CZ09_Proceedings/Abstract%20PDFs/Oral.Crowell.pdf. A 2010 power point presentation of this study is found at http://www.norfma.org/conference/2010/090810_conf/090810/estimate_us_cooling.pdf.

[17] See J. Scott Holladay and Jason A. Schwartz, "Flooding the Market: The Distributional Consequences of the NFIP," New York University School of Law, Institute for Policy Integrity, April 2010, at http://policyintegrity.org/documents/ Floodingthemarket.pdf.

[18] See CRS Report R41752, *Locally Operated Levees: Issues and Federal Programs*, by Natalie Keegan et al.

[19] The states affected by Hurricane Sandy include Connecticut, Delaware, District of Columbia, Maine, Maryland, Massachusetts, New Hampshire, New Jersey, New York, North Carolina, Ohio, Pennsylvania, Rhode Island, Virginia, and West Virginia.

[20] These states include Arkansas, Illinois, Kentucky, Louisiana, Mississippi, Missouri, and Tennessee.

[21] National Oceanic and Atmospheric Administration, National Weather Service, "United States Flood Loss Report – Water Year 2011," at http://www.nws.noaa.gov/hic/summaries/ WY2011.pdf.

[22] Ibid.

[23] Ibid.

[24] American Academy of Actuaries, "The National Flood Insurance Program: Past, Present ... and Future?, July 2011, at http://www.actuary.org/pdf/casualty/AcademyFloodInsurance_ Monograph_110715.pdf.

[25] National Science and Technology Council, Climate Change Science Program and the Subcommittee on Global Change Research, *Weather and Climate Extremes in a Changing Climate Regions of Focus: North America, Hawaii, Caribbean, and U.S. Pacific Islands*, June 2008, at http://www.climatescience.gov/Library/sap/sap3-3/final-report/ sap3-3-final-all.pdf.

[26] U.S. Commission on Ocean Policy, "An Ocean Blueprint for the 21st Century," September 2004, at http://oceancommission.gov/documents/full_color_rpt/000_ocean_full_report.pdf.

[27] Lloyds of London and Risk Management Solutions, *Coastal Communities and Climate Change: Maintaining Insurability*, 2008, at http://www.lloyds.com/NR/rdonlyres/ 38782611-5ED3-4FDC-85A4-5DEAA88A2DA0/0/ FINAL360climatechangereport.pdf.

[28] Properties not financed by federally insured or guaranteed mortgages usually fall outside of the NFIP's insurance regulatory framework. Although there is no requirement to purchase flood insurance to protect the property as collateral, the property owner might be subject to land-use development and zoning and construction ordinances.

[29] James Anderson, "Economic Regulation," *Encyclopedia of Policy Studies*, Stuart S. Nagel, ed. (New York: Dekker Publishers), 1994, p. 404.

[30] 42 U.S.C. § 4001(a); § 4012(a)-(b).

[31] Dan R. Anderson, "The National Flood Insurance Program: Problem and Potential," *The Journal of Risk and Insurance*, 1974, vol.16 (4), p. 579-599.

[32] P.L. 93-234, 87 Stat. 975.

[33] P.L. 103-325, 108 Stat. 2255.

[34] P.L. 108-264, 118 Stat. 712.

[35] Before FEMA began its map modernization programs, many FIRMs were 20 to 25 years old and did not accurately reflect residual risk behind or below flood control structures, giving residents living behind them a false sense of security.

[36] FEMA designates flood-risk zones on a flood insurance rate according to risk level. The codes are Zones A, AO, A1- A30, AE, AR, AR/AO, AR/A1-A30, AR/AE, AR/AH, AR/A99, A99, AH, VO, V1-V30, VE, and V. These zones are highly susceptible to flooding and, therefore, subject to mandatory flood insurance purchase requirements. V-lettered zones are also subject to wave action. Older maps use Zones B and C to represent areas of moderate- and low-flood risk. Newer maps have replaced these designations with Zone X (shaded) and Zone X (unshaded), respectively.

[37] A *stage-damage curve* is an estimate of damages as a percentage of value based on the depth of flooding experience.

[38] See Department of Homeland Security, Federal Emergency Management Agency, "Risk MAP 2010-2014 Multi- Year Plan," at http://www.fema.gov/library/viewRecord.do?id=3587.

[39] These unusual flood loss years were 1978, 1979, 1980, 1983, 1989, 1995, 2004, 2005, and 2008.

[40] It appears unlikely that the $17.75 billion in debt to the U.S. Treasury, as of June 30, 2012, will be repaid within the next 10 years given annual interest payments of about $1 billion and annual premium income of approximately $3.5 billion.

[41] P.L. 112-141; 126 Stat. 916, Sec. 100212.

[42] Ibid, Sec. 100211.

[43] Buildings constructed after December 31, 1974, or after the publication of a flood insurance rate map (FIRM), are charged an actuarial premium that reflects the property's risk of flooding. Subsidized rates, on the other hand, are determined by a statutory mandate that requires rates to be affordable so individuals are encouraged to participate. Owners of properties built prior to the issuance of a community's flood hazard map or January 1, 1974 (Pre-Firm structures), usually pay subsidized rates and are exempted from the NFIP's floodplain management standards. Even properties that are remapped into higher-risk areas pay the subsidized rates—a situation that exacerbates the financial challenges facing the NFIP.

[44] U.S. Government Accountability Office, FEMA's Rate-Setting Process Warrants Attention," GAO-09-12, October 31, 2008.

[45] In contrast, commercial insurance premiums are typically set at a level that covers expected losses and expenses plus an amount for a profit margin. A portion of each premium dollar collected is then set aside in loss reserves, which are invested and used to pay claims and expenses.

[46] Federal Emergency Management Agency, "Actuarial Rate Review: In Support of the October 1, 2010, Rate and Rule Changes," July 2010, p. 22.

[47] P.L. 112-141; 126 Stat. 916, Sec. 100211.

[48] Ibid., Sec. 100236.

[49] Ibid., Sec. 100212.

[50] A repetitive loss property (RLP) is defined as an insured property that experiences two or more flood losses greater than $1,000 within any 10-year period. A subset of RLPs, called severe repetitive loss properties (SRLP), have incurred at least four NFIP claim payments of at least $5,000 each or the cumulative amount of such claims payments exceeds $20,000 or for which at least two separate claims have been made with the cumulative amount of the building portion of such claims exceeding the market value of the building.

[51] U.S. Department of Homeland Security, Office of Inspector General, *FEMA's Implementation of the Flood Insurance Reform Act of 2004*, OIG-09-45, March 26, 2009, p. 4, at http://www.dhs.gov/xoig/assets/mgmtrpts/OIG_09- 45_Mar09.pdf.

[52] P.L. 108-264; 118 Stat. 712.

[53] P.L. 112-141, Sec. 100225.

[54] CRS Report RS22945, *Flood Insurance Requirements for Stafford Act Assistance*, by Edward C. Liu.

[55] Howard C. Kunreuther, "The Changing Societal Consequences of Risks from Natural Hazards." *Annals of the American Academy of Political and Social Science* 1979, vol. 443, pp. 104-116.

[56] Rand Institute for Civil Justice, "The National Flood Insurance Program's Market Penetration Rate: Estimates and Policy Implications," 2006, available at http://www.rand.org/pubs/technical_reports/2006/RAND_TR300.pdf.

[57] P.L. 112-141; Sec. 100208.

[58] Ibid, Sec. 100216.

[59] Ibid, Sec. 100218.

[60] Ibid. Sec. 100243.

[61] 44 CFR 59.21.

[62] National Wildlife Federation, *Heavy Rainfall and Increased Flooding Risk: Global Warming's Wake-up Call for the Central United States*, 2008, at http://www.nwf.org/extremeweather/pdfs/Heavy_Rainfall_and_Increased_Flooding- Wake-Up_Call_for_Central_U.S2.pdf.

[63] U.S. Government Accountability Office, GAO-08-504, *National Catastrophe Insurance: Analysis of Proposed Combined Federal Flood and Wind Insurance Program*, April 25, 2008.

[64] P.L. 112-141; Sec. 100252.

[65] Testimony of Craig Fugate, administrator of Federal Emergency Management Agency, before the Senate Committee on Banking, Housing, and Urban Affairs, *National Flood Insurance*

Program Reform, June 9, 2011, p. 3, located at http://banking.senate.gov/public/index.cfm?FuseAction=Files.View&FileStore_id=c6f08bf5-5daa-4406-b461- 1781159ec9c1.

[66] U.S. President Jimmy Carter, "Floodplain Management" Executive Order 11988, *Federal Register,* May 24, 1977, p. 26951, at http://www.fema.gov/plan/ehp/ehplaws/attachments-laws/eo11988.pdf.

[67] Government disaster assistance is usually available only for uninsurable damages. The recipients of disaster assistance do not bear direct cost for remittances. However, the availability of disaster assistance could produce a moral hazard problem. It could reinforce vulnerabilities and provide little incentive to reduce risky behavior. Moreover, disaster assistance could reduce the direct costs associated with risky behavior, where costs are shifted to taxpayers.

[68] Association of State Flood Plain managers, *Floodplain Management 2050: A Report of the 2007 Assembly of the Gilbert F. White National Flood Policy Forum*, November 6-7, 2007.

[69] For more information see Carolyn Kouky and Howard Kunreuther, "Improving Flood Insurance and Flood Risk Management: Insights from St. Louis, Missouri," *Resources for the Future*, February 2009, at http://www.rff.org/rff/ documents/rff-dp-09-07.pdf.

[70] Federal Emergency Management Agency*, National Flood Insurance Program: Discussion of Financial Stabilization Possibilities*, FEMA Unpublished Internal Document, November 20, 2000.

[71] P.L. 112-141; Sect.100232.

[72] Ibid., Sec. 100247.

[73] P.L. 112-141; Sect. 100232(b).

[74] See, Comments of David M. Rowe, President, David M. Rowe Risk Advisory, before the *NAIC/CIRP Luncheon Panel on Financing Home Ownership*, November 30, 2012, located at http://www.marketcore.com/media/Marketcore- David_Rowe-Press_Release.pdf.

[75] See Eric Nordman, Financing Home Ownership: Origins and Evolution of Mortgage Securitization - Public Policy, Financial Innovations and Crises, located at http://www.naic.org/documents/ cipr_120812_white_paper_financing_home_ownership.pdf.

[76] H.R. 2555 (111th Congress): Homeowners' Defense Act of 2010.

[77] See Department of Homeland Security, Federal Emergency Management Agency, "FEMA's Risk Mapping, Assessment, and Planning (Risk MAP), Fiscal Year 2012 Report To Congress," February 23, 2012, at http://www.fema.gov/library/viewRecord.do?id=5924.

[78] Under 44 CFR 65.10 regulations, FEMA removes areas protected from certified 100-year levees from the flood map. Individuals are then not required to purchase flood insurance and floodplain management standards are not applicable in these areas. If a levee is not certified, FEMA will designate the area behind the levee as a risk and the mandatory purchase requirement will apply.

[79] P.L. 112-141, 126 Stat. 916.

[80] Id., Sec. 100205.

[81] Ibid.

[82] Ibid

[83] Ibid.

[84] Ibid, Sec. 100236.

[85] Ibid, Sec. 100232.

[86] Ibid.

[87] Ibid.

[88] Ibid., Sec. 100247.

[89] Ibid., Sec. 100212.

[90] Ibid., Sec. 100213.

[91] Ibid., Sec. 100215.

[92] Ibid., Sec. 100218.

[93] Ibid., Sec. 100216.

[94] Ibid., Sec. 100218.

[95] Ibid., Sec. 100253.
[96] Ibid., Sec. 100225.
[97] Ibid., Sec. 100220.
[98] Ibid., Sec. 100221.

INDEX

D

G

H

I

J

L

M

Q

R

S

T

U

V

W

Y